CLINICAL APPLICATIONS OF ZINC METABOLISM

Proceedings of the International Symposium

Case Western Reserve University Medical School
Cleveland Metropolitan General Hospital
Cleveland, Ohio

CLINICAL APPLICATIONS OF ZINC METABOLISM

Edited by

WALTER J. PORIES, M.D.

WILLIAM H. STRAIN, Ph.D.

JENG M. HSU, Ph.D.

RAYMOND L. WOOSLEY, M.D., Ph.D.

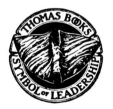

CHARLES C THOMAS • PUBLISHER
Springfield • Illinois • U.S.A.

Published and Distributed Throughout the World by

CHARLES C THOMAS • PUBLISHER

Bannerstone House

301-327 East Lawrence Avenue, Springfield, Illinois, U.S.A.

© 1974 *by* CHARLES C THOMAS • PUBLISHER

ISBN 0-398-02968-7

Library of Congress Catalog Card Number: 73-18378

*With THOMAS BOOKS careful attention is given to all details of
manufacturing and design. It is the Publisher's desire to present books
that are satisfactory as to their physical qualities and artistic possibilities
and appropriate for their particular use. THOMAS BOOKS will be true
to those laws of quality that assure a good name and good will.*

Printed in the United States of America

EE-11

PARTICIPANTS

KNUT HAEGER, M.D.
Assistant Professor of Surgery
Vascular Surgery Section
Department of Surgery
University Hospital
Malmö, Sweden

ROBERT I. HENKIN, M.D., Ph.D.
National Heart Institute
National Institutes of Health
Bethesda, Maryland

JOHN H. HENZEL, M.D.
Department of Surgery
University of Missouri
Columbia, Missouri

JOHN B. HERRMANN, M.D.
Professor & Chief of Surgery
Worcester City Hospital
University of Massachusetts
Medical School
Worcester, Mass.

JENG M. HSU, Ph.D.
Chief, Biochemistry Research Laboratory
Veterans Administration Hospital
Department of Biochemistry
Johns Hopkins University
Baltimore, Maryland

LUCILLE S. HURLEY, Ph.D.
Department of Nutrition
University of California
Davis, California

S. LATAFAT HUSAIN, M.B.
Department of Dermatology
Royal Infirmary
Glasgow C. 4
Scotland

Participants

DUANE L. LARSON, M.D.
Shriners Burns Institute
University of Texas Medical Branch
Galveston, Texas

WALTER MERTZ, M.D.
Human Nutrition Research
Agricultural Research Service
United States Department of Agriculture
Beltsville, Maryland

BOYD O'DELL, Ph.D.
Professor of Agricultural Chemistry
University of Missouri
Columbia, Missouri

CARL C. PFEIFFER, M.D., Ph.D.
Director, Brain Bio Center
Princeton, N. J.

WALTER J. PORIES, M.D.
Professor & Chief of Surgery
Cleveland Metropolitan General Hospital
Case Western Reserve University
Cleveland, Ohio

ANANDA S. PRASAD, M.D.
Professor of Medicine
Chief of Hematology
Wayne State University
School of Medicine
Detroit, Michigan

FREDRIC W. PULLEN II, M.D. F.A.C.S.
Director, Division of Neuro-otology
University of Miami
School of Medicine
Miami, Florida

HOSSAIN RONAGHY, M.D.
Professor of Community Medicine
Pahlavi University
School of Medicine
Shiraz, Iran

HAROLD H. SANDSTEAD, M.D.
Human Nutrition Laboratory
United States Department of Agriculture
Grand Forks, North Dakota

JAMES F. SMITH, D.D.S., Ph.D.
Professor of Pathology and Oral Surgery
University of Tennessee
College of Dentistry
Memphis, Tennessee

HERTA SPENCER, M.D.
Chief, Metabolic Section
Veterans Administration Hospital
Hines, Illinois

WILLIAM H. STRAIN, Ph.D.
Director of Surgical Laboratories
Cleveland Metropolitan General Hospital
3395 Scranton Road
Cleveland. Ohio

JAMES F. SULLIVAN, M.D.
Professor of Medicine
Creighton University
Omaha, Nebraska

BERT L. VALLEE, M.D.
Cabot Professor of Biological Chemistry
Harvard Medical School, Harvard University
25 Shattuck Street
Boston, Massachusetts

CONTRIBUTORS

James Bell, M.D.
Rodney G. Bessent, Ph.D.
Diane A. Bronzert, B.A.
Milos Chvapil, M.D., Ph.D.
Allan Cott, M.D.
Arthur Flynn, Ph.D.
William T. Friedewald, M.D.
Knut Haeger, M.D.
Robert I. Henkin, M.D., Ph.D.
John H. Henzel, M.D.
John B. Herrmann, M.D.
Jeng M. Hsu, Ph.D.
Lucille S. Hurley, Ph.D.
S. Latafat Husain, M.D.
Elizabeth H. Jenney, M.S.
Lois Kramer, B.S.
Erik Lanner, Leg. Apot.
Duane L. Larson, M.D.
Edgar L. Lichti, Ph.D.
Per-Olow Magnusson, Leg. Apot.
Walter Mertz, M.D.
W. Jack Miller, Ph.D.
Donald Oberleas, Ph.D.
Boyd O'Dell, Ph.D.
Dace Osis
Joshp Paone, B.S.
Carl C. Pfeiffer, M.D., Ph.D.
Walter J. Pories, M.D.
Ananda S. Prasad, M.D.
Fredric W. Pullen II, M.D.
Morton S. Raff, M.A.
Hossain Ronaghy, M.D., M.P.H.

Harold H. Sandstead, M.D.

Paul J. Schecter, M.D.

William Shepard, M.A.

James F. Smith, D.D.S., Ph.D.

Herta Spencer, M.D.

Paul E. Stake, M.S.

William H. Strain, Ph.D.

James F. Sullivan, M.D.

Marjorie W. Terhune, M.S.

Bert L. Vallee, M.D.

Emilie Wiatrowski, B.S.

Raymond L. Woosley, M.D., Ph.D.

Charles F. Zukoski, M.D.

FOREWORD

To the casual observer an International Symposium on the Clinical Applications of Zinc Metabolism would not seem to be a particularly unusual event, but to the initiated, it is a remarkable first of its kind. The importance of zinc to clinical medicine is just beginning to emerge from long and tedious efforts in basic and applied research of the past: in succession, its biological effects were viewed as mostly harmful, questionable and now essential.

It is just one hundred years ago that zinc was found to be biologically indispensible. In 1869 Raulin first discovered that *Aspergillus niger* fails to grow in its absence. Its presence in plants and animal tissues was established within a decade. Thereafter, despite the rapid growth of biological science during the next half century, almost no progress was made in regard to the nature of its biolgical role. It may be timely to recall that the impetus for renewed interest in the 1920's came from industrial toxicology: zinc fumes proved to be toxic to exposed workers. Remarkably, the perspicacious investigators of metal fume fever were the ones to revive the hypothesis that zinc has an essential biological function. Indeed, nutritionists demonstrated its critical importance to the growth of rodents soon thereafter.

A discrete biochemical role for zinc was established in the early forties. Keilin and Mann discovered that zinc is part of the active site of the enzyme carbonic anhydrase documenting the metal's direct participation in catalysis. In the recent past, zinc has been shown, of course, to be a part of the active sites of enzymes of various types in virtually all forms of life. In addition, it stabilizes the structures of proteins and enzymes, affecting their functions indirectly, and further it controls important biochemical pathways.

Ever since nutritional studies indicated the importance of zinc in biology, the arrest of growth has been the outstanding manifestation of its deficiency in microorganisms, plants, animals and man. Such data have long implied that it also exercises a dominant role in the metabolism and structures of nucleic acids and, hence, in protein synthesis, and that this might prove to be the basis of its effects on normal growth and development. Biochemical investigations are progressively verifying such conclusions.

The advent of highly sensitive and precise instrumental methods for the analysis of zinc, better means to ascertain the consequences of its nutritional deficiency and advances in biochemical techniques have all hastened appreciation of its biological importance but also of the complexity of its mode of action. The latter point is exemplified by the fact that other metals can markedly antagonize its normal metabolic action. Porcine parakeratosis, the first zinc-deficient disease discovered in animals, is actually a *conditioned deficiency*. Zinc intake of calcium causes a *relative* deficiency with characteristic symptoms which are reversed completely by augmenting the supply of zinc. There are analogous relationships between zinc and calcium in enzymes, microorganisms and plants, and a conditioned deficiency has been postulated to account for some aspects of human cirrhosis, though its nature requires much further study. The importance of zinc in growth and reproduction of animals and man and to the integrity of the integument, liver, gastrointestinal tract and gonads and to the formation of normal offspring are now well established. Clearly, the three grams of the element long known to be a component of an adult human being do not reflect "passive contamination," as was once thought.

It is, indeed, remarkable that the delineation of the biological importance of this element should have been delayed so long. Though therapeutic applications are beginning to emerge, the benefits for medicine yet to be reaped are not fully apparent, even now.

Much of the medical information to be presented may remain incomplete for some time, though the means to establish its biological basis are clearly at hand. The effective exchange of information among scientists, physicians and surgeons fostered here will no doubt greatly hasten medical progress by integrating emerging biochemical understanding with that gained from clinical trial.

BERT L. VALLEE

ACKNOWLEDGMENTS

Clinical Applications of Zinc Metabolism is comprised of the papers presented at an International Symposium on Zinc Metabolism held at Cleveland Metropolitan General Hospital, Case Western Reserve University School of Medicine, Cleveland, Ohio, October 29-30, 1971. The Symposium was supported in part by an educational grant from the Division of Medical Research, Meyer Laboratories, Detroit, Michigan, and Fort Lauderdale, Florida.

The Cleveland Symposium forms a continuum with previous symposia held on zinc metabolism. The first symposium was held at Wayne State University Medical School, Detroit, Michigan, 1964. The papers presented in Detroit were published by Charles C Thomas, Publisher in 1966 as the monograph *ZINC METABOLISM*, compiled and edited by Doctor Ananda S. Prasad, who organized and directed the symposium. Another symposium on zinc metabolism, also organized and edited by Doctor Prasad, appeared in the *American Journal of Clinical Nutrition,* Vol. 22, September, 1969. Interest in zinc metabolism and therapy is growing at such a vigorous pace that other symposia may be expected, both on zinc itself and on zinc in relation to other elements, enzymes and complexing agents.

Zinc medication appears to be the oldest form of therapy. Topical application of calamine, an impure zinc oxide, was described in the Ebers Papyrus (1550 B.C.), and several recipes are given in the translation by Priboam. Calamine is still widely employed, even though topical steroids have replaced some applications of this ancient remedy. Use of pharmacopea grade of zinc oxide and of other zinc salts for topical therapy probably stems from the good results obtained with calamine.

Systemic administration of zinc apparently began in Western Europe during the period of the American Revolution. Flowers of zinc, or zinc oxide, were employed for the treatment of convulsive disorders. Although reportedly successful at first, the therapy fell into disfavor with the passage of years. Uncertainty of the composition of the medication may have contributed to the waning of interest, but the lack of suitable analytical procedures to follow the therapy and to document the results must have contributed greatly to the uncertainties. Currently, zinc in combination with taurine is being advocated.

In 1955, the Australian physicist Allan Walsh, perfected atomic absorption spectroscopy and this analytical procedure has provided a very sensitive and exact method for determining zinc and many other mineral elements. Atomic absorption spectroscopy had been proposed by Kirchoff in 1859, but was an unreliable method for over a century. Just as flame photometry and radioisotopic methods established potassium and sodium metabolism and therapy, atomic absorption spectroscopy and zinc radio-isotopes have made it possible to study zinc metabolism and the benefits of zinc therapy. As a consequence, the new understanding of zinc metabolism has indicated the many clinical applications of zinc therapy summarized in this monograph. Much more is to be learned, however, because zinc seems to be critical for growth and repair, two basic metabolic processes.

Many contributed to the success of the Cleveland Symposium. The essayists presented stimulating papers with enthusiasm to an audience that participated wholeheartedly. There was a free flow of ideas in both the structured and informal meetings. The magnificent weather contributed to the appreciation and enjoyment of the many cultural, educational and technical institutions of Cleveland before and after the meetings. Unfortunately, various factors contributed to delay publication of the papers. Fortunately, the chapters have been updated where necessary, particularly by the addition of references that contribute to the development of the growing boundaries of knowledge.

WALTER J. PORIES
WILLIAM H. STRAIN
JENG M. HSU
RAYMOND L. WOOSLEY

CONTENTS

CLINICAL APPLICATIONS OF ZINC METABOLISM

SECTION A
ROLE OF ZINC IN PROTEIN SYNTHESIS

INTRODUCTION

BOYD L. O'DELL

PROTEIN IS NOT STORED in the animal body in the same sense that fat and glycogen are stored. Except for a limited quantity of secretory protein, net protein synthesis or accretion is associated with true growth, i.e. increase in cell size or number. For this reason impaired growth and tissue regeneration are associated with a depressed rate of protein synthesis. Since a cardinal symptom of zinc deficiency is failure of growth in young animals, it almost surely follows that there is a decreased rate of protein synthesis. Whether or not the growth failure results primarily from a specific effect of zinc on protein synthesis is not clear.

There are a multitude of factors that may affect protein synthesis. Probably the most common cause of failure is a lack of free amino acids in the tissues. Some of the amino acids can be synthesized but the essential ones must be derived from food. Perhaps an even more fundamental cause of failure is a lack of energy. Since a source of utilizable energy is primary to life, even amino acids will be converted to energy if energy is limiting. Besides the fundamental building blocks and the energy needed to put them together, various biocatalysts or enzyme cofactors must be supplied by the diet. These include the vitamins and trace elements.

Zinc deficiency could affect protein synthesis by a direct effect on appetite and thus on the energy supply and the amino acid pool size. A deficiency could prevent DNA replication and thus mitosis and production of new cells. As a consequence protein synthesis would soon cease. It could also be involved in transcription and RNA synthesis or in the translation process.

According to the central dogma of protein synthesis, there is a progression of information transfer from template deoxyribonucleic acid (DNA) to messenger ribonucleic acid (m-RNA) to the polypeptide chain, eventually giving rise to a protein structure of specific conformation. The latter may involve a metal ion to form a metallo-protein, e.g. a zinc metalloenzyme. This concept may be depicted schematically as follows:

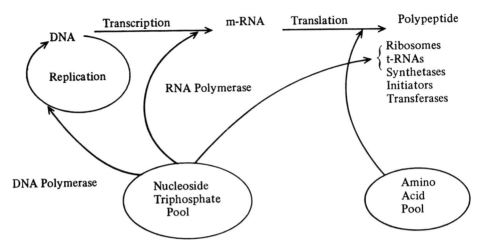

STRUCTURE 1. Schematic representation of polypeptide and protein synthesis.

Does zinc play a specific role in this process? If so, where?

Replication and DNA Synthesis

There is evidence for a direct and specific involvement of zinc in the process of replication, or more specifically in DNA biosynthesis. Without DNA replication, growth and protein synthesis are severely limited. Lieberman et al.[3] and Fujioka and Lieberman[1] provided some of the first evidence that zinc is essential for DNA synthesis in kidney and liver cells. The chelating agent, EDTA, prevented the incorporation of thymidine into DNA and the effect was corrected specifically by zinc. RNA synthesis was not affected. Sandstead and Renaldi[6] have shown that zinc deficiency in young rats decreases DNA synthesis of nuclear DNA in liver parenchymal cells and Swenerton and Hurley[10] have demonstrated that maternal zinc deficiency impairs DNA synthesis in the rat embryo. Weser et al.[13] also observed that zinc deficiency impairs DNA but not RNA synthesis in regenerating rat liver. Williams and Chesters[15] found a significantly reduced thymidine incorporation into DNA of rat liver, kidney and spleen before there was clear evidence of reduced growth rate or food consumption. The most convincing evidence that zinc has a specific effect on DNA synthesis comes from the observations of Slater et al.[9] that DNA polymerases from E. *coli* and sea urchins contain zinc in stoichiometric proportions, 2 and 4 atoms of Zn per mole, respectively.

In spite of this evidence there are reports that zinc deficiency has no effect on DNA synthesis. However, it must be noted that, in part, different species were involved. Wacker[12] and Schneider and Price,[7] using Euglena gracilis, observed a marked decrease in RNA concentration but an increased concentration of DNA per unit cell volume. It appeared that mitosis was blocked but that DNA synthesis proceeded until the amount per cell was doubled. Thus, synthesis of DNA *per se* was not impaired. Zinc deficiency in the chick did not affect the DNA or RNA content of the liver,[11] and zinc deficiency in the rat had no effect on DNA content or rate of synthesis in the testes.[4] Although the bulk of evidence suggests an effect of zinc on DNA synthesis, one must carefully assess whether the effect is specific or whether zinc deficiency simply decreases cell division and only, by another mechanism, secondarily decreases DNA synthesis.

Transcription and RNA Synthesis

As mentioned above Wacker[12] and Schneider and Price[7] observed a decreased rate of RNA synthesis in *Euglena gracilis* grown in zinc deficient media. Wegener and Romano[14] made similar observations in *Rhizopus nigricans.*

On the other hand the work of Fujioka and Lieberman,[1] Turk,[4] Macapinlac et al.,[4] Weser et al.[13] and O'Neal et al.,[5] which dealt with the zinc deficient rats and chicks, failed to show an effect of zinc on RNA synthesis. These differences between the lower and higher life forms are clear cut and appear to be species differences.

The strongest evidence for direct involvement of zinc in RNA synthesis comes from the observation of Scrutton et al.[8] that highly purified preparations of DNA-dependent RNA polymerase from *E. coli* contains 2 g atoms of tightly bound zinc per mole (370,000 M.W.) of enzyme. Initiation of RNA synthesis was specifically inhibited by 1, 10-phenanthroline. These results confirm the earlier observations that zinc plays a role in RNA synthesis in microorganisms.

Overall Protein Synthesis

There are no data that relate zinc directly to the translation process, but the incorporation of labeled amino acids into tissue proteins has been used as an index of the rate of overall protein synthesis in higher animals.

Macapinlac et al.[4] found that zinc deficiency has no effect on the incorporation of leucine into testis protein while O'Neal et al.[5] observed no effect in brain protein. Similarly Hsu and Anthony[2] observed no difference in the incorporation of cystine-^{35}S into liver, kidney and testis protein between zinc deficient and pair-fed control rats. On the other hand, they observed strikingly less incorporation into skin protein. There was higher incorporation into bones and muscle and markedly higher urinary excretion of ^{35}S in the zinc deficient animals. In these studies there seems to be a high degree of tissue specificity. This fact suggests that another undefined factor plays a role. For example, zinc may influence the delivery of the amino acid to the cells of certain tissues.

In summary, it may be concluded that zinc plays a specific role in both DNA and RNA synthesis but there is species specificity. Zinc deficiency decreases the rate of protein synthesis, in higher animals, at least in some tissues, but the specific role is unclear at this time.

REFERENCES

1. Fujioka, M., and Lieberman, L.: A Zn^{++} requirement for synthesis of deoxyribonucleic acid by rat liver. *J Biol Chem*, 239:1164, 1964.

2. Hsu, J. M., and Anthony, W. L.: Impairment of cystine-^{35}S incorporation into skin protein by zinc-deficient rats. *J Nutr*, 101:445, 1971.

3. Lieberman, I., Abrams, R., Hunt, N., and Ove, P.: Changes in the metabolism of ribonucleic acid preceding the synthesis of deoxyribonucleic acid in mammalian cells cultured from the animal. *J Biol Chem*, 238:2141, 1963.

4. Macapinlac, M. P., Pearson, W. N., Barney, G. H., and Darby, W. J.: Protein and nucleic acid metabolism in the testes of zinc-deficient rats. *J Nutr*, 95:569, 1968.

5. O'Neal, R. M., Pla, G. W., Fox, M. R. S., Gibson, F. S., and Fry, B. E., Jr.: Effect of zinc deficiency and restricted feeding on protein and ribonucleic acid metabolism of rat brain. *J Nutr*, 100:491, 1970.

6. Sandstead, H. H., and Rinaldi, R. A.: Impairment of deoxyribonucleic acid synthesis by dietary zinc deficiency in the rat. *J Cell Physiol*, 73:81, 1969.

7. Schneider, E., and Price, C. A.: Decreased ribonucleic acid levels: A possible cause of growth inhibition in zinc deficiency. *Biochim Biophys Acta*, 55:406, 1962.

8. Scrutton, M. C., Wu, C. W., and Goldthwaite, D. A.: The presence and possible role of zinc in RNA polymerase obtained from *Escherichia Coli*. *Proc Natl Acad Sci USA*, 68:2497, 1971.

9. Slater, J. P., Mildvan, A. S., and Loeb, L. A.: Zinc in DNA polymerase. *Biochem Biophys Res Commun*, 44:37, 1971.

10. Swenerton, H., Shrader, R., and Hurley, L. S.: Zinc-deficiency embryos: Reduced thymidine incorporation. *Science*, 166:1014, 1969.

11. Turk, D. E.: Nucleic acid metabolism and zinc deficiency in the chick. *Poult Sci* 45:608, 1966.

12. Wacker, W. E. C.: Nucleic acids and metals. Three changes in nucleic acid, protein and metal content as a consequence of zinc deficiency in *Euglena gracilis*. *Biochemistry*, 1:859, 1962.

13. Weser, O., Hübner, L., and Jung, H.: Zn^{2+} induced stimulation of nuclear RNA synthesis in rat liver. *FEBS Letters* 7:356, 1970.

14. Wegner, W. S., and Romano, A. H.: Zinc stimulation of RNA and protein synthesis in *Rhizopus nigricans*. *Science*, 142:1669, 1963.

15. Williams, R. B., and Chesters, J. K.: The effects of early zinc deficiency on DNA and protein synthesis in the rat. *Br J Nutr*, 24:1053, 1970.

Chapter 1

ZINC DEFICIENCY: EFFECT ON THE ACTIVITY OF LIVER RNA POLYMERASE, SUCROSE DENSITY GRADIENTS AND *IN VIVO* URIDINE INCORPORATION

HAROLD H. SANDSTEAD[*]

AND

MARJORIE W. TERHUNE[†]

~~~~~~

INTRODUCTION

THE ROLE OF ZINC IN METABOLISM has intrigued nutritionists since 1934 when Todd et al.[1] first produced zinc deficiency in the rat. Since then, zinc has been shown to be essential for the function of many enzymes[2] and to influence the conformation of nucleic acids.[3-6] Presumably these two aspects of the role of zinc in homeostasis are interrelated, and account for the effects of zinc deficiency on the synthesis of proteins[7-10] and nucleic acids.[11-14] More grossly they are thought responsible for the effect of zinc on wound healing[15,16] and the role of zinc in growth and sexual maturation.[17]

Zinc influences so many aspects of metabolism that it is difficult to ascribe to it a primary role analogous to that of iron in oxygen transport. Even so, the effect of zinc deficiency on RNA of *Euglena gracilis* prompted Schneider and Price[18] to suggest that impaired synthesis or metabolism of RNA in zinc deficiency may be central to many of the manifestations of the deficiency. The observations of others noted above have since increased the attractiveness of this hypothesis. The studies reported in this manuscript were done to further evaluate the role of zinc in mammalian metabolism of ribonucleic acid.

Materials and Methods

Rats and mice were raised in a temperature and light-controlled relatively zinc-free environment in plastic cages and given glass distilled drinking water. The diet contained less than 0.5 ppm zinc, 20 percent sprayed egg white and was enriched with biotin.[13] Animals were divided into

[*]Supported By A Future Leaders Award from the Nutrition Foundation to Harold H. Sandstead and a National Science Foundation Fellowship to M. W. Terhune and the Human Nutrition Research Division of the Agricultural Research Service, U. S. Department of Agriculture.

[†]*Acknowledgements:* The technical assistance of Mr. David Gillespie and Mr. William Holloway is gratefully acknowledged.

groups of three. One animal in each group was fed the diet alone. The second animal (pair-fed control) was fed an amount of diet equivalent to what the deficient animal ate on the previous day and was injected intraperitoneally with 160 µg of zinc sulfate every other day, if a rat or was given 20 µg of zinc per ml of drinking water, if a mouse. The third animal was fed the diet ad libitum (ad lib control) and supplemented with zinc in the same manner as the pair-fed control animal.

For studies of the effect of zinc deficiency on liver nuclear DNA dependent RNA polymerase, pregnant dams were fed the diet from the eighteenth day of gestation. Thus suckling pups, nursed by dams receiving the diet alone, became zinc deficient, and pups nursed by pair-fed dams were starved due to poor milk production.[19] The litters were sampled at intervals by removing three to eleven pups for assay. The number of pups required for assay was greatest soon after delivery, the usual number in each sample being five or six.

Pups were decapitated, their livers rapidly removed and pooled in ice cold 0.32 M/sucrose containing 3 mM magnesium chloride. A nuclear suspension was prepared by the method of Widmell and Tata[20] and assayed for RNA polymerase activity by the method of Weiss.[21] The deoxyribose content of the nuclear suspension was assayed by the Giles and Meyers modification of Burton's diphenylamine method.[22] The activity of RNA polymerase was expressed as the average ^{14}C counts (from ^{14}C-ATP) per minute per milligram of deoxyribose per milliliter of nuclear suspension.

Assessment of the method for reproducibility and for quantitative differences in activity between pups of the same age and treatment revealed that the method was highly reproducible and that the activity of the enzyme in the livers of pups of the same age and treatment was similar.

The effect of zinc deficiency on the liver deoxycholate treated postmitochondrial supernatant was assessed in weanling and adult male rats. The *in vivo* incorporation of ^{3}H-uridine into fractions of the supernatant was measured in adult mice.

When rats fed the diet alone showed clinical evidence of deficiency, they and their control *mates* were fasted overnight (16 hours) and decapitated in the morning. Their livers were rapidly removed and a portion homogenized in a solution containing 0.005 M Tris buffer, 0.025 M KCl, 0.005 M Mg Cl₂, 0.25 M sucrose at pH 7.7 (0°C.) with a glass-teflon homogenizer. The remaining liver was promptly frozen at −140°F for subsequent conformation of findings on the initial gradient.

The liver homogenates were centrifuged for 15 minutes at 11,000 × g at 0°C. Ten percent Na-deoxycholate was added to the supernatants to a final concentration of 1 percent and the solutions were centrifuged at 105,000 × g for two hours at 0°C. The pellets were then suspended in the buffer solution and centrifuged at 11,000 × g for 15 minutes at 0°C. The optical densities of the supernatant were determined at 260 mμ and one to two OD units of each supernatant was placed on a 15 to 30 percent four centimeter sucrose gradient above a 50 percent sucrose cushion. The gradients were centrifuged for two hours at 105,000 × g at 0°C and then pumped through an ISCO ultra-violet analyzer with 65 percent sucrose containing 3 mM potassium acid phthalate at wave length 250 mμ.

The *in vivo* incorporation of uridine into fractions of the liver post-mitochondrial supernatant was assessed in adult mice by the intraperitoneal injection of 10 to 50 μc of ³H-uridine 16 to 17 hours prior to decapitation. Livers of two mice of the same age, sex and treatment were pooled for each assay. Following passage of the density gradients through the U.V. analyzer, they were collected in fractions with an automatic device and the radioactivity in each fraction assayed by liquid scintillation counting.

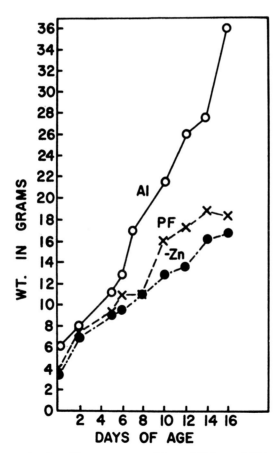

FIGURE 1-1. Growth of suckling rats nursed by ad libitum (AL), pair-fed (PF) and zinc deficient (—Zn) dams from delivery.

Results and Discussion

The effects of maternal zinc deprivation, pair feeding and ad libitum feeding on the growth of suckling rats are shown in Figure 1-1. While the average weight gain of the pups nursed by ad libitum-fed dams was rapid, the gain of pups nursed by pair-fed and zinc-deficient dams was slow. Pups of dams deprived of zinc or pair fed from the eighteenth day of gestation weighed, on the average, two grams less than those born to the ad libitum-fed dams. Growth of zinc-deficient and pair-fed pups generally paralleled growth of ad libitum pups until five days of age, after which it fell behind. The retardation in growth of the pups nursed by pair-fed dams reflected the decrease in milk production which occurs in starvation.[19] The patterns of growth observed were similar to those previously reported in pups nursed by dams fed in this manner.[19,23]

The RNA polymerase activities of the isolated liver nuclei from the suckling rats are summarized in Table 1-I and presented graphically in Figure 1-2.

TABLE 1-I°

Age (days)	Zinc Deficient	Pair fed Control	Ad Libitum fed Control
2	83.0[a]	81.5	78.6
4	85.9[a]		90.9
5		91.5	
6	85.0	87.0	94.8
7			103.5
8		98.9	105.0[a]
10	91.2	111.3[a]	
11			115.9[a]
12	80.4	114.4[a]	112.8
14	70.0	112.1	115.4[b]
15	64.8	111.1[a]	112.8[a]
16	60.4	107.8	107.4

°Expressed as ¹⁴C cpm/mg deoxyribose/ml
[a]Average of two sets of pups.
[b]Average of three sets of pups.

By inspection, it can be seen that there were striking differences in the activity of the enzyme in the liver nuclei obtained from the zinc-deficient pups compared to liver nuclei from pups nursed by pair-fed or ad libitum-fed dams. Statistically the differences were highly significant from the tenth day ($P < 0.001$). In addition, the activity of the enzyme in nuclei from the control pups progressively increased during the initial ten days of the experiment while it did not in the zinc-deficient pups.

From these findings it is not possible to specify whether the decrease in enzyme activity occurred because of an impairment in synthesis of the enzyme or was due to a requirement of zinc for activity of the enzyme.

The effect of zinc deficiency on the sedimentation characteristics of

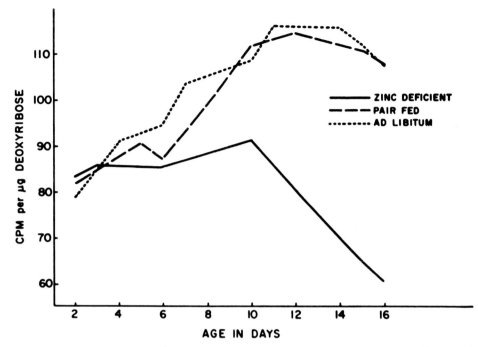

FIGURE 1-2. Effect of maternal zinc deficiency on the activity of liver nuclear DNA dependent RNA polymerase of suckling rats.

RNA in the deoxycholate-treated post-mitochondrial fraction of liver from adult rats is shown in Figure 1-3. In this and all subsequent figures, the top of the gradient is on the left. A consistent feature of the gradients of

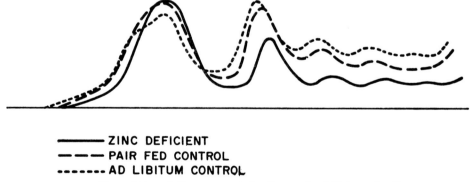

FIGURE 1-3. Effect of Zinc deficiency, pair-feeding and ad libitum feeding on sucrose density gradients of liver deoxycholate treated, postmitochondrial supernatent of representative adult rats. The top of the gradient is on the left. The first peak represents monomers of RNA. Polymers of RNA are represented on the right. The apparent decrease in RNA polymers in postmitochondrial supernatent from the zinc deficient animal is obvious.

the zinc-deficient livers was an increase in the first peak (monosomes), and a decrease in all subsequent peaks. In contrast, the monosomal peak of the control livers was lower, as was the area under the monosomal peak, relative to the area under the second and subsequent peaks.

Because this abnormality of RNA sedimentation was a consistent finding in the zinc-deficient rats, and injection of 100 µg of zinc into a zinc-deficient rat the day before decapitation was followed by a shift in the pattern to one similar to that of the pair-fed control animal, the effect of zinc deficiency on the *in vivo* uridine incorporation into fractions of the post-mitochondrial supernatant was studied. Seven days after initiation of the diet, the incorporation was decreased in the zinc-deficient mice (Fig. 1-4). Prior to this time, the incorporation was greater in the zinc-deficient compared to the pair-fed pups.

After ten days of deficiency, the differences in incorporation were even

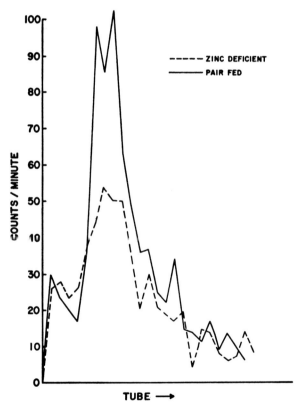

FIGURE 1-4. Effect of zinc deficiency and pair-feeding on the *in vivo* incorporation of ³H-uridine into the liver deoxycholate treated postmitochondrial supernatent of mice fed the diet for seven days. The top of the gradient is on the left.

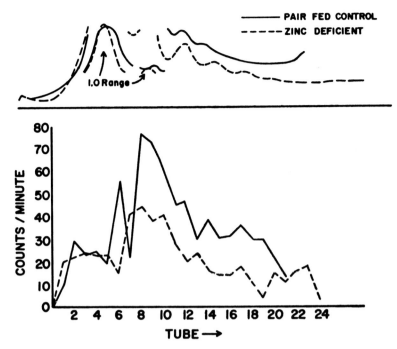

FIGURE 1-5. Effect of zinc deficiency and pair-feeding on the sucrose density gradient profile and the *in vivo* ³H-uridine incorporation of liver deoxycholate treated post-mitochondrial supernatent from mice fed the diet ten days. The top of the gradient is on the left.

greater between pair-fed and zinc-deficient animals (Fig. 1-5). Also, the density gradient pattern showed a decrease in heavier polymers.

Figure 1-6 shows the incorporation of uridine after fourteen days. No radioactivity was found in fractions heavier than monosomes. The density-gradient pattern was consistent with this finding. In contrast, the net uridine incorporation into heavier RNA polymers of the control livers was not decreased.

The cause of the decreased incorporation of uridine into liver RNA of the zinc-deficient animals and their abnormal density-gradient patterns is unclear. The decreased RNA polymerase activity found in zinc-deficient suckling rats suggests that impaired synthesis of RNA may account, in part, for the findings. On the other hand, degradation of RNA may have been increased. It is possible that both phenomena may have occurred. Studies in microorganisms[7,18] and the rat[12] support the suggestion that RNA synthesis was decreased. The second possibility is supported by the finding of an increased RNA polymerase activity in testes of zinc-deficient rats.[25] Inadequate amounts of zinc for maintenance of tertiary structure of

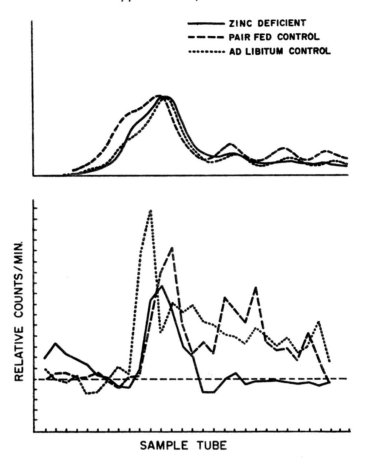

FIGURE 1-6. Effect of zinc deficiency, pair-feeding and ad libitum feeding on the sucrose density gradient profile and the *in vivo* incorporation of ³H-uridine into the liver deoxycholate treated postmitochondrial supernatent of mice fed the diet for fourteen days. The top of the gradient is on the left.

RNA[3,4,6] and possibly for formation of polymers of RNA through covalent binding might result in an increase in the concentration monomers as well as increase in susceptibility to RNA polymerase.

Because of the role of polysomes in protein synthesis,[26] the findings we have reported may help explain why zinc-deficient animals demonstrate impaired incorporation of amino acids into protein[9,10,24] and of thymidine into DNA.[11,13,14] In any case, our observations support the hypothesis of Schneider and Price,[18] and suggest that additional investigation of this molecular aspect of zinc deficiency may prove fruitful.

SUMMARY

1. Zinc deficiency in suckling rates results in a decreased activity of liver nuclear DNA dependent RNA polymerase.
2. The sedimentation characteristics of the deoxycholate treated liver post-mitochondrial supernatant RNA are altered by zinc deficiency. Monomers are increased, while heavier polymers are decreased.
3. The net 16-hour *in vivo* incorporation of uridine into RNA of the liver postmitochondrial supernatant is decreased by zinc deficiency.

REFERENCES

 1. Todd, W. R., Elvejhem, C. A., and Hart, E. B.: Zinc in the nutrition of the rat. *Am J Physol, 107*:146, 1934.
 2. Mikac-Devic, D.: Methodology of zinc determinations and the role of zinc in biochemical processes. In Bodansky, O., and Stewart, C. P. (Eds.): *Advances in Clinical Chemistry*. New York, Academic Press, 1970, Vol. 13, pp. 271-333.
 3. Wacker, W. E. C., and Vallee, B. L.: Nucleic acids and metals. I. Chromium, manganese, nickel, iron and other metals in ribonucleic acid from diverse biological sources. *J Biol Chem, 234*:3257, 1959.
 4. Altmann, H., Fetter, F., and Kaindl, K.: Untersuchungen über den Einfluss von Zn-Ionen auf die M-RNS-Synthese in Chlorellazellen. *Z Naturforsh, 23b*:395, 1968.
 5. Shin, Y. A., and Eichorn, G. L.: Interactions of metal ions with polynucleotides and related compounds. XI. The reversible unwinding and rewinding of deoxyribonucleic acid by zinc (II) ions through temperature manipulation. *Biochemistry,* 7:1026, 1968.
 6. Tal, M.: Metal ions and ribosomal conformation. *Biochim Biophys Acta, 195*:76, 1969.
 7. Wacker, W. E. C.: Nucleic acids and metals. III. Changes in nucleic acids, proteins and metal content as a consequence of zinc deficiency in *Euglena gracilis*. *Biochemistry, 1*:859, 1962.
 8. Theuer, R. C., and Hoekstra, W. G.: Oxidation of ^{14}C-labeled carbohydrate, fat and amino acid substrates by zinc deficient rats. *J Nutr, 89*:448, 1966.
 9. Hsu, J. M., Anthony, W. L., and Buchanan, P. J.: Zinc deficiency and incorporation of ^{14}C-labeled methionine into tissue proteins of rats. *J Nutr, 99*:425, 1969.
10. Hsu, J. M., and Anthony, W. L.: Zinc deficiency and urinary excretion of taurine-^{35}S and inorganic sulfate-^{35}S following cystine-^{35}S injection in rats. *J Nutr, 100*:1189, 1970.
11. Fujioka, M., and Lieberman, I.: A Zn^{+2} requirement for synthesis of deoxyribonucleic acid by rat. *J Biol Chem, 239*:1164, 1964.
12. Williams, R. B., Mills, C. F., Quartman, J., and Dalgarno, A. C.: The effect of zinc deficiency on the *in vivo* incorporation of ^{32}P into rat liver nucleotides. *Biochem J, 95*:29P, 1965.
13. Sandstead, H. H., and Rinaldi, R. A.: Impairment of deoxyribonucleic acid synthesis by dietary zinc deficiency in the rat. *J Cell Physiol, 73*:81, 1969.
14. Swenerton, H., Schrader, R., and Hurley, L. S.: Zinc deficient embryos: Reduced thymidine incorporation. *Science, 166*:1014, 1969.

15. Pories, W. J., Henzel, J. H., Rob, C. G., and Strain, W. H.: Acceleration of wound healing in man with zinc sulfate given by mouth. *Lancet, i*:121, 1967.
16. Sandstead, H. H., Lanier, V. C., Shepard, G. H., and Gillespie, D. D.: Zinc and wound healing: Effects of zinc deficiency and zinc supplementation. *Am J Clin Nutr, 23*:514, 1970.
17. Sandstead, H. H., Prasad, A. S., Schulert, A. R., Farid, Z., Miale, A. Jr., Bassilly, S., and Darby, W. J.: Human zinc deficiency, endocrine manifestations and response to treatment. *Am J Clin Nutr, 20*:422, 1967.
18. Schneider, E., and Price, C. A.: Decreased ribonucleic acid levels: A possible cause of growth inhibition in zinc deficiency. *Biochim Biophys Acta, 55*:406, 1962.
19. Mutch, P. B., and Hurley, L. S.: Zinc deficiency in suckling rats. *Fed Proc, 30*: 2501, 1971 (Abstract).
20. Widnell, C. C., and Tata, J. R.: A procedure for the isolation of enzymatically active rat liver nuclei. *Biochem J, 92*:313, 1964.
21. Weiss, S. B.: Enzymatic incorporation of ribonucleoside triphosphates into the internucleotide linkages of ribonucleic acid. *PNAS, 46*:1020, 1960.
22. Giles, K. W., and Meyers, A.: An improved diphenylamine method for estimation of deoxyribonucleic acid. *Nature, 206*:93, 1965.
23. Sandstead, H. H., Gillespie, D. D., and Brady, R. N.: Zinc deficiency: Effect on brain of the suckling rat. *Ped Res, 6*:119, 1972.
24. Lema, O., and Sandstead, H. H.: Zinc deficiency: Effect on epiphyseal growth. *Clin Res, 18*:458, 1970 (Abstract).
25. Somers, M., and Underwood, E. J.: Ribonuclease activity and nucleic acid and protein metabolism in the testes of zinc deficient rats. *Aust J Biol Sci, 22*:1277, 1969.
26. Wittman, J. S., and Miller, O. N.: Functional nature of the polysomes as indicated by the influence of insulin-glucose and adrenalectomy-cortisol on rat liver polysomes *in vivo. Am J Clin Nutr, 24*:770, 1971.

DISCUSSION

Dr. Vallee: I think there is some new information in this week's issue of the Proc. of the National Academy of Sciences, 68:2497 (1971), which you will like. It was shown that DNA dependent RNA polymerase is a zinc dependent enzyme.

Dr. Sable: Is it possible that there is any change in the incorporation of uridine?

Dr. Sandstead: If you mean incorporation of uridine *in vitro*, we have not tried that experiment. It should be done. I left Vanderbilt about the time these things were going on and have not been able to continue these studies. A lot of things need to be looked at.

Chapter 2

BIOCHEMICAL EFFECTS OF ZINC DEFICIENCY IN EXPERIMENTAL ANIMALS*

ANANDA S. PRASAD

AND

DONALD OBERLEAS

INTRODUCTION

ZINC IS AN ESSENTIAL MICRONUTRIENT for the growth of plants, animals and man.[1] Various studies by Vallee[2] have shown that zinc is an essential constituent for activity of a number of metallo-enzymes. One may suggest, therefore, that the level of zinc in cells controls the physiological processes through the formation and/or regulation of activity of zinc-dependent enzymes. Until 1966, evidence of support for this concept in experimental animals did not exist in the literature.[3] During the past five years, we have analyzed various tissues of zinc-deficient rats and pigs for zinc and activities of several enzymes. The results of our analyses[4-7] will be summarized in this paper.

Some investigators have suggested that zinc may play a role in the polymeric organization of macromolecules such as ribonucleic acid (RNA) and deoxyribonucleic acid (DNA).[18] In micro-organisms, results have been obtained which show that the primary effect of zinc may be on RNA and protein synthesis.[9,10] Macapinlac et al.[11] have observed a consistent decrease in RNA content of the testis in zinc-deficient rats as compared to their pair-fed controls, but Theuer[12] failed to show any reduction in RNA content of the rat liver in zinc-deficient state. We, therefore, assayed RNA, DNA and protein content of various tissues in zinc-deficient pigs in order to investigate some of the metabolic effects of zinc.

MATERIALS AND METHODS

Experiments in the rats

Two sets of experiments were carried out in the rats. In the first set, weanling male albino rats (Holtzman strain) were maintained in stainless steel cages and given distilled water in glass bottles. Diets were fed ad libitum except in the pair-feeding study, in which the animals were kept in individual cages and the control animals received an amount of diet equal to the mean consumed daily by the deficient animals. The animals were weighed weekly for 6 weeks.

*Supported in part by a grant from the Detroit General Hospital Research Corporation.

19

The basal diet (low zinc) contained the following (grams per kg): glucose hydrate (cerelose), 666; corn oil, 90; C-1 assay protein, 150; minerals,* 50; phytic acid (54.3 percent), 7.3; vitamins and methionine.† This diet was calculated to contain 12 percent crude protein, 1.6 percent calcium, 0.6 percent inorganic phosphorus and 1 percent phytate. The zinc content was determined to be 10 mg/kg. For the normal (high zinc) diet, 55 mg/kg of zinc as the carbonate were added to the basal diet.

In the first experiment, 18 rats served as ad libitum controls and 18 received a diet deficient in zinc for 6 weeks. Ten rats received zinc-deficient diet for 3 weeks, after which they received zinc supplement for 2 weeks (repleted group); in the sixth week they were sacrificed for tissue analysis. In the second experiment, 6 rats served as pair-fed controls and 6 were made zinc deficient for 6 weeks.

The animals were sacrificed by cardiectomy after ether anesthesia. The tissues were removed, washed several times with deionized water, and placed in metal-free polyethylene containers. The samples were lyophilized‡ for 3 days. The lyophilized dry weight was taken, and the tissues were placed in micro-kjeldahl flasks with re-distilled nitric acid§ and digested until solution was complete. The digested materials were diluted 1:5 with deionized water for most analyses. Analysis for zinc was performed by atomic absorption spectrophotometry‖ according to methods reported previously.[4]

Tissues from different groups of rats were analyzed histochemically for enzyme activities. We studied NADH diaphorase and lactic, malic, alcohol and succinic dehydrogenases. Small pieces of tissue were frozen in a test tube and immersed in dry ice and acetone at $-65°C$. They were transferred to a Linderstrom-Lang cryostat and cut and maintained at $-25°C$ until ready to be immersed in the substrate. The substrate for NADH diaphorase consisted of 5 mg NADH in 12 ml phosphate buffer (0.2 M, pH 7.5) and 3 ml of nitro blue tetrazolium (2 mg per ml H_2O).

---

*The following minerals were supplied (grams per kilogram diet):
$CaCo_3$, 10.6; $CaHPO_4·2 H_2O$, 16.5; $MgCO_3$, 1.0; $MgSO_4·7 H_2O$, 1.2; NaCl, 5.0; KCl, 0.8; $FePO_4$ (soluble), 1.6; KH_2PO_4, 12.5; $MnSO_4· H_2O$, 0.8; $CuSO_4·5 H_2O$, 0.06; AlK $(SO_4)_2·12 H_2O$, 0.01; KIO_3, 0.03; $CoCl_2·6 H_2O$, 0.002; NaF, 0.04.

†Vitamins were supplied at the following levels per kilogram diet:
Vitamin A, 20,000 IU; vitamin D, 3,000 IU; menadione, 10 mg; α-tocopheryl acetate, 30 mg; thiamine HCl, 16 mg; riboflavin, 16 mg; pyridoxine HCl, 16 mg; Ca pantothenate, 40 mg; biotin, 0.2 mg; folacin, 5 mg; cyanocobalamin, 0.05 mg; choline chloride, 1,000 mg; methionine, 2.0 g. The antioxidant, butylated hydroxyanisole was supplied at 100 mg per kg.

‡Virtis mechanically refrigerated Freeze Mobile, Virtis Co., Gardiner, N. Y.

§G. F. Smith, Columbus, Ohio.

‖Model 303, Perkin-Elmer Corp., Norwalk, Conn., equipped with a model SRL Recorder, E. H. Sargent Co., Detroit, Mich.

The substrate solution for lactic dehydrogenase consisted of 5 ml Ca L-(+)-lactate (0.2 M) and 5 mg NAD in 7 ml Tris buffer (0.2 m, pH, 7.4), and 3 ml nitro blue tetrazolium (2 mg per ml H_2O). The substrate for malic dehydrogenase consisted of L-malic acid (0.25 M) and 5 mg NAD in 7 ml Tris buffer (0.2 M, pH 7.4). The substrate solution for succinic dehydrogenase consisted of 5 ml disodium salt of succinic acid (0.1 M) in 7 ml phosphate buffer (0.2 M, pH 7.5) and 3 ml of nitro blue tetrazolium (2 mg per ml H_2O). The incubation solution for alcohol dehydrogenase was prepared according to the method published by Pearse.[13]

The slides with the affixed tissues were incubated at 25°C for 15 minutes for NADH diaphorase and 30 minutes for malic, lactic and succinic dehydrogenases. The slides for ADH were incubated for 3 hours. In the presence of appropriate tissue enzymes and added co-enzymes, the tetrazolium was reduced to form a colored insoluble formazan, which precipitated at the sites of enzymes in the tissues. The mean formazan intensities were visually evaluated from 1 to 4 plus by three investigators independently.

Alkaline phosphatase reaction was determined histochemically by a method reported by Wolf et al.[14] Fresh frozen and cold acetone-fixed sections were incubated in solutions containing para-toluidinium 5-bromo-4-chloro-3-indolyl phosphate, or para-toluidinium 5-bromo-6-chloro-3-indolyl phosphate, depending on the desired color of the end product. The solutions were made specific for alkaline phosphatase by varying the pH of the buffer used for incubation. The incubating solution employed for alkaline phosphatase was as follows: 14.0 ml (0.1 M) Tris buffer (pH 8.4) containing 4.0 mg of spermadine trihydrochloride, 1.0 ml (0.05 M in dimethyl formamide) of substrate (paratoluidinium 5-bromo-4-chloro-3-indolyl phosphate), and 1.0 ml of 0.005 M $MgCl_2$. After incubation for 2 hours the slides were washed briefly in tap water and mounted in glycerol gel for microscopic examination.

In the second set of experiments, 12 weanling male albino rats (Holtzman strain) from each treatment group were maintained in stainless steel cages and were given distilled water automatically from polyethylene jugs by polyvinyl chloride pipe (Upjohn Carematic°). The diet was presented to the pair-fed animals in a time-controlled feeder similar to Mills and Chesters'.[15] Dietary treatments were for 5 weeks prior to sacrifice.

The basal diet (low zinc) contained the following (g/kg): glucose hydrate (cerelose), 623.5; corn oil, 100; soybean assay protein washed with ethylenediaminetetraacetate (EDTA), 200; minerals, 50; phytic acid, 6.5; calcium carbonate, 20; vitamins and methionine. The basal

°Upjohn Carematic, Kalamazoo, Mich.

deficient diet contained 8 mg/kg of zinc. For the controls, 110 mg/kg zinc as carbonate were added to the basal diet.

Liver, kidney, testis, pancreas, bone (tibia) and thymus were analyzed for their zinc content by means of atomic absorption spectrophotometry.[4] For enzyme analysis, liver, kidney, testis, and pancreas were appropriately diluted with 0.02 M tris buffer and homogenized in a Potter-Elvehjem glass homogenizer.* The bone was pulverized in the frozen state to a homogenous powder using a Thermovac tissue pulverizer† cooled in an acetone dry ice bath. The powder was then weighed and appropriately extracted with 0.02 M tris buffer. For the analysis of alcohol dehydrogenase, alkaline phosphatase, aldolase and lactic dehydrogenase, supernate was obtained by centrifuging the whole homogenate for 30 minutes at 8000g in an International refrigerated centrifuge‡ equipped with a high speed head.

Alcohol dehydrogenase was measured by a modified method of Bonnichsen and Brink[16] as reported by Mezey et al.[17] Optimum substrate level was established for each tissue in the control samples by varying the final concentration of ethanol between 1×10^{-1} to 4×10^{-2}M. .01M Na pyrophosphate, pH 10.3 was used as a buffer. A blank control containing no substrate was included with each test. The enzyme activity was expressed as ΔOD (change in optical density) at 340 nmμ/min/mg protein.

Alkaline phosphatase activity was determined by a method described by Linhardt and Walter[18] using p-nitrophenyl-phosphate substrate. Optimum substrate levels were determined for each tissue in the control group. as ΔOD (change in optical density) at 340 nmμ/min/mg protein.

The activity of aldolase was determined by a spectrophotometric method as reported by Bruns and Bergmeyer.[19] Lactic dehydrogenase activity was measured spectrophotometrically by the modified method of Bergmeyer et al.[20] Optimum substrate level for controls was determined for each tissue by varying the concentration of pyruvate from 3.3×10^{-5} M to 1.7×10^{-3} M.

Succinic dehydrogenase activity was measured at optimum substrate level by the method of Cooperstein et al.[21] Carboxypeptidase activity was determined by the method of Ravin and Seligman.[22] For each test, tissue homogenate inactivated for 5 minutes in boiling water, was used as a blank.

The effect of additional zinc in the final concentrations ranging from 1×10^{-5} M to 1×10^{-4} M on the activities of various enzymes was determined when the substrate levels were optimal. In separate experiments, EDTA was added in the final concentrations ranging from 2×10^{-4} M to

*Kontes Glass Co., 9943 Franklin Ave., Franklin Park, Ill.
†Thermovac Industries Corp., 41 Decker Street, Copiagne, N. Y. 11726.
‡International Equipment Co., 1284 Soldier's Field Rd., Boston, Mass.

1×10^{-1} M and its effect determined on the enzyme activities. Protein content of tissue homogenate was determined by a method reported by Inchiosa.[23]

Experiments in the pigs

Two sets of experiments were performed in the pigs. In the first set of experiments, 28 baby pigs from four crossbred Yorkshire-Hampshire litters were taken from their dams at 3 days of age and reared in stainless steel cages with trays underneath, which made it possible to estimate food wastage. During the next 4 day adjustment period, all pigs received a purified diet (Table 2-I) containing 12 ppm of zinc. At 1 week of age the pigs were allotted to two groups with an attempt to equalize for sex, litter, and weight. The zinc-deficient group received the basal diet containing 12 ppm of zinc while the controls received the same diet supplemented with zinc to a dietary concentration of 90 ppm. All pigs were supplied with diet daily for ad-libitum intake. The control pigs were

TABLE 2-I

COMPOSITION OF DRY PURIFIED DIET

Ingredient	%	Vitamins	Parts per Million in Diet
Isolated soy[a]	30.0	Thiamine-mononitrate	3
DL-Methionine	0.3	Riboflavin	6
α-Cellulose	5.0	Nicotinamide	40
Lard	5.0	Calcium pantothenate	30
Cerelose[b]	50.7	Pyridoxine hydrochloride	2
Mineral mixture	6.0	Para-aminobenzoic acid	13
Corn oil with fat-			
soluble vitamins	1.0	Ascorbic acid	80
Mineral mixture		α-Tocopheryl acetate	10
KCl	10.0	Inositol	130
KI	0.002	Choline chloride	1,300
			Parts per Billion in Diet
$FeSO_4 2H_2O$	0.7	Pteroylglutamic acid	260
$CuSO_4$	0.1	Biotin	1,000
$CoCO_3$	0.1	Cyanocobalamin	100
$MnSO_4 H_2O$	0.1	2-Methyl-1, 4-naphtho-	40
$ZnSO_4 H_2O$[c]	0.0[d] (0.4)[e]	quinone	
$MgCO_3$	2.0	Vitamin A palmitate	1,500
$NaHCO_3$	25.0	Vitamin D_2	12.5
$CaHPO_4 2H_2O$	36.0		
$CaCO_3$	12.5		
Cerelose	13.098		
Total	100.000		

[a]Soya assay protein, General Biochemicals Co., Chagrin Falls, Ohio. [b]Glucose monohydrate, cerelose, Corn Products Co., Argo, Ill. [c]The analysis revealed the zinc content of deficient diet to approximate 12 ppm, whereas of the control diet, 90 ppm. [d]Zn-deficient diet. [e]Control diet.
Source: Prasad et al., *Am J Clin Nutr*, 22:628, 1969.

limited to about the daily mean intake of the zinc-deficient pigs. The pigs were allowed free access to drinking water (zinc content less than 0.1 ppm). Weight was recorded weekly.

Pigs were sacrificed on the 23rd day. Tissues were removed by blunt dissection and quickly frozen for further analysis. Tissues were analyzed for zinc, and activities of various enzymes were measured histochemically according to methods discussed earlier.

In the second set of experiments, 16 baby pigs were used. The dietary treatments were similar to the previous set of experiments. Pigs were sacrificed on the thirtieth day.

Liver, kidney, pancreas and bone (rib) were analyzed for their zinc content, and activities of various enzymes in tissue homogenates were determined by using methods as discussed earlier (see second set of experiments of rats). DNA and RNA were measured spectrophotometrically by the Schmidt-Thannheuser method as modified by Monroe and Fleck.[24]

RESULTS

Experimental Results in Rats

Table 2-II shows the results of zinc analysis in various tissues of rats, in the first set of experiments. Zinc content of the bone, testis, muscle, esophagus and kidney was significantly decreased in the deficient animals as compared to their pair-fed controls. Figure 2-1 shows the changes in

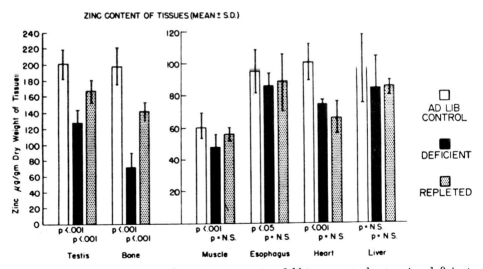

FIGURE 2-1. Zinc content of various tissues in ad libitum control rats, zinc-deficient rats and a repleted group of rats (3 weeks on zinc-deficient diet followed by zinc supplementation for 2 weeks). Comparison of means between ad libitum controls and the deficient group and the repleted group were indicated by the p values.

TABLE 2-II

ANALYSIS OF VARIOUS TISSUES FOR ZINC IN PAIR-FED CONTROLS
AND ZINC-DEFICIENT RATS*

Tissue	Rats	Zinc (mcg/g dry wt.)†
Liver	Control	101 ± 13
	Deficient	89 ± 12
Bone	Control	168 ± 8
	Deficient	69 ± 6
		$p < 0.001$
Testis	Control	176 ± 12
	Deficient	132 ± 16
		$p < 0.001$
Muscle	Control	45 ± 5
	Deficient	31 ± 6
		$p < 0.01$
Esophagus	Control	108 ± 17
	Deficient	88 ± 10
		$p < 0.05$
Heart	Control	73 ± 16
	Deficient	67 ± 9
Lung	Control	81 ± 3
	Deficient	77 ± 9
Spleen	Control	105 ± 13
	Deficient	92 ± 5
Kidney	Control	91 ± 3
	Deficient	80 ± 3
		$p < 0.001$
Thyroid	Control	63 ± 7
	Deficient	58 ± 9
Adrenal	Control	66 ± 15
	Deficient	66 ± 20

*Tissues for analysis were obtained from six pair-fed controls and six zinc-deficient rats. All determinations were done in duplicate. Where the differences between the means were found to be statistically significant, p values have been included.
†Mean ± standard deviation.

the zinc content of the various tissues of the ad-libitum controls, the zinc-deficient group and the repleted group. The zinc content of the testis, bone, muscle, esophagus, and heart was decreased in the zinc-deficient rats compared to the ad-libitum controls. On repletion with zinc in the deficient group, the zinc content of the testis and bone increased significantly.

The activities of LDH, MDH, ADH and NADH diaphorase were reduced in the testes of the zinc-deficient rats compared to the controls (ad libitum and pair-fed), as determined histochemically. In the repleted group, the activities of the above enzymes in the testes were increased. The activities of LDH, MDH, ADH, NADH diaphorase, and alkaline phosphatase in the bone were reduced in the zinc-deficient rats compared

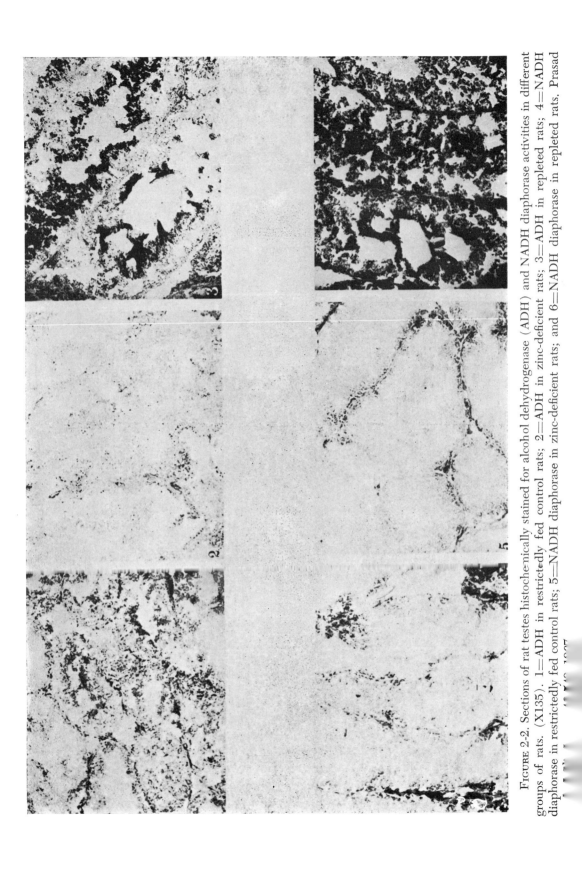

FIGURE 2-2. Sections of rat testes histochemically stained for alcohol dehydrogenase (ADH) and NADH diaphorase activities in different groups of rats. (X135). 1=ADH in restrictedly fed control rats; 2=ADH in zinc-deficient rats; 3=ADH in repleted rats; 4=NADH diaphorase in restrictedly fed control rats; 5=NADH diaphorase in zinc-deficient rats; and 6=NADH diaphorase in repleted rats. Prasad

to the controls (pair-fed and ad libitum). In the repleted group, these enzymes showed increased activities. The activities of MDH, ADH and NADH diaphorase in the esophagus were decreased in the zinc-deficient rats compared to the controls. Increased activity of NADH diaphorase in the esophagus was noted in the repleted group. In the kidneys, the activities of MDH and alkaline phosphatase were decreased in the zinc-deficient rats compared to the controls. After zinc supplementation, the activities of LDH, MDH, and NADH diaphorase increased in the kidneys. Figure 2-2 shows the enzyme activities as determined histochemically in the testes of rats.

Tissues such as liver, muscle, heart, lung, spleen, thyroid, and adrenal failed to show any consistent changes in the activities of the above mentioned enzymes in the deficient rats. No consistent change in the activity of SDH (an iron dependent enzyme) in the testis, bone, esophagus and kidneys was noted in the different groups of rats.

The results obtained in the second set of experiments in rats are summarized in Tables 2-III, 2-IV and 2-V. The zinc content and the activity of alcohol dehydrogenase and alkaline phosphatase in the kidney, testis and bone were significantly decreased in the deficient animals as compared to their ad-libitum and pair-fed controls.

The zinc content of the liver, pancreas and thymus was significantly decreased in the deficient rats as compared to their pair-fed controls, but was not significantly different when compared to the ad-libitum controls. The activities of alcohol dehydrogenase in the liver, carboxypeptidase and alkaline phosphatase in the pancreas and alkaline phosphatase in the thymus were significantly reduced in the deficient rats in comparison to both the ad-libitum and pair-fed controls.

The zinc content of some tissues (liver, bone and thymus) and the specific activities of certain zinc-dependent enzymes (aldolase in liver, alkaline phosphatase in kidney, and alcohol dehydrogenase and alkaline phosphatase in bone), were significantly higher in the pair-fed rats in comparison to the ad-libitum controls.

The activities of isocitric dehydrogenase (manganese dependent enzyme) and succinic dehydrogenase (iron dependent enzyme) remained essentially unaltered in the three groups of animals in various tissues with one exception. In the testis, the activity of isocitric dehydrogenase was highest in the zinc-deficient animals and lowest in the case of the pair-fed rats.

The effects of exogenous zinc and addition of EDTA to homogenates of the kidney from six pair-fed controls and six zinc-deficient rats, on the activities of alcohol dehydrogenase, alkaline phosphatase, and lactic dehydrogenase, were investigated. Exogenous zinc (1×10^{-5} M) significantly

TABLE 2-III

ZINC AND THE ACTIVITIES OF ENZYMES IN TISSUES OF CONTROLS AND ZINC-DEFICIENT RATS

	Zinc μg/g dry wt.	Activity of Enzymes*					Alkaline Phosphatase Sigma Units /mg Protein
		ADH	Aldolase	LDH	ICDH	SDH	
		ΔOD/min/mg protein					
Liver							
A	91.7±4.7	.021±.022	0.107±.0064		.43±.02	.151±.012	
B	107.3±3.1	.022±.0013	0.134±.0098		.38±.03	.152±.017	
C	87.6±3.5	.013±.008	0.124±.0010		.38±.02		
Comparison of Means							
A vs B	p<.025	NS	p<.05		NS		
A vs C	NS	p<.00	NS		NS		
B vs C	p<.001	p<.001	NS		NS	NS	
Kidney							
A	93±2.2	.0031±.00025	.20±.01	2.9±.27	.57±.03	.188±.0075	3.3±.22
B	87±.8	.0031±.0002	.22±.01	2.67±.07	.48±.03	.187±.0056	4.5±.25
C	80±.9	.0014±.0003	.21±.01	2.53±.04	.49±.04		2.3±.17
Comparison of Means							
A vs B	NS	NS	NS	NS	NS		p<.005
A vs C	p<.001	p<.001	NS	NS	NS		p<.005
B vs C	p<.001	p<.001	NS	NS	NS	NS	p<.001
Testis							
A	191.0±3.1	.022±.0018	.161±.0034	1.20±.08	.063±.0067	.128±.0048	2.75±.11
B	197.1±2.9	.028±.0030	.161±.0047		.046±.0052	.127±.0054	2.80±.10
C	114.7±4.9	.012±.0014	.164±.0112	1.22±.09	.090±.0076		1.70±.10
Comparison of Means							
A vs B	NS	NS	NS	NS	p<.025		NS
A vs C	p<.001	p<.001	NS		p<.025		p<.001
B vs C	p<.001	p<.001	NS	NS	p<.001	NS	p<.001

Values are: Mean ± S.E.

A—Ad libitum-fed controls, B—Pair-fed controls, C—Zinc-deficient rats NS—Not significant (p>0.05)

* ADH—alcohol dehydrogenase, LDH—lactic dehydrogenase, ICDH—isocitric dehydrogenase, SDH—succinic dehydrogenase

TABLE 2-IV

ZINC AND THE ACTIVITIES OF ENZYMES IN BONE AND THYMUS OF CONTROLS AND ZINC-DEFICIENT RATS

	Zinc g/g dry wt.	Activity of Enzymes*			Alkaline Phosphatase Sigma units /mg protein
		ADH	Aldolase	LDH	
			AOD/min/mg Protein		
Bone					
A	180±7.7	.0020±.0001	.128±.009	0.82±.04	3.46±.23
B	211±5.4	.0026±.0001	.068±.006	0.76±.04	4.69±.16
C	139±9.6	.0009±.0001	.078±.009		2.69±.14
Comparison of Means					
A vs B†	p<.01	p<.001	p<.001		p<.001
A vs C	p<.01	p<.001	p<.001		p<.025
B vs C	p<.001	p<.001	NS	NS	p<.001
Thymus					
A	83.7±1.9		.079±.008	4.41±.34	6.2±0.54
B	98.8±3.5		.080±.006	3.78±.52	5.7±0.32
C	81.1±2.2		.077±.005		3.5±0.25
Comparison of Means					
A vs B	p<.005		NS		NS
A vs C	NS		NS		p<.001
B vs C	p<.005		NS	NS	p<.001

Values are: Mean ± S.E.

A—Ad libitum-fed conrols; B—Pair-fed controls; C—Zinc-Deficient rats; NS—Not significant (p>0.05)

* ADH, alcohol dehydrogenase, LDH, lactic dehydrogenase

† Comparison of means

TABLE 2-V

ZINC AND THE ACTIVITIES OF ENZYMES IN PANCREAS OF CONTROLS AND ZINC-DEFICIENT RATS

	Zinc μg/g dry wt.	ICDH* ΔOD/min/mg Protein	Alkaline Phosphatase Sigma units /mg protein	CPD μ Moles β Naphthol Liberated /mg protein
Pancreas				
A	79.5 ± 3.2	.18 ± .02	1.8 ± .18	64.8 ± 11.2
B	88.9 ± 3.7	.16 ± .02	1.7 ± .11	61.19 ± 10.3
C	74.4 ± 3.2	.14 ± .01	1.4 ± .05	10.69 ± 3.43
Comparison of Means				
A vs B†	NS	NS	NS	NS
A vs C	NS	NS	$p < .05$	$p < .001$
B vs C	$p < .01$	NS	$p < .025$	$p < .001$

Values are: Mean ± S.E.
A—Ad libitum-fed controls; B—Pair-fed controls; C—Zinc-deficient rats
NS—Not significant ($p > 0.05$)
ICDH—isocitric dehydrogenase, CPD—carboxypeptidase
† Comparison of means

reduced the activity of alcohol dehydrogenase ($p<0.01$) but had no significant effect on the activity of alkaline phosphatase. In a concentration of
5×10^{-6} M, zinc had no significant effect on the activity of lactic dehydrogenase.

Addition of EDTA (5×10^{-2} M) to renal homogenate inhibited completely the activities of alcohol dehydrogenase and alkaline phosphatase. In
a concentration of 1×10^{-2} M EDTA, the activity of lactic dehydrogenase,
($\Delta OD/min/mg$ protein) in the pair-fed controls increased from a control
level of $2.67 \pm .07$ to $3.09 \pm .11$ (mean $\pm$ S.E.), whereas in the case of
zinc-deficient animals the activities before and after addition of EDTA
were $2.53 \pm .04$ and $2.69 \pm .09$ respectively. Following addition of EDTA
(5×10^{-2} M), the pair-fed controls showed a significantly higher activity
of lactic dehydrogenase as compared to the zinc-deficient animals
($p<0.025$).

Experimental Results in Pigs

In both sets of experiments, the growth of zinc-deficient pigs was
retarded and the feed-efficiency ratio was half of the control pigs (Table
2-VI). Parakeratosis of skin became moderately severe by the end of the
second week.

TABLE 2-VI

BODY WEIGHT, DAILY GAIN, FEED-EFFICIENCY RATIO, SERUM ZINC AND
ALKALINE PHOSPHATASE OF CONTROLS AND ZINC DEFICIENT PIGS

Groups	Final Body Weight (kg)	Daily Gain (gm)	Gain/Food Consumed	Serum Zinc mcg%	Serum Alkaline Phosphatase Sigma Units
Control	6.56 ± 0.3	151 ± 5.34	0.71 ± 0.01	61 ± 2	5.8 ± 0.8
Deficient	4.57 ± 0.32	75.8 ± 6.31	0.37 ± 0.02	13 ± 0.4	1.2 ± 0.3
p†	<0.01	<0.01	<0.01	<0.01	<0.01

Values are:
   Mean $\pm$ S.E.
   †Comparison of means between pair-fed controls and deficient pigs.
   Source: Prasad et al., *Am J Clin Nutr*, 22:628, 1969.

Most organs of zinc-deficient pigs were reduced in size proportionate
to the decrease in total body weight. Whereas the kidneys and adrenals
were proportionately larger in the deficient animals, the thymus was
markedly reduced in size in relation to body weight in the deficient animals
(Table 2-VII).

Table 2-VIII shows the zinc content of various tissues in the first set of
experiments. Zinc content of the bone, pancreas, and liver was decreased
in the deficient pigs as compared to the pair-fed controls.

As determined histochemically, the activities of LDH, MDH, ADH and

TABLE 2-VII

ORGAN WEIGHTS OF PIGS*

	Body wt. g	Liver g	Kidney g	Spleen g	Pancreas g	Thyroid mg	Adrenal mg	Pituitary mg	Testes g	Thymus g
Control	6,377 ±282	169.9 ±5.1	32.2 ±1.?	10.4 ±0.5	12.2 ±0.6	844.1 ±83.0	755.5 ±38.6	61.1 ±2.0	8.0 ±0.6	12.7 ±1.0
% of body weight		2.66	0.?	0.16	0.19	0.01	0.01	0.001	0.12	0.20
Deficient	4,274 ±247	118.7 ±7.6	28.9 ±1.6	7.3 ±0.9	6.9 ±0.6	503.6 ±29.4	718.2 ±33.5	53.8 ±1.7	4.8 ±0.8	4.4 ±1.0
% of body weight		2.77	0.68	0.17	0.16	0.01	0.02	0.001	0.11	0.10
P†	0.001	0.001	NS	0.01	0.001	0.001	NS	0.025	0.005	0.001

Values: NS—Not significant
* Mean and standard error
† Probabilities are for weight differences

TABLE 2-VIII

ZINC IN TISSUES OF PAIR-FED CONTROLS AND ZINC-DEFICIENT PIGS, mcg/g DRY WEIGHT

	Bone	Pancreas	Liver	Kidney	Intestine	Esophagus	Testis	Pituitary	Adrenals	Thyroid
Zinc										
A	95.0 ± 1.8 (14)	139 ± 4.0 (14)	150.8 ± 12.0 (8)	97.8 ± 3.0 (8)	89.3 ± 3.0 (8)	88.1 ± 3.0 (8)	54 ± 2.0 (7)	161 ± 21.0 (11)	61.3 ± 1.0 (6)	58.2 ± 2.0 (6)
B	47.4 ± 1.6 (14)	88.3 ± 4.0 (14)	96.1 ± 8.0 (8)	90.8 ± 4.0 (8)	96.6 ± 6.0 (8)	97.6 ± 5.0 (8)	59 ± 2.0 (7)	199.6 ± 32.0 (11)	60.2 ± 2.0 (6)	50.8 ± 1.0 (6)
	p<0.001	p<0.001	p<0.005	p, NS	p, NS	p, NS	p, NS	p, NS	p, NS	p, NS

Values are:
Mean ± S.E.
A—pair-fed controls, B—Zinc deficient, NS—Not significant.
Numbers in parentheses indicate the number of animals in each group.

alkaline phosphatase were reduced in the bone of the zinc-deficient pigs as compared to the pair-fed controls. In the pancreas, LDH, MDH, and ADH; in the skin, LDH and MDH; in the esophagus, LDH, MDH, and ADH; in the pituitary, LDH, MDH, and ADH; and in the testis, LDH and ADH, revealed decreased activities in the zinc-deficient pigs as compared to the controls. SDH revealed no changes in the two groups. Adrenals, thyroid, and kidneys revealed no significant differences in their enzyme activities between the deficient and the control groups. Figure 2-3 shows the enzyme activities as determined histochemically in the bone of the pigs.

Table 2-IX shows the data obtained in the second set of experiments. In the liver, zinc and RNA content were significantly reduced in the deficient animals as compared to their pair-fed controls, whereas DNA content showed no significant change. The activities of alcohol dehydrogenase and aldolase were significantly reduced in the deficient group.

Zinc, RNA and protein were decreased in the deficient tissues in the kidney. The activities of ADH, aldolase, and alkaline phosphatase were decreased in the deficient group, whereas those of SDH and ICDH showed no differences between the 2 groups of animals. Exogenous zinc did not affect significantly the activities of any of the enzymes investigated. Following addition of EDTA, no activity of ADH or alkaline phosphatase could be measured; but under similar conditions, aldolase was not affected significantly.

Zinc, RNA and protein were significantly reduced in the bone in the zinc-deficient animals in comparison to their pair-fed controls. The activities of ADH, alkaline phosphatase, and LDH were also significantly decreased in the zinc-deficient bone. Addition of exogenous zinc *in vitro* to tissue homogenates had no statistically significant effect on the enzyme activities. No activity of ADH and alkaline phosphatase could be measured following addition of EDTA to tissue homogenates. However, under similar conditions, activities of LDH and aldolase remained unaffected.

Zinc and RNA were reduced in the pancreas of deficient animals as compared to their pair-fed controls. No significant changes were observed in the DNA content. The activity of carboxypeptidase was reduced, but that of LDH remained unaltered in the deficient animals as compared to their pair-fed controls. Exogenous zinc had no significant effect on carboxypeptidase or LDH activity. Following addition of EDTA, the activity of carboxypeptidase declined significantly, but under similar conditions, LDH was not affected.

DISCUSSION

Our studies demonstrate that in the zinc-deficient rats, the content of zinc and activities of certain enzymes in the bones, testis, esophagus, and

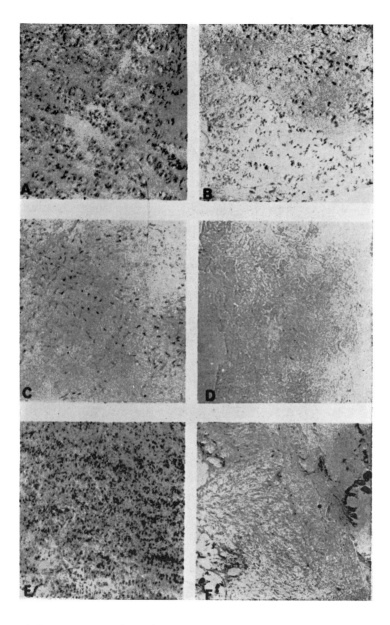

FIGURE 2-3. Sections of bone histochemically stained for alcohol dehydrogenase (ADH), alkaline phosphatase, and malic dehydrogenase (MDH) activities in different groups of pigs. X135. A—ADH in restrictedly fed control pig; B—ADH in zinc-deficient pig; C—Alkaline phosphatase in restrictedly fed control pig; D—Alkaline phosphatase in zinc-deficient pig; E—MDH in restrictedly fed control pig; F—MDH in zinc-deficient pig. Prasad et al., *Am J Clin Nutr*, 22:628, 1969.

TABLE 2-IX

ZINC, DNA, RNA AND PROTEIN CONTENT AND THE ACTIVITIES OF VARIOUS ENZYMES IN TISSUES OF PAIR-FED CONTROLS AND ZINC-DEFICIENT PIGS*

	Zinc μg/g dry wt.	DNA μg/mg wet wt.	RNA μg/g DNA	Protein mg/mg DNA	Activities of Enzymes† OD/min/mg of DNA					AP Sigma U/mg of DNA	CPD μg/μg DNA
					ADH	LDH	ALD	SDH	ICDH		
Liver											
A	150.8±12	4.2±0.42	3.5±0.34	40±2.9	6.4±0.69	46±4	5.7±0.7				
B	96.1±8	5.1±0.3	2.5±0.18	35±1.9	3.6±0.39	50±4	3.0±0.2				
p†	<0.005	NS	<0.005	NS	<0.005	NS	<0.005				
Kidney											
A	97.8±2.6	3.7±0.16	1.4±0.06	23.4±0.8	0.162±0.009		2.54±0.11	1.6±0.17	6.9±0.72	154.8±16.4	
B	87.0±2.8	3.9±0.20	1.1±0.05	21.2±1.0	0.123±0.008		1.86±0.09	1.7±0.19	7.2±0.19	80.2±9.5	
p†	<0.025	NS	<0.005	<0.05	<0.025		<0.001	NS	NS	<0.005	
Bone											
A	98.5±2.08	0.53±0.07	3.04±0.26	57.5±5	2.30±0.35	81±10	21±3.4			2640±420	
B	48.1±2.74	0.83±0.13	1.81±0.22	36.8±5	0.64±0.07	44±7	12±2.5			480±120	
p†	<0.001	<0.1>0.05	<0.005	<0.025	<0.001	<0.025	<0.1>0.05			<0.001	
Pancreas											
A	133.3±6	4.7±0.28	5.0±0.15	25±1.8		14±1.6					2.8±0.1
B	96.8±4	4.0±0.30	4.1±0.1	22±2.2		14±1.0					1.3±0.2
p†	<0.001	0.2>0.	<0.05	NS		NS					<0.001

Values:

* Mean ± S.E.

† ADH, alcohol dehydrogenase; ALD, aldolase; SDH, succinic dehydrogenase; CPD, carboxypeptidase; LDH, lactic dehydrogenase; ICDH, isocitric dehydrogenase; and AP, alkaline phosphatase

A—Pair-fed controls, B—Zinc deficient

† Comparison of means

kidneys are decreased as compared to their ad-libitum and pair-fed controls. The zinc content of the liver, pancreas, and thymus was decreased in zinc-deficient rats as compared to the pair-fed controls, but showed no significant difference when compared to the ad-libitum controls. Since the pair-fed controls were restricted with respect to calories and their growth was much less in comparison to the ad-libitum controls, it is possible that a higher zinc concentration in the former was a result of an overloading with zinc for their body size. The pair-fed control rats showed higher specific activity of aldolase in the liver, and ADH and alkaline phosphatase in the bone (Tables 2-III & 2-IV). The higher activities of some of the zinc-dependent enzymes in the pair-fed as compared to ad-libitum controls thus seem to correlate with the zinc level in the tissues. Recently, Reinhold et al.[25] observed a significant correlation between activities of ADH in the liver, alkaline phosphatase in the intestinal mucosa, and zinc concentration in rats maintained on a controlled regimen of zinc-deficient or zinc-supplemented diets. No such changes were observed in the cases of ICDH (manganese dependent enzyme) or SDH (iron dependent enzyme) under similar conditions in our experiments.

Although the zinc content of the liver, pancreas, and thymus showed no statistically significant change in the deficient state as compared to their ad-libitum controls, the activity of ADH in the liver, alkaline phosphatase and carboxypeptidase in the pancreas and alkaline phosphatase in the thymus decreased in comparison to the controls, suggesting that these enzymes were sensitive to zinc depletion.

In the pigs, the zinc content and RNA/DNA ratios of the bone, pancreas, liver, and kidney were significantly decreased in comparison to their pair-fed controls. Only zinc-dependent enzymes revealed significantly reduced activities in zinc-deficient tissues; exceptions were LDH in the liver and pancreas, and aldolase in the bone. Addition of small amounts of EDTA to tissue homogenates significantly reduced activities of ADH, AP and CPD, but not that of LDH and aldolase, thus revealing the differences in affinity for zinc in the various enzymes.

Hsu et al.[26] and Mills et al.[27] have previously reported a decrease in the activity of carboxypeptidase in the pancreas of zinc-deficient rats, and our results confirm their findings. Whereas Hsu et al.[26] reported no changes in the activity of alcohol dehydrogenase in the liver of zinc-deficient rats, Kfoury et al.[28] demonstrated a decrease in the activity of alcohol dehydrogenase in homogenate of perfused liver and alkaline phosphatase in the intestinal mucosa and kidney of zinc-deficient rats, as compared to their pair-fed controls. Swenerton and Hurley[29] found no differences in the activities of various enzymes such as pyridoxal phosphokinase, glutamic dehydrogenase and lactic dehydrogenase in the homogenate of unperfused liver between controls and zinc-deficient rats. In another study by Hurley et al.[30] in which lactic dehydrogenase, malic dehydrogenase, and carbonic anhydrase were assayed in 21-day-old rat fetuses of zinc-deficient mothers, no differences were observed in comparison to their controls. From our results, one would conclude that testis, bone, and kidney of rats are some of the more sensitive tissues inasmuch as these tissues show a decrease in zinc content; and, concomitantly, some of zinc metallo-enzymes showed decreased activities as a result of zinc deficiency in comparison to their pair-fed and ad-libitum controls.

Enzyme activity in tissue homogenate has classically been expressed as units per mg of protein or wet weight of tissue. Since one of the major effects of zinc deficiency happens to be growth retardation, one may conclude that the protein content of the cell is being decreased concomitantly and, therefore, the expression of enzyme activity in the traditional manner may not be satisfactory. However, if one were to examine the specific activity of the enzymes (activity of enzyme per mg of protein), it becomes clear that only the zinc-dependent enzymes show a definite reduction in the specific activity, suggesting a specific effect of zinc nutriture in such enzymes.

In the experiments with pigs, the DNA content of the tissues per mg of wet weight was determined to be the same in zinc-deficient pigs and their pair-fed controls and, therefore, the expression of the enzyme activity in terms of tissue DNA may be satisfactory. The differences in activity of zinc-dependent enzymes between the zinc-deficient pigs and their pair-fed controls when expressed as activity per mg of DNA were highly significant and approached the level of significance observed by histochemical methods.[4,5] However, in view of a recent report that DNA synthesis is also affected as a result of zinc deficiency,[31] it appears that this may not be an ideal way to express the enzyme activity.

The likelihood of detecting any biochemical changes is greatest in tissues that are sensitive to zinc depletion. Unfortunately, most investigators in the past have not selected the proper tissues in experimental animals for the determination of enzyme activities. Some investigators have studied those enzymes which are not zinc dependent and obtained negative results, which is not at all surprising. Also, one should not expect that all zinc-dependent enzymes would be affected similarly in all tissues of zinc-deficient animals. Obviously, the differences in susceptibility of the enzymes may be caused by differences in the affinity for zinc of the various zinc-dependent enzymes and on the turnover rate of the cells of tissues involved. Thus from the studies reported so far, glutamic dehydrogenase and carbonic anhydrase would appear to be much less susceptible to zinc deficiency,

Methods of Biochemical Analysis. New York, Interscience, 1966, vol. 14, p. 113.

25. Reinhold, J. G., Pascoe, E., Arslanian, M., and Bitar, K.: Relations of zinc metallo-enzyme activities to zinc concentrations in tissues. *Biochim Biophys Acta, 215:* 430, 1970.

26. Hsu, J. M., Anilane, J. K., and Scalon, D. E.: Pancreatic carboxypeptidase activities in zinc-deficient rats. *Science, 153:*882, 1966.

27. Mills, C. F., Quarterman, J., Williams, R. B., Daigarno, A. C., and Panic, B.: The effects of zinc deficiency on pancreatic carboxypeptidase activity and protein digestion and absorption in the rat. *Biochem J, 102:*712, 1967.

28. Kfoury, G. A., Reinhold, J. G., and Simonian, S. J.: Enzyme activities in tissues of zinc-deficient rats. *J Nutr, 95:*102, 1968.

29. Swenerton, H., and Hurley, L. S.: Severe zinc deficiency in male and female rats. *J Nutr, 95:*8, 1968.

30. Hurley, L. S., Dreosti, I. E., and Swenerton, H.: Studies on zinc enzymes and nucleic acid synthesis in relation to congenital malformations in zinc-deficient rats. *Proceedings Western Hemisphere Nutrition Congress,* San Juan, Puerto Rico, Aug. 1968, p. 39.

31. Sandstead, H. H., and Rinaldi, R. A.: Impairment of deoxyribonucleic acid synthesis by dietary zinc deficiency in the rat. *J Cell Physiol, 73:*8, 1969.

DISCUSSION

Dr. Reussner: Did you try to determine the enzyme activities in the prostate and seminal vesicles?

Dr. Prasad: We have not done anything with the prostate so far. We have no idea what zinc is doing in the prostate. For that matter, I do not know what is happening in the eyes either, and these are some of the other aspects that one has to look into.

Dr. Reussner: A second question: Did you look to the adrenal weights? What happened to corticoid levels?

Dr. Prasad: I did not show this since most of this has been published previously: If I recall correctly, the weight of the adrenals in the deficient animals was, in terms of body weight, proportionately larger as compared to the controls. There were two organs, the testes and the thymus that were smaller in the zinc deficient animals than in the controls. The other organs were reduced proportionately to the body size, again suggesting that perhaps the testes and thymus are indeed sensitive tissues.

Dr. Chvapil: I was surprised that in your zinc deficient animals the depletion of zinc in tissues was not more pronounced. Do you have any evidence for the character of this stable form of zinc in tissues?

Dr. Prasad: This is a good question. So far as the decrease is concerned, you have to consider one thing. If you are talking about the total zinc, all you have to do is to look at the rat. The rat is very small and the total zinc is low. If you express all the zinc content in terms of the organ weight, you don't even have to do an assay. You can just predict this. But what we are trying to do is to express this in terms of mcg per g of tissue weight and see if there is a significant decrease. The results are significant and we can say that this is decreasing faster than if you were to restrict the weight by reducing calories for instance. It is a very difficult problem to determine the most appropriate way in which to express the data.

Dr. Spencer: It is very interesting that the adrenal enlarged while the thymus was smaller. This again infers that there is apparently a thymus-adrenal axis. It is very interesting and has many implications. In your experiment where you gave 100 mg of zinc, was there a difference in rate of growth when compared to controls?

Dr. Prasad: I don't remember the exact rate and I will have to look this up. However, we were not impressed with a marked increase. They were perhaps comparable, but you know from one experiment to the other you do see some difference. Dr. Don Oberleas has found a difference in the weight of the animals who are supplemented 55 vs. 110 ppm, and this brings up the question "what is optimum?" This is another area which we should discuss later perhaps.

Dr. Hurley: I just wanted to raise an issue of terminology. One of the questioners and Dr. Prasad both referred to "depletion of zinc" in your experimental animals, and I would like to suggest that this was not **deple-tion** but rather reduced incorporation of zinc, since you were dealing with young growing animals. I think this is not only a question of semantics, but is an important concept.

Dr Prasad: This would be true for "chemically zinc deficient" diets. However, when phytate is present, endogenous intestinal zinc may also be complexed and made unavailable.

Dr. Larson: Have you looked at carbonic anhydrase? We have made standard skin wounds in rabbits and looked at all of the compounds presently used in the treatment of burns. We find that if, we put sulfamylon on the wound, healing requires 40 days, whereas, control rabbits require only 20 days. If we take another set of rabbits and give them zinc by mouth, we can bring our healing time almost back to normal. As far as I know, the only thing we know about sulfamylon is that it is a carbonic anhydrase inhibitor.

Dr. Prasad: A very good question. We have not looked at carbonic anhydrase. However, I believe someone has determined this in the chicken or red cells. It is my impression that carbonic anhydrase has not been shown to be affected and I would suspect that this would be the case since zinc is much more tightly bound to carbonic anhydrase than other enzymes. Therefore, this will be one of the last enzymes to be affected. However, I have no data in support of this hypothesis.

Chapter 3

METABOLIC STUDIES IN RAT SKIN DURING ZINC DEFICIENCY

Jeng M. Hsu

THE ROLE OF ZINC in regulating metabolic events at the molecular level is becoming evident, but it is not yet possible to correlate biochemical function to the pathology of deficiency. The development of skin lesions in experimental zinc-deficient animals and the beneficial effects of zinc on wound healing suggest that this ion is essential in the maintenance of normal performance of the skin. It is the purpose of this presentation to describe studies from the author's laboratory concerning the incorporation of labeled amino acids into skin proteins and to reveal other metabolic changes which are linked in the regulation of protein synthesis.

Incorporation of Cystine-^{35}S into Skin Protein

Studies from the author's laboratory using isotope administration have demonstrated that metabolic fate of labeled cystine is altered in zinc-deficient rats.[1,2,3] After intramuscular injection of DL-cystine-1-^{14}C, zinc-deficient rats had an enhanced excretion of radioactivity in expired CO_2 within 6 hours. An increase of total ^{35}S in 24 hours urinary specimens was also observed in zinc-deficient rats after L-cystine-^{35}S injection. The increase in urinary radioactivity was primarily due to the increase of ^{35}S-labeled inorganic sulfate and ^{35}S-labeled taurine. Conversely, the uptake of ^{35}S by the skin of zinc-deficient rats was markedly reduced as compared to zinc-supplemented pair-fed controls. The latter findings prompted us to study cystine incorporation into skin protein.

Results in Table 3-I indicate that at 4 hours the specific activity present in the skin protein of zinc-deficient rats was one seventh of that of ad libitum fed zinc-supplemented rats, and one fifth of that of pair-fed controls. Although more cystine-^{35}S was incorporated into skin protein of zinc-deficient animals at 8 hours than at 4 hours, the amounts were still only 35 percent of the normal value. Similar trends were found between zinc-supplemented and zinc-deficient rats at the end of 16 and 24 hours of cystine-^{35}S incorporated into skin protein.

Incorporation of Cystine-^{35}S into Other Tissue Proteins

Results of the effect of zinc deficiency on the incorporation of cystine-^{35}S into other tissue proteins are given in Table 3-II. No significant differences

TABLE 3-I

INCORPORATION OF L-CYSTINE-^{35}S INTO SKIN PROTEIN

Type of Diet	Days of Feeding	No. of Rats	Hrs After Injection	Specific Activity dpm/mg Protein
Zn-supplemented (ad lib)	14	7	4	1302 ± 585[1, ° °]
Zn-supplemented (pair-fed)	14	5	4	881 ± 319°
Zn-deficient	14	6	4	174 ± 66
Zn-supplemented (ad lib)	16	5	8	1444 ± 136° °
Zn-supplemented (pair-fed)	16	6	8	1337 ± 108°
Zn-deficient	16	5	8	506 ± 118
Zn-supplemented (ad lib)	16	6	16	1080 ± 227° °
Zn-deficient	16	6	16	352 ± 83
Zn-supplemented (ad lib)	15	5	24	1267 ± 112° °
Zn-supplemented (pair-fed)	15	5	24	1117 ± 295°
Zn-deficient	15	5	24	306 ± 155

[1]Mean ± SD.
° °Difference between Zn-supplemented (ad lib) and Zn-deficient rats is statistically significant ($p < 0.01$).
°Difference between Zn-supplemented (pair-fed) and Zn-deficient rats is statistically significant ($p < 0.01$).

TABLE 3-II

TWENTY-FOUR HOURS' INCORPORATION OF L-CYSTINE-^{35}S
INTO OTHER TISSUE PROTEIN

Type of Diet	Specific Activity				
	Pancreas	Liver	Kidney	Testes	Muscle
	dpm/mg protein				
Zn-supplemented (ad lib)	341 ± 35[1, °]	213 ± 39	397 ± 48	301 ± 38	120 ± 32
Zn-supplemented (pair-fed)	458 + 82°	210 ± 28	382 ± 9	304 ± 24	129 ± 44°
Zn-deficient	587 ± 64	201 ± 46	382 ± 61	257 ± 61	84 ± 28

[1]Mean ± SD. Six rats in each group were on experimental diet for 15 days.
°Difference between Zn-supplemented (ad lib and pair-fed) and Zn-deficient rats is statistically significant ($p < 0.05$).

were observed in the proteins-^{35}S activity of the liver, kidney, testes and muscle between the two groups. However, more cystine-^{35}S was incorporated into pancreatic protein of zinc-deficient rats than of those fed the diet containing an adequate level of zinc.

The increase of cystine-^{35}S incorporation into pancreatic protein of zinc-deficient rats was unexpected. This appears to be true regardless of the time of isotope injection. Similar findings have been documented in the pancreas of zinc-deficient rats 2 hours after ^{14}C-methionine administration.[4] Since the increased specific activity of pancreatic protein in zinc-deficient rats is abolished in animals previously treated with non-radioactive methionine, we believe that a depletion of methionine may occur in the pancreas of zinc-deficient animals. Whether this possibility is also true for cystine has not been investigated. It is clear that under the experimental conditions we have employed zinc deficiency in rats results in various degrees of damage in different tissues.

Incorporation of Amino Acid-^{14}C into Skin Protein

To obtain more information about the biological role of zinc on skin function, the incorporation of other labeled amino acids was studied. Figure 3-1 shows that in 24 hours the assimilation of five nonessential amino acids (glycine-2-^{14}C, L-cystine-3-^{14}C, L-proline-U-^{14}C, L-glutamic acid-U-^{14}C and DL-alanine-1-^{14}C) into skin protein was significantly less in zinc-deficient rats than in zinc-supplemented controls.

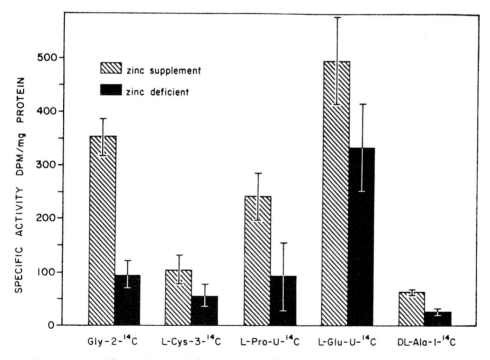

FIGURE 3-1. Effects of zinc deficiency on 24 hours' incorporation of 5 nonessential amino acids into skin protein. The heights of the solid bars and the cross bars represent the mean specific activity of 6 zinc-supplemented and 6 zinc-deficient rats. Vertical lines denote standard deviations.

Similarly, there was a reduced incorporation of 3 essential amino acids (L-histidine-2-^{14}C, L-lysine-U-^{14}C and L-methionine-2-^{14}C) into skin protein of zinc-deficient rats as compared with that of zinc-supplemented rats (Figure 3-2). Thus, zinc-deficient rats may have a common defect in the utilization of amino acids for the synthesis of skin proteins.

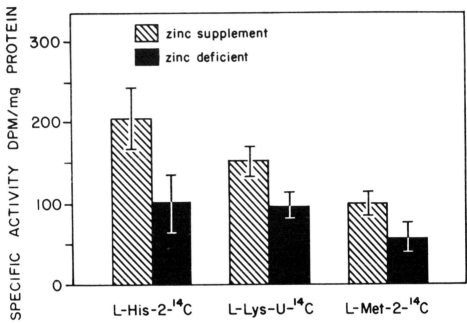

FIGURE 3-2. Effects of zinc deficiency on 24 hours' incorporation of 3 essential amino acids into skin protein. The heights of the solid bars and the cross bars represent the mean specific activity of 6 zinc-supplemented and 6 zinc-deficient rats. Vertical lines denote standard deviations.

Incorporation of L-arginine-^{14}C into Skin Protein

Table 3-III demonstrates that a significant decrease of radioactive protein was formed from both L-arginine-guanido ^{14}C and L-arginine-U-^{14}C in the skin of the zinc-deficient rats when compared with pair-fed controls. As shown by Swick and Handa,[5] L-arginine-guanido-^{14}C is not subject to isotope reutilization in liver because of the large amount of arginase, which hydrolyzes the label to urea. If this is also true in skin, it would indicate that the decreased incorporation of amino acids into skin protein of zinc-deficient rats is not attributable to amino acid reutilization.

Zinc Repletion and Skin Protein

The effect of zinc repletion on cystine-^{35}S and glycine-2-^{14}C incorporation into skin protein was determined by daily intraperitoneal injections of

TABLE 3-III

INCORPORATION OF ^{14}C-ARGININE INTO SKIN PROTEIN

Type of Diet	Isotope Used	Sp. A DPM/mg Protein	No. of Rats	Hours After Injection
Zn-supplemented	Arginine-guanido-[14]C	418 ± 22[1,*]	4	4
Zn-deficient	Arginine-guanido-[14]C	220 ± 102	4	4
Zn-supplemented	Arginine-U-[14]C	262 ± 15*	5	24
Zn-deficient	Arginine-U-[14]C	63 ± 12	5	24

[1]Mean ± SD.
*$p<0.01$.

400 µg of zinc as zinc chloride on the last 3 days of the experiment. Results summarized in Table 3-IV indicate that skin protein in zinc-repleted rats had the same radioactivity as zinc-supplemented pair-fed rats. The defects in incorporation observed in zinc-deficient rats seemed to be readily reversible.

TABLE 3-IV

ZINC REPLETION ON 24 HOURS' INCORPORATION OF LABELED
AMINO ACIDS INTO SKIN PROTEIN

Type of Diet	No. of Rats	Isotope Injected	Sp. A. DPM/mg Protein
Zn-supplemented	6	L-cystine-[35]S	343 ± 53[2]
Zn-deficient & repleted[1]	6	L-cystine-[35]S	309 ± 86
Zn-supplemented	7	Glycine-2-[14]C	279 ± 74
Zn-deficient & repleted	6	Glycine-2-[14]C	311 ± 35

[1]400 mcg zinc daily on last 3 days of 18-day experiment.
[2]Mean ± SD.

Incorporation of ^{14}C-labeled Amino Acid into Skin Collagens

The findings of reduced incorporation of labeled glycine and proline, two major precursors of collagen, into skin protein of zinc-deficient rats indicate that zinc might be involved in collagen synthesis. To test this possibility, insoluble and soluble skin collagens were isolated[6] and their specific activities were determined after an injection of labeled amino acid. Table 3-V shows the results of the incorporation of ^{14}C-amino acid into skin collagens. The radioactivity recovered as insoluble fraction was markedly reduced in the skin of zinc-deficient rats regardless of the origin of isotope used. The ratios between zinc-supplemented and zinc-deficient rats were approximately 5.0, 2.5, 1.5 and 1.7 after injection of glycine-2-^{14}C, L-proline-U-^{14}C, L-glutamic acid-U-^{14}C and L-histidine-2-[14]C. Table 3-V also shows zinc-deficient rats incorporated significantly less labeled glycine and

TABLE 3-V

TWENTY-FOUR HOURS' INCORPORATION OF AMINO ACID-^{14}C
INTO SKIN COLLAGEN

Type of Diet	Amino Acid-^{14}C Injected	No. of Rats	Skin Collagens DPM/100mcg Hydroxyproline	
			Insoluble	Soluble
Zn-supplemented	Glycine-2-^{14}C	6	267 ± 28[1,**]	993 ± 79**
Zn-deficient	Glycine-2-^{14}C	6	50 ± 18	412 ± 141
Zn-supplemented	L-Glutamic-U-^{14}C	6	450 ± 169*	1630 ± 536
Zn-deficient	L-Glutamic-U-^{14}C	5	274 ± 39	1450 ± 302
Zn-supplemented	L-Proline-U-^{14}C	7	290 ± 39**	879 ± 135**
Zn-deficient	L-Proline-U-^{14}C	6	139 ± 32	446 ± 222
Zn-supplemented	L-Histidine-2-^{14}C	5	78 ± 16**	....
Zn-deficient	L-Histidine-2-^{14}C	5	44 ± 11	....

[1]Mean ± SD.
**$p < 0.01$.
*$p < 0.05$.

proline into the soluble fraction of skin collagens. The above finding is of great interest because it points out that the biological role of zinc is specifically involved in one type of protein, namely skin collagen. Furthermore, these observations provide some explanation in regard to the beneficial effect of zinc on wound repair.

A general question arises concerning the causes of this impairment of amino acid incorporation into rat skin during zinc deficiency. Hormones have long been known to have profound effects on the growth, development and metabolism of higher organisms. Accordingly, we injected growth hormone and insulin into zinc-deficient rats and their corresponding pair-fed controls to study glycine-2-^{14}C incorporation into skin collagens. Results are presented in Table 3-VI. The treatment of insulin appeared to have a greater effect than that of growth hormone in incorporation of labeled glycine into both soluble and insoluble fractions. There was a significant increase in the formation of labeled collagens by insulin-injected zinc-deficient rats as compared to zinc-deficient rats without hormone injection. Whether these findings are related to a decreased plasma insulin in zinc-deficient rats as shown by Quartman, Mills and Humphries[7] remains to be studied. That the treatment of insulin results in an enhancement of collagens synthesis in zinc-supplemented rats indicates that insulin has its own action *in vivo* regardless of the status of zinc.

Oxidation of ^{14}C-labeled Amino Acids

Increased oxidation of ^{14}C-labeled amino acids in zinc-deficient rats has been reported by Theuer and Hoekstra[8] and Hsu et al.[9] It seemed reasonable to suppose that observed defects in amino acid catabolism in zinc-deficient rats might be associated with alteration in the rate of protein

TABLE 3-VI

ZINC DEFICIENCY AND HORMONE EFFECT ON 4 HOURS' INCORPORATION
OF GLYCINE-2-14C INTO SKIN COLLAGEN

Type of Diet	Hormone Treatment	Skin Collagens DPM/100mcg Hydroxyproline	
		Insoluble	Soluble
Zn-supplemented	None	136 ± 18[3],**	1043 ± 99**
Zn-deficient	None	49 ± 30	582 ± 303
Zn-supplemented	Growth hormone[1]	205 ± 74**	1356 ± 375**
Zn-deficient	Growth hormone	75 ± 23	500 ± 104
Zn-supplemented	Insulin[2]	236 ± 73*	1848 ± 787*
Zn-deficient	Insulin	153 ± 56	1025 ± 261

[1]Each received 0.1 mg of NIH GH B14 subcutaneously daily for last 6 days of 14-day experiment.
[2]Each received 0.5U of Iletin (insulin injection, Lilly and Co., Indianapolis, Ind.) subcutaneously daily for 15-day experiment.
[3]Mean ± SD.
**$p < 0.01$.
*$p < 0.05$.

synthesis in rat skin. To substantiate this possibility we examined the oxidation of several 14C-labeled amino acids in zinc-deficient rats. The results in Table 3-VII reveal that zinc deficiency increased the oxidation of glycine-1-14C, DL-cystine-1-14C and L-leucine-U-14C but had no effect on the conversion of DL-methionine-2-14C and L-glutamic-1-14C to respiratory 14CO2. Since the incorporation of the last two amino acids into skin protein was significantly less in zinc-deficient rats, it is difficult to believe that an enhancement of amino acid oxidation is the primary cause in the impairment of protein synthesis.

TABLE 3-VII

14C-LABELED AMINO ACIDS TO 14CO2 BY ZN-DEFICIENT
AND ZN-SUPPLEMENTED RATS

Type of Diet	No. of Rats	14C-Amino Acid	Hours After Injection	% Injected Dose
Zn-supplemented	4	DL-methionine-2-14C	4	14.3 ± 4.74[1]
Zn-deficient	4	DL-methionine-2-14C	4	14.4 ± 5.60
Zn-supplemented	4	L-glutamic-1-14C	3	59.8 ± 1.74
Zn-deficient	4	L-glutamic-1-14C	3	56.3 ± 3.22
Zn-supplemented	5	L-leucine-14C (U)	2	7.7 ± 0.1*
Zn-deficient	5	L-leucine-14C (U)	2	15.1 ± 1.8
Zn-supplemented	4	Glycine-1-14C	2	14.9 ± 2.5**
Zn-deficient	4	Glycine-1-14C	2	24.9 ± 5.2
Zn-supplemented	4	DL-cystine-1-14C	6	40.6 ± 5.86**
Zn-deficient	4	DL-cystine-1-14C	6	51.9 ± 2.86

[1]Mean ± SD.
*$p < 0.01$.
**$p < 0.05$.

Zinc Content in the Skin

Zinc concentration in various tissues has been shown to be reduced in rats receiving zinc-deficient diet. Whether the amount of zinc is directly involved in the protein metabolism is not clear. It is interesting that the pancreas of zinc-deficient rats possessed a reduced zinc content but had an enhancement of labeled methionine into acid insoluble protein.[4] Nevertheless, zinc content in rat skin was determined. Results of the effect of zinc deficiency on the content of zinc and other minerals in rat skin are given in Table 3-VIII. It appears that the skin of zinc-deficient rats contained less zinc than that of zinc-supplemented rats. A statistical significance was reached between zinc-deficient rats and zinc-supplemented ad libitum animals.

TABLE 3-VIII

EFFECT OF ZN DEFICIENCY ON THE SKIN CONTENT OF
ZN, CU, MN, NA AND K

Type of Diet	Skin Content			Skin Content	
	Zn	Cu	Mn	Na	K
	μg/ dry wt			mg/g dry wt	
Zn-supplemented (ad lib)	41.28 ± 3.25[1],°°	7.76 ± 1.34	7.19 ± 2.36	2.89 ± 0.61	3.48 ± 0.77
Zn-supplemented (pair-fed)	36.21 ± 9.02	7.83 ± 3.39	7.74 ± 1.81	3.01 ± 0.77	3.85 ± 1.04
Zn-deficient	28.13 ± 5.11	12.52 ± 6.71	10.17 ± 3.18	3.33 ± 1.32	2.95 ± 0.66

[1]Mean ± SD. Six rats in each group were on experimental diet for 15 days.
°°Difference between Zn-supplemented (ad lib) and Zn-deficient rats is statistically significant ($p < 0.01$).

DNA Synthesis in Rat Skin

The evidence of a zinc requirement for DNA synthesis by rat liver has been shown by several investigators.[10,11,12] Recent findings of a zinc-containing DNA polymerase[13] suggests that a further study of relationship between zinc and nucleic acid is needed. Our investigations have been concerned primarily with the rate of DNA synthesis from ^{3}H-labeled thymidine in rat skin. The changes of skin DNA synthesis as affected by zinc deficiency are shown in Table 3-IX. The suppression of skin DNA formation was clearly demonstrated in rats receiving a zinc-deficient diet. The decrease was found to be 20 percent of normal value when the specimens were obtained one hour after thymidine injection. After 2 hours, the rate of skin DNA formation of zinc-deficient rats was approximately 44 percent of the value obtained from zinc-supplemented pair-fed controls. The direct involvement of zinc in DNA synthesis is further strengthened by the findings of our autoradiographic study. In Table 3-X, uptakes of thymidine-

TABLE 3-IX

INCORPORATION OF THYMIDINE-C³H₃ INTO SKIN DNA

Type of Diet	No. of Rats	Hours After Injection	DNA Conc. mcg DNAP/g Wet Wt	Sp. A. DPM/100mcg DNA
Zn-supplemented	5	1	151 ± 10[1]	696 ± 140°
Zn-deficient	6	1	139 ± 26	150 ± 75
Zn-supplemented	5	2	171 ± 5	527 ± 47°
Zn-deficient	6	2	164 ± 9	230 ± 58

[1]Mean ± SD.
°$p < 0.01$.

TABLE 3-X

UPTAKE OF THYMIDINE-C³H₃ BY THE SKIN OF ZN-SUPPLEMENTED
AND ZN-DEFICIENT RATS

Type of Diet	No. of Rats	Uptake of Thymidine-C³H₃ DPM/mg Wet Weight	% Labeling Index
Zn-supplemented	6	607 ± 57[1],°	17.1 ± 3.4°°
Zn-deficient	6	537 ± 13	7.4 ± 0.8

[1]Mean ± SD.
°$p < 0.05$.
°°$p < 0.01$.

C³H₃ by the skin of zinc-supplemented and zinc-deficient rats are illustrated. Incorporation of labeled thymidine into the skin of deficient rats was significantly lower than that of zinc-supplemented rats. The skin thymidine labeling index (LI), the number of cells labeled in the cell population, in zinc supplemented animals was considerably higher than in zinc deficient rats. Although more detailed studies are necessary to prove that DNA synthesis in the liver, kidney, spleen, and thymus is depressed under these conditions, the data presented here conclusively show that dietary zinc deficiency impairs DNA synthesis in rat skin.

Uptake of Thymidine C³H₃ and Wound Repair

If zinc deficiency impairs DNA synthesis in skin of intact rats, a quantitative difference would be expected in thymidine incorporation into the nuclei of epidermal cells covering a small wound. For this purpose, zinc-deficient rats and their controls were prepared in the same manner as described in a previous study.[9] After experimental feeding of 10 to 14 days, a one inch linear incision was made on the back of each rat. Two, 4 and 6 days after wounding, each animal received a single intramuscular injection of thymidine-C³H₃. One hour later, biopsy specimens were obtained from wound site and fixed in Orth's fluid for autoradiography. Results are presented in Figure 3-3 (A, B, C, D). Wounding resulted in

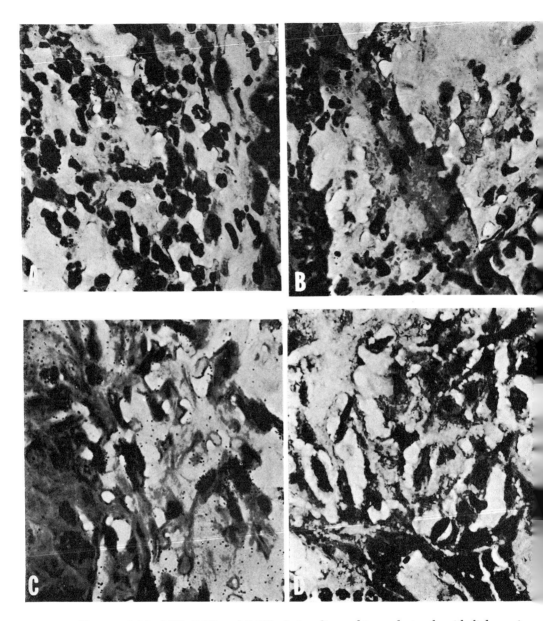

FIGURES 3-3A, 3-3B, 3-3C and 3-3D. Autoradiographic analysis of epithelial repair X 1040. A and B are sections 2 days after wounding; C and D, section 4 days after wounding. Animals A and C are zinc-supplemented; B and D zinc-deficient. Proliferative activity of epithelial cells is much more intense in the zinc-supplemented animals, as shown by number of labeled nuclei. Such activity leads to a quicker and better organized repair of the tissue. See text.

destruction of a large number of cells at the lesion site. However, 2 days after wounding, repair was evident; labeled cells, signifying cell proliferation, appeared in the wound site. In histological sections, there were obviously more labeled nuclei in zinc-supplemented tissue (Figure 3-3A) than in zinc-deficient tissue (Figure 3-3B). After 4 days, histological sections revealed re-epithelization of the skin with rudimentary restoration of the strata in zinc-supplemented animals, but this was not seen in zinc-deficient rats (Figure 3-3C, 3-3D).

The thymidine labeling indices (L.I.) after two days of wound healing shown in Figure 3-4 were 29.4 ± 1.2 and $26.3 \pm 1.1\%$ for zinc-supplemented and zinc-deficient rats respectively. By the 4th day the rate of healing was markedly accelerated for zinc-supplemented rats as reflected by increasing

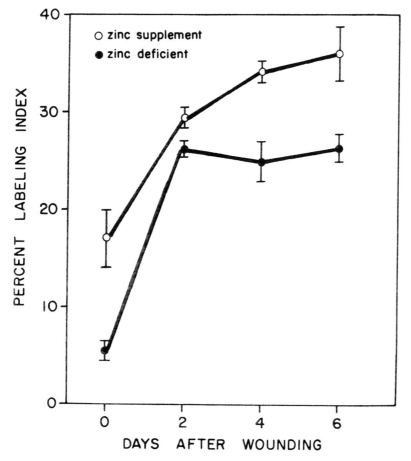

FIGURE 3-4. Percent labeling indices for zinc-supplemented and zinc-deficient rats. Labeling indices for nonwounded animals are shown at day 0, and represents the normal situation. Wounded animals show a much higher labeling index.

L.I. to about 34 percent whereas it was plateaued at about 25 percent for zinc-deficient rats. Further increase of L.I. to 36 percent was noted for zinc-supplemented rats after 6 days of wound healing, but L.I. of zinc-deficient rats remained around 26 percent. Thus, it appears that a zinc-deficient condition creates a slower rate of epithelial cell renewal as demonstrated by a decrease of thymidine incorporation into DNA and a decrease of amino acid incorporation into skin proteins.

SUMMARY

The biosynthesis of DNA and protein is indeed intricate and interrelated processes, the exact controls of which are not fully understood. A major question, one which cannot be answered at this time, is whether the primary limiting factor lies in the reduced synthesis of DNA, of protein, or of both. Numerous enzymes are essential in the reactions leading to DNA synthesis. A decrease in protein production which limits the availability of these necessary enzymes would then diminish the production of nucleic acid. The exact mechanisms of action of zinc in regulating protein and nucleic acid metabolism are far from clear. It is hoped that these answers will be forthcoming in the near future.

REFERENCES

1. Hsu, J. M., Anthony, W. L., and Buchanan, P. J.: Zinc deficiency and the metabolism of labelled cystine in rats. In Mills, C. F. (Ed.): *The Proceedings of the First International Symposium on Trace Element Metabolism in Animals.* Edinburgh, Livingstone, 1970, p. 151.
2. Hsu, J. M., and Anthony, W. L.: Zinc deficiency and urinary excretion of taurine-^{35}S and inorganic sulfate-^{35}S following cystine-^{35}S injection in rats. *J Nutr, 100*:1189, 1970.
3. Hsu, J. M., and Anthony, W. L.: Metabolic fate of labeled cystine in zinc-deficient rats. In Hemphill, D. D. (Ed.): *Trace Substances in Environmental Health—IV.* Columbia, U Mo. Pr, 1970, p. 222.
4. Hsu, J. M., Anthony, W. L., and Buchanan, P. J.: Zinc deficiency and incorporation of ^{14}C-labeled methionine into tissue proteins in rats. *J Nutr, 99*:425, 1969.
5. Swick, R. W., and Hana, D. T.: The distribution of fixed carbon in amino acids. *J Biol Chem, 218*:577, 1956.
6. Kao, K. Y. T., Hitt, W. E., Dawson, R. L., and McGavack, T. H.: Connective tissue VII Changes in protein and hexosamine content of bone and cartilage of rats at different ages. *Proc Soc Exp Biol Med, 110*:538, 1962.
7. Quartman, J., Mills, C. F., and Humphries, W. R.: The reduced secretion of and sensitivity to insulin in zinc deficient rats. *Biochem Biophys Res Commun, 25*: 354, 1966.
8. Theuer, R. C., and Hoekstra, W. G.: Oxidation of ^{14}C-labeled carbohydrate, fate and amino acid substrates by zinc-deficient rats. *J Nutr, 89*:448, 1966.

9. Hsu, J. M., Anthony, W. L., and Buchanan, P. J.: Zinc deficiency and oxidation of L-methionine-methyl-^{14}C in rats. *J Nutr, 97*:279, 1969.

10. Fujioka, M., and Lieberman, I.: A Zn^{++} requirement for synthesis of deoxyribonucleic acid by rat liver. *J Biol Chem, 239*:1164, 1964.

11. Sandstead, H. H., and Rinaldi, R. A.: Impairment of deoxyribonucleic acid synthesis by dietary zinc deficiency in the rat. *J Cell Physiol, 73*:81, 1969.

12. Weser, U., Seeber, S., and Warnecke, P.: Reactivity of zn^{2++} on nuclear DNA and RNA biosynthesis of regenerating rat liver. *Biochim Biophys Acta, 179*:422, 1969.

13. Slater, J. P., Mildvan, A. S., and Loeb, L. A.: Zinc in DNA polymerase. *Biochem Biophys Res Commun, 44*:37, 1971.

DISCUSSION

Dr. Sable: You showed a difference in a couple of your slides between oxidation of cystine and oxidation of cysteine. Do you think that is because you have the disulphide form versus the thio-amino acid or was it because of a difference in the position of the label?

Dr. Hsu: It was a difference in the label. The carboxyl label is increased, but not the form with the label on position 3.

Dr. Sable: That is the only difference?

Dr. Hsu: That is all.

Dr. Pfeiffer: I have a question which intrigues us and I can illustrate by three quick pictures. The first picture shows in a woman, stria gravidarum, and we note that the stria occur on the abdomen at a time when copper is high and zinc is low. Namely, when the abdomen is extended, stria are evident there, I think. As a woman says, she has these stretch marks all over her "kangaroo pouch." We also have a picture of her breast, and she has, because of the period of lactation when copper is high and zinc is low, stretch marks on the breast. The next slide is that of a weight lifter, a schizophrenic boy, and he has stretch marks all over the volar surface of his arms, deltoid and pectoral muscles and with inadequate elastin or collagen formation. We think when we see these on the young people that it is a sign of perhaps zinc deficiency. In other words, they have increased their muscles, and increased their hip size, at a time when zinc is low. This is of interest because all women do not get stretch marks on their abdomen at the time of pregnancy, only some. There must be a diet factor or some other factor in the occurrence of so-called "stretch marks." I have asked Dr. Prasad about this and he cannot recall observing this in the dwarfs he has studied previously. They did not see stretch marks in these patients. However, we called this to the attention of our psychiatrists and they now notice these stretch marks in many of their patients.

Dr. Prasad: The only thing that we saw in our patients is that they did have a protuberant abdomen, but had no ascites and I do not recall having seen the stria. Drs. Sandstead and Ronaghy will have to bear me out. However, I must say that I was not looking for this and it could have been easily missed, but I remember Dr. Pfeiffer sent me these photographs and I was quite intrigued. Certainly, I do not have a ready explanation on this point.

Dr. O'Dell: It is not clear to me why you picked out the lack of zinc as being the cause of this stria. Why do you think it might be related to zinc?

Dr. Pfeiffer: We have a problem in our schizophrenic patients of high iron and copper and as we give zinc and manganese then the copper and iron may go to a higher level and then go down after a period of four or five months. We have a similar situation, we think, in the late months of pregnancy where the copper is high and the zinc is low. The analogy between our young people and those in the final period of pregnancy is evident, to us at least. Whether this is due to excess copper which is also needed to produce the cross bonds in elastin, we don't know. But in the formation of elastin and collagen there is certainly an interplay of trace metals.

Dr. Larson: Just one quick comment. In burned patients which are low in zinc, over a period of three to six months even these patients, we do not see stria on their body.

Dr. Husain: The common belief about stria is that those people who are obese and later lose weight or when the abdomen is stretched after pregnancies, get this type of stria. We believe this is a stretching mechanism. May I ask Dr. Pfeiffer, what is his criteria for zinc deficiency. Did you measure tissue or blood?

Dr. Pfeiffer: Blood.

Chapter 4

ZINC AND ITS INFLUENCE ON DEVELOPMENT IN THE RAT*

LUCILLE S. HURLEY

INTRODUCTION

A LTHOUGH ZINC has been known for over one-hundred years to be an essential element for plants and for higher animals for almost forty years,[2] its influence on embryonic development has only recently received attention.[3] This chapter reviews published work from the laboratory on the effects of zinc deficiency on prenatal and postnatal development in the rat. Since these studies led to investigation of the problem of availability of zinc from tissue deposits, this subject is also discussed. In addition, some current unpublished work is described.

The primary goal of these studies was elucidation of the role of zinc in prenatal mammalian development, but the effect of zinc deficiency in the nonpregnant rat has also been investigated. This was done in order to test diets and other procedures, and also to provide a model other than the maternal-fetal organism in which to examine various mechanisms apparently operating in zinc-deficient animals.

The basic procedures of diet composition, diet preparation, and environmental control that were developed in this laboratory have been followed in all the work that is summarized in this review.

The ration used had the following percentage composition: isolated soybean protein,† 30.0; sucrose, 57.3; corn oil, 8.0; salts,‡ 4.0; and DL-methionine, 0.7. The zinc content of the soybean protein was reduced by treatment with the tetrasodium salt of ethylenediaminetetraacetic acid by a modification of the method described by Davis et al.[5] Crystalline vitamins were given separately.§ The basal zinc-free ration used in

---

*Supported in part by the National Institute of Child Health and Human Development Research Grant HD-01743.

†ADM C-1 Assay Protein (Archer-Daniels-Midland Company, Cincinnati) or Purina Assay Protein RP-100 (Ralston Purina Company, St. Louis, Mo.).

‡Composition of the basal salt mix: (in grams): $CaCO_3$, 600; $Ca(H_2PO_4)_2 \cdot H_2O$, 220; K_2HPO_4, 650; $NaCl$, 336; $MgSO_4 \cdot 7H_2O$, 250; $FeSO_4 \cdot 7H_2O$, 50; $MnSO_4 \cdot H_2O$, 4.6; KI, 1.6; $CuSO_4 \cdot 5H_2O$, 0.6.

§A mixture of crystalline vitamins in glucose was given three times each week in amounts to provide the following intake in micrograms, per day: Ca pantothenate, 500; p-aminobenzoic acid and riboflavin, each 100; pyridoxine•HCl, thiamin•HCl, and nicotinic acid, each 300; menadione, 250; folic acid, 6; biotin, 2.5; vitamin B_{12}, 0.3; choline chloride, 10 mg; inositol, 5 mg; ascorbic acid, 1 mg; α-tocopheryl acetate, 1.2 IU; vitamin A palmitate, 150 IU, and vitamin D_3, 15 IU. During pregnancy the vitamin supplement was doubled.

the various experiments contained from 0.20 to 0.60 ± 0.05 ppm of zinc as determined by atomic absorption spectroscopy. Zinc-supplemented control animals received the same basal diet except that zinc carbonate was added to the salt mix providing a total content in the diet of 40, 60, or 100 ppm of zinc. In the studies of reproduction, 60 or 100 ppm were used for the control diet.

Stainless steel cages and racks were used in all experiments, and all rats were housed individually, except for the brief periods when a male was introduced into the cage for breeding purposes. Deionized water was given in Pyrex bottles with vinyl plastic stoppers and stainless steel mouthpieces. Aluminum and stainless steel feed cups were used. Throughout the experimental work, careful attention was given to the prevention of zinc contamination from the environment as well as from the diet.[4]

ZINC DEFICIENCY IN NON-PREGNANT RATS

General

In both male and female weanling rats, a specific and severe zinc deficiency was produced which resulted in extreme retardation of growth.[4,6] Other signs of deficiency were also striking. These included alopecia, dermal lesions, emaciation, and an abnormal "kangaroo-like" posture. Zinc-deficient females had abnormal estrous cycles, as seen by examination of daily vaginal smears. Repletion with zinc rapidly increased body weight and produced a normal rate of growth. The females developed normal estrous cycles and were able to produce normal young.

Leukocyte Changes

In zinc-deficient animals, there was a change in the ratio of types of leukocytes in the blood. Although the total white blood cell count remained normal, the ratio of polymorphonuclear neutrophils to lymphocytes changed from 0.2 to 1.5 in weanling males after 21 days of the deficiency regime. Inanition controls (pair-fed or paired-weight) showed no increase in the ratio. Zinc content of the leukocytes, however, was normal. Similar changes were found in pregnant females.[7]

The effects of zinc deficiency on the enzyme histochemistry of leucocytes in the peripheral blood and bone marrow of young growing male rats were investigated. The previously reported increase in the ratio of polymorphonuclear leucocytes to lymphocytes in zinc-deficient rats was confirmed. In addition, hypersegmentation, increased reactivity of acid and alkaline phosphatases, leucine aminopeptidase and naphthol-AS-D chloroacetate esterase, and decreased reactivity of γ-glutamyl transpeptidase were observed in the neutrophils of peripheral blood and bone marrow in zinc-deficient rats.[8]

Plasma Protein

In zinc-deficient weanling males, there was a reduction in total plasma protein from 7.67 to 5.95 g/100 ml after four weeks on the experimental diet. Zinc deficiency also resulted in alterations in plasma protein patterns obtained by disc gel electrophoresis. These results were due to zinc deficiency *per se* and not to inanition since neither pair-fed nor pair-weight controls showed these changes.[9]

Histopathological Changes

Dietary zinc deficiency in the rat produces atrophy of the testis and hyperplasia of the esophageal mucosa.[10,11,12] The development and reversibility of testicular and esophageal changes produced by zinc deficiency were investigated in young rats. Weanling males developed characteristic esophageal and testicular lesions as early as day 7. By day 14, all the rats showed such changes. Weight of the testis appeared to be relatively more reduced than was body weight. Following 28 days of depletion, repletion with zinc resulted in a partial reversal after 6 days and complete disappearance of the lesions after 15 days. Thus, esophageal mucosa and testicular tubules appear to be highly sensitive to dietary zinc content and respond rapidly to its deficit or presence.[13]

Thus, zinc deficiency appears to have a marked effect on growing or proliferating tissues. This is exemplified by the extreme retardation or cessation of growth shown by young weanling rats, and the complete arrest of both ovarian maturation in the female and spermatogenesis in the male.

ZINC DEFICIENCY IN PREGNANT RATS

Teratogenic Effects

GENERAL: The deleterious effect of zinc deficiency on rapidly growing tissues is also evident in the embryo. Hens which were fed a zinc-deficient diet produced chicks which were weak and died shortly after hatching.[14] Other workers, using a more severely deficient diet, observed gross malformations in chick embryos including skeletal defects, brain abnormalities, and herniation of viscera.[15,16]

In pregnant rats, zinc deficiency resulted in a high rate of embryonic death, severe retardation of intrauterine growth, and a high incidence of congenital malformations affecting every organ systems.[17,18] The observation of congenital malformations from zinc-deficient rats has since been confirmed by Mills et al.,[19] Warkany and Petering,[20] and Wilkins and

TABLE 4-I

EFFECT OF SHORT-TERM AND TRANSITORY ZINC DEFICIENCY ON REPRODUCTION IN RATS

Period of Deficiency, Days of Gestation	Number* of Rats	Net Weight Change During Gestation	Rats With Living Young	Implantation Sites, Dead or Resorbed	Implantation† Sites Affected	Full-term Fetuses			
		g	%	%	%	No.	Number‡ per Litter	Mean§ Weight	Mal-formed
								g	%
None (control)	15	+76 ± 5	100	4.3	4.9	176	11.7 ± 0.5	5.2	0.6
0-6	14	+66 ± 4	100	5.9	7.0	160	11.4 ± 0.6	5.1	1.2
0-8	13	+58 ± 5	100	5.5	7.3	155	11.9 ± 0.6	5.0	1.9
0-10	17	+63 ± 4	82	25	42	133	7.8 ± 1.2	4.8	22
0-12	15	+47 ± 5	93	49	77	97	6.5 ± 1.0	4.1	56
0-14	20	+42 ± 3	70	55	89	103	5.2 ± 1.0	3.6	76
0-16	20	+29 ± 4	70	57	91	103	5.1 ± 1.0	3.6	80
0-18	17	+18 ± 4	76	52	92	96	5.6 ± 1.0	3.4	82
0-21	15	-21 ± 7	93	41	94	101	6.7 ± 1.0	2.7	90
4-10	10	+71 ± 5	100	9.5	18	105	10.5 ± 0.6	5.1	10
6-10	10	+84 ± 5	100	1.6	9.0	120	12.0 ± 0.8	5.0	8
4-12	11	+56 ± 3	100	12	38	106	9.6 ± 1.0	4.5	29
6-12	15	+50 ± 5	87	24	37	129	8.6 ± 1.2	4.8	18
8-12	15	+66 ± 5	73	37	43	116	7.7 ± 1.3	5.0	9
4-14	12	+46 ± 8	92	24	79	103	8.6 ± 1.0	4.2	73
6-14	13	+61 ± 4	100	5.6	49	151	11.6 ± 0.9	4.4	46
8-14	14	+65 ± 5	86	27	43	129	9.1 ± 1.2	4.9	22

Source: L. S. Hurley, J. Cowan, and H. Swenerton, "Teratogenic Effects of Short-Term and Transitory Zinc Deficiency in Rats," Teratology, 4:199, 1971.

*Number of rats with implantation sites.
†Implantation sites with either a resorption or a malformed fetus.
‡Implantation sites with implantation sites.
§Means include all females with implantation sites.
§In every instance standard errors were less than ± 0.1 g.

Dreosti.[21] In our studies, when female rats were given a zinc-deficient diet during pregnancy (days 0 to 21), even though they had been fed a normal diet adequate in zinc until the beginning of gestation, 41 percent of the implantation sites were resorbed. Full-term young weighed about half that of controls, and 90 percent of the fetuses showed gross malformations affecting every organ system (see Table 4-I). The fetal malformations were specifically due to a maternal dietary deficiency of zinc rather than to reduced food intake since females fed restricted amounts of a zinc-supplemented diet had normal young. Shorter periods of deficiency were also teratogenic. With a zinc-deficient diet from days 0 to 12, 56 percent of the full-term fetuses were malformed. When the zinc deficiency regime was imposed from days 6 to 14 of pregnancy, almost half the young were abnormal. Transitory periods of deficiency altered the incidences of the anomalies observed in accordance with the developmental events occurring at the time the deficiency was imposed. The rapid and severe effects of even relatively short periods of zinc deficiency on fetal development suggested that the pregnant rat cannot mobilize zinc from body stores in amounts sufficient to supply the needs of developing fetuses.

Histological studies were made of these small, malformed, full-term fetuses. The congenital anomalies were found to consist of stunting and tissue defects devoid of necrosis and inflammation. Hyperplasia of the esophageal mucosa occurred in all these fetuses. The appearance of this lesion is sufficiently characteristic to be used as a histological indicator of the deficiency state. Somewhat similar fetal mucosal lesions were found in the tongue, pharynx, and forestomach.[22]

CENTRAL NERVOUS SYSTEM: In fetuses from zinc-deficient pregnant rats, there was a high incidence of malformations of the central nervous system. When the deficient diet was fed from day 0 to day 21 of pregnancy, 47 percent of the fetuses had gross malformations of the brain, including hydrocephalus (42%), anencephalus (36%), and exencephalus (11%) (see Fig. 4-1). Under these conditions, 3 percent of the fetuses had frank spina bifida, and 42 percent had micro- or anophthalmia.

BRAIN: In a study of the incorporation of tritiated thymidine in the neural cells of the zinc-deficient rat embryo,[23] the developing brain of 12-days zinc-deficient rat was found to consist of an extremely thin-walled tube. The number of its cells, as well as those incorporating thymidine, was significantly reduced in comparison with controls. At days 14 and 15 of gestation, the brains of zinc-deficient rats also showed the same pattern: a thin-walled tube surrounding distended vesicles and lacking the degree of differentiation and organization typical of the developing brain at this stage. Particularly evident was the lack of normal flexion and the disproportionate narrowness of the elongated heads.[24]

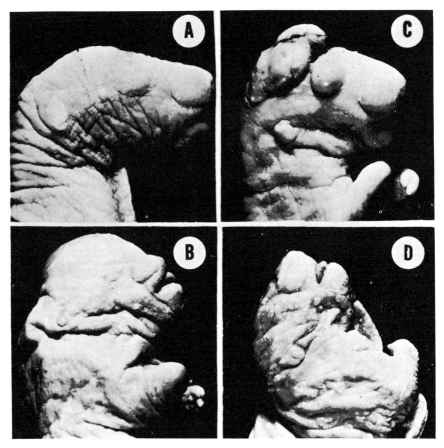

FIGURE 4-1. Gross malformations of the brain in full-term fetuses from female rats fed a zinc-deficient diet during pregnancy as compared with normal control. A. Normal, B. Hydrocephalus, C. Exencephalus, D. Anencephalus. (Razor cuts on the head were made for examination of brain.) Photographic magnification 3X.

By day 17 of gestation, the pattern of abnormal brain development characteristic of the malformed rats at term could be identified. Possibly as a result of the abnormal flexion of the head, the communicating passage between the caudal end of the third ventricle and the aqueduct was forked, stenosed, or even completely obliterated with consequent dilation of the anterior ventricles. Neopallial differentiation was partially or completely suppressed, and portions of the differentiating prosencephalon seemed to have undergone compression changes or shifts in location.

At 21 days of gestation, abnormalities of the brain again involved closure of the opening between the third ventricle and the aqueduct. Concomitant distention of the third and lateral ventricles occurred with resultant alterations in the telencephalic and diencephalic derivatives. In many instances there was also moderate distention of the fourth ventricle and cerebellar hypoplasia.

CORD: In the spinal cords of zinc-deficient fetal rats, marked reduction of cellularity coupled with disorganization of the cells lining the central canal was characteristic of the animals in the youngest age groups. In animals 17 days or older the central canal was widely distended in animals showing distention of the fourth ventricle, and stenosis and forking of the central canal were seen in others in which drainage from the fourth ventricle appeared unimpaired. Derangement of the cells of the mantle layer and discontinuity of the ependyma were also commonly encountered.

OPTIC TRACT: The most consistent pattern of optic tract malformation involved the lack of a demonstrable optic cup, or its organized derivatives, and the absence of a discrete optic chiasm or of optic nerves peripheral to the brain. The identifiable optic components consisted characteristically of a malformed lens buried at a variable depth beneath the skin and connected to the surface of the head by an epithelial-lined tube or cord. Some few ocular muscle bundles could occasionally be identified in the vicinity of these tubular structures.

OLFACTORY TRACT: A peculiar malformation of the olfactory nerve was observed in many of the zinc-deficient fetuses in which development of the olfactory lobe of the telencephalon was abnormal. In these animals nerve fibers from the olfactory epithelium formed twisted knots in a mass which occupied the space rostral to the basal portion of the telencephalon normally filled by the olfactory lobe. These fibrous masses were not incorporated into an organized olfactory bulb, but terminated in the lateral and basal brain substance in a seemingly random manner. The sensory epithelium of the nasal passages was frequently immature.

Prenatal zinc deficiency thus affected many derivatives of the developing basal, alar, and roof plates of the primitive neural tube and resulted in malformations of brain, cord, eye, and olfactory tract. The nature of these malformations, as well as their diverse origins, suggests that the action of zinc is on fundamental rather than secondary processes. Development of defects of the anterior brain in zinc-deficient rats appeared primarily to involve closure of the aqueduct. This is a common lesion in hydrocephalus. Abnormal but recognizable lens structures were observed in the absence of organized retinal components. This appears to be a unique malformation. Defective development of the primitive neural tube may have resulted in both optic and olfactory-tract malformations in zinc-deficient rat embryos. The present evidence suggests that asynchronous development of the central nervous system may be fundamental to the pathology of brain, cord, eye, and olfactory tract. This concept would concur with the results of studies with tritiated thymidine in which large numbers of cells appeared to be in mitotic arrest.[23]

The basic assumption underlying this hypothesis is that zinc influences development through its effect on nucleic acid synthesis.[25,23] Prolongation of the mitotic interval and reduction in the number of neural tube cells early in development could combine to produce a wide range of abnormalities. The specific nature of the defect would thus depend on the state of activity in the presumptive area of the primitive tube when a developmental process was initiated.

EFFECT OF EDTA: Congenital malformations similar in type and quantity to those produced by maternal dietary zinc deficiency also resulted from ingestion of a chelating agent ethylenediaminetetraacetic acid (EDTA). When EDTA (3% of the diet) was fed to pregnant rats from days 6 to 21 of gestation, all the full-term young had gross congenital malformations. These effects were prevented by simultaneous supplementation with 1,000 ppm of dietary zinc. These findings suggest that the congenital anomalies caused by EDTA were due specifically to zinc deficiency.[26]

BASIC DEFECT IN ZINC DEFICIENCY

Enzyme Studies

Studies were undertaken to investigate the mechanisms bringing about disturbances in embryonic development and the lesions of zinc deficiency in weanling rats. Several liver enzymes were assayed in severely zinc-deficient weanling rats. Pyridoxal phosphokinase activity was not significantly different in livers from zinc-deficient rats than from those of controls. Liver glutamic dehydrogenase activity was also normal in zinc-deficient weanlings. Lactic dehydrogenase (LDH) activity was significantly lower in the livers of deficient animals than in those of rats fed the control diet ad libitum; a similar decrease was, however, also observed in the livers of pair-fed controls. Thus, the alteration of liver lactic dehydrogenase activity could have resulted from reduced food intake rather than from zinc deficiency *per se*.[4]

Lactic dehydrogenase and malic dehydrogenase (MDH) were assayed in liver of fetuses at 21, 19, and 17 days of gestation, and in the placentas of these animals. In addition, carbonic anhydrase was assayed in whole blood of 21-day-old fetuses. No differences were seen between controls and zinc-deficient animals in any of the groups.[27]

LDH and MDH were also studied in testes of severely deficient young males with signs of testicular lesions including arrest of spermatogenesis.

These enzymes were measured by both spectrophotometric and histochemical methods. There was no difference between zinc-deficient rats and controls in the activities of LDH or MDH of the supernatant fraction of testis homogenates. Neither did the intensity of histochemical reactivity of the enzymes differ in the two groups. However, some differences in cellular localization of enzyme reactivity were seen, due apparently to differences in the populations of the cells in the two groups.[28] Prasad et al.[29] have reported that LDH and other enzymes were reduced in testis as a result of zinc deficiency. Perhaps in milder but more prolonged deficiency states, degenerative changes altering the types of cells present in the tissue bring about apparent reductions in certain enzymes because the cells containing them are absent.

In addition to the chemical assays of enzyme activity described above, histochemical studies were made of the occurrence, distribution, and localization of the following enzymes: glucose-6-phosphate dehydrogenase, acid and alkaline phosphatase, ATP'ase, succinic dehydrogenase, malic dehydrogenase, lactic dehydrogenase, glutamic dehydrogenase, DPN and TPN diaphorase, non-specific esterase, leucine aminopeptidase, and γ-glutamyl transpeptidase. These enzymes were studied in zinc-deficient and control fetuses of various ages from 14 to 21 days of gestation.

In general, it appeared that the intensity of enzyme activity was a function of the cell types present, not of zinc deficiency, and that enzyme changes are probably not causative factors in producing the congenital malformations of zinc deficiency.

Nucleic Acid Synthesis

Several investigations have demonstrated a requirement of zinc ion for DNA synthesis in partially hepatectomized rats[25,30] and in young growing rats.[31] In zinc-deficient embryos DNA synthesis was studied by examining the uptake of tritiated thymidine injected intravenously into pregnant rats.

The 12-day-old embryos of rats with a deficiency of zinc showed a reduced uptake of tritiated thymidine when compared with controls, as shown by both liquid scintillation and autoradiography. The high incidence of gross congenital malformations resulting from zinc deficiency may thus be caused by impaired DNA synthesis.[23]

AVAILABILITY OF ZINC AND ITS MOVEMENT IN THE BODY

Plasma Zinc

An outstanding aspect of zinc deficiency both in young growing animals and in embryos is the rapidity with which it occurs. The extremely rapid effect of zinc deficiency arises from the need for a constant extraneous source of zinc in order to maintain plasma levels of the element. When rats were given a zinc-deficient diet at the beginning of pregnancy, plasma zinc concentration dropped sharply. After only 24 hours of the deficiency regime, plasma zinc fell by approximately 38 percent (from 96 to 60 mcg/ 100 ml), and a plateau was reached at about 30 mcg/100 ml after 14 days. Similar observations were made with weanling rats subjected to the zinc-deficiency regime.[7] Mills et al.[19] have also found decreases of plasma zinc in zinc-deficient calves and lambs after only a short period of deficiency. Thus, there appears to be little homeostatic control of plasma zinc levels.

Bone and Liver Zinc

The rapid effect of the zinc-deficiency regime in pregnant rats was brought about by lack of mobilization of zinc from maternal stores. This was shown by examining the effect of pregnancy on the zinc content of maternal bone and liver in rats fed either a zinc-deficient or a zinc-supplemented purified diet.[32] Although the zinc content of fetuses from deficient females was lower than that of fetuses from zinc-supplemented controls, the zinc content of maternal liver and bone was not significantly lower at term than that of nonpregnant rats fed the same diet for 21 days (see Table 4-II).

During the 21 days of the experiment, there was no significant bone growth in any group, but both pregnant and nonpregnant rats on the zinc-deficient regimen had slightly lower concentrations of zinc in the femur at the end of the experiment. However, since pregnant females fed the zinc-deficient diet did not have a lower concentration of zinc in their femurs than did nonpregnant females fed the same diet, pregnancy itself did not result in a release of zinc from the maternal skeleton, even in the presence of teratogenic zinc deficiency in the fetuses. These results suggest that the reduction observed in bone zinc after 21 days of the zinc-deficient diet was not due to withdrawal of zinc from skeletal stores but rather to reduced incorporation of zinc during bone formation in the normal turnover of bone tissue. Bone thus cannot be considered a storage reservoir for zinc, since the zinc in bone is not readily available to the rat even in the face of demonstrated need.

In the zinc-deficient animals, liver growth was prevented while concentration of zinc in the liver was maintained. This is consistent with the suggestion that soft-tissue levels of zinc are maintained at the expense of growth and proliferation of new tissue,[33] and with the recent findings that zinc may be involved in the normal synthesis of DNA.[23] Concentrations of zinc were not reduced in the livers of pregnant females as compared to nonpregnant females in either the zinc-deficient or the zinc-supple-

TABLE 4-II

BONE AND LIVER ZINC IN PREGNANT AND NONPREGNANT RATS

Group	No. of Rats	Body Wt Female		Femur				Liver			
					Zinc Content				Zinc Content		
		Zero Time	Net Change* After 21 Days	Wet Wt Femur	Per Femur	Per g Wet Wt	Per g Ash	Wet Wt Liver	Per Liver	Per g Wet Wt	Per g Dry Wt
		g	g	mg	mcg	mcg	mcg	g	mcg	mcg	mcg
Zero time controls	6	245 ± 6†		684 ± 24	116 ± 4	170 ± 4	391 ± 7				
After 21 days zinc-supplemented control diet											
Nonpregnant	6	241 ± 8	+31 ± 5	692 ± 30	128 ± 8	185 ± 9	413 ± 22	9.0 ± 0.4	252 ± 16	27.7 ± 1.2	91.9 ± 4.6
Pregnant	6	239 ± 8	+61 ± 6§	710 ± 10	119 ± 4	168 ± 5	392 ± 16	11.8 ± 0.5§	311 ± 12	26.6 ± 1.2	91.6 ± 4.3
After 21 days zinc-deficient diet											
Nonpregnant	6	244 ± 5	−19 ± 2§	689 ± 18	106 ± 2	157 ± 3§	344 ± 5	6.7 ± 0.4§	174 ± 13§	24.9 ± 0.6	83.9 ± 2.0
Pregnant	6	249 ± 6	−37 ± 6‖	701 ± 28	106 ± 4	152 ± 4‡	354 ± 13	7.0 ± 0.5‖	189 ± 8‖	27.0 ± 1.1	90.1 ± 5.6

Source: L. S. Hurley, and H. Swenerton, "Lack of Mobilization of Bone and Liver Zinc under Teratogenic Conditions of Zinc Deficiency in Rats." *J Nutr, 101*:597, 1971.

*Net change in body weight is the difference in body weight of the female between days 0 and 21 minus the total weight of the fetuses.

†Means ± standard errors.

‡Significantly different from zero time controls (P<0.02).

§Significantly different from zinc-supplemented nonpregnant controls (P<0.02).

‖Significantly different from zinc-supplemented pregnant controls (P<0.02).

mented group. Thus, neither liver zinc nor bone zinc was available to the zinc-deficient rat during pregnancy.

Under conditions of severe deficiency, more zinc was found in the fetuses than could be accounted for by calculation of dietary zinc intake. It is possible that because of the marked loss in body weight of females fed the zinc-deficient diet, some recycling of tissue zinc may have contributed to the zinc content of the fetuses. Nevertheless, when there is a severe deficiency of dietary zinc, body deposits cannot maintain normal plasma-zinc levels nor support normal fetal development.

Effect of Calcium Deficiency

Because of these findings, we postulated that zinc could be removed from the skeleton (which contains a large proportion of the body zinc[34,35]) only under conditions in which there is a breakdown of bone itself. This hypothesis was tested by experiments in which a diet lacking in calcium as well as in zinc was fed to pregnant rats, and its effects on various parameters of fetal development were compared with those of a diet deficient in zinc alone. Since calcium-deficient diets cause increased bone resorption in order to maintain normal plasma-calcium levels,[36] it was postulated that such a diet would bring about release of zinc from bone, making additional amounts of the element available to the animal. In almost every parameter measured, there was better reproduction in females receiving the zinc-deficient-calcium-deficient diet than in those receiving the zinc-deficient diet.[37] In pregnant females deprived of both zinc and calcium, the resorption rate was lower (17 percent of implantation sites as compared with 56 percent), and the number of live young per litter was higher than in females lacking zinc alone (9.6 as compared with 4.8). Furthermore, only 57 percent of living young at term showed gross malformations in the zinc-deficient-calcium-deficient group, while 83 percent of term fetuses from females receiving the zinc-deficient diet were malformed. Thus, in the zinc-deficient group, 93 percent of all implantation sites were affected (dead, resorbed, or malformed), while in the zinc-deficient-calcium-deficient group, only 65 percent were affected. In females fed the zinc-deficient-calcium-deficient diet, the percentage of ash in the femur and its zinc content and concentration were all lower than in females given the zinc-deficient ration. In the former group, furthermore, the total amount of calcium per bone and its concentration on a wet weight basis were lower than in the zinc-deficient animals.

These results show that the teratogenic effect of zinc deficiency was alleviated by feeding a diet deficient in both zinc and calcium during pregnancy, and support the hypothesis that conditions bringing about resorption of bone increase the availability of skeletal zinc.

INFLUENCE OF LEVEL OF DIETARY ZINC

The experiments cited above were all made under extreme conditions of dietary deprivation of zinc. It was also of interest to correlate the level of zinc in the diet with the incidence of malformations and to determine the concentration of dietary zinc that would prevent such malformations. This was done by feeding pregnant females (again under strict conditions to avoid zinc contamination) diets containing various levels of zinc. When the diet contained between 0 and 1 ppm zinc, almost all the fetuses were malformed (see Fig 4-2); with 2.5 ppm, 67 percent were malformed; and with 6.5 ppm, 21 percent showed malformations. Nine or 18 ppm dietary zinc produced fetuses that were essentially normal on a gross morphological basis. It is thus evident that morphogenesis in the rat embryo is sensitive to dietary zinc, not only with respect to the timing of the deficiency period but also in terms of the amount of zinc available from the maternal diet.[38]

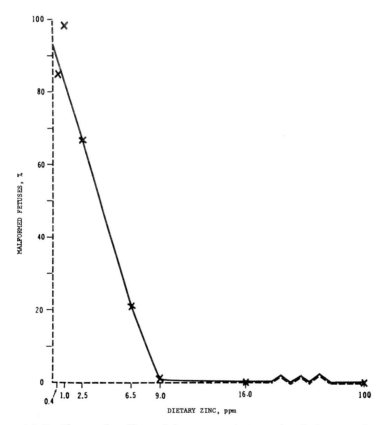

FIGURE 4-2. Incidence of malformed fetuses in relation to level of zinc in the maternal diet during pregnancy. Abcissa: zinc in maternal diet, in parts per million. Ordinate: full-term fetuses showing gross malformations, in percent of live young.

MATERNAL ZINC DEFICIENCY AND POSTNATAL DEVELOPMENT

Mild Deficiency (9 ppm Zinc)

Although a level of 9 ppm of dietary zinc did not cause gross congenital malformations visible at birth, it was possible that there might exist in these offspring more subtle abnormalities which could affect postnatal life. Accordingly, the effect on postnatal survival of a prenatal diet (days 0-21) containing 9 ppm of zinc was examined. Before breeding, and after parturition, the females were given stock diet.* Females given the diet containing 9 ppm zinc during pregnancy had a high rate of stillbirths (28 percent as compared to 1 to 5 percent in controls) and birth weight was reduced. Postnatal survival of young born to mothers getting 9 ppm zinc was markedly affected. By day 7 after birth, all young in this group were dead. In controls fed ad libitum, 84 percent of young alive at birth survived to day 21, and in controls restricted in food intake to the amount eaten by the low-zinc group, 24 percent survived to day 7, and nine percent to day 21. Thus, a diet containing 9 ppm of zinc did not support normal postnatal life, even though few effects were apparent at birth. Part of the postnatal mortality was caused by inanition, but there was also a specific zinc effect, especially in the neonatal period.[39]

Transitory Deficiency

Another aspect related to postnatal development was the effect of a relatively short transitory deficiency during prenatal life on subsequent postnatal development. The effect on postnatal survival of a zinc-deficient diet (< 1 ppm) from day 6 to day 14 of gestation was studied. Although birth weight was normal, only 46 percent of young survived to 21 days after birth, as compared with 92 percent of controls. This occurred despite normal zinc levels in the milk, and in the blood plasma of the newborn. Maternal plasma zinc was also normal except for a short period during pregnancy. After only two days of the zinc-deficient regimen (day 8 of gestation), the plasma-zinc level of the experimental females dropped to only 39 percent that of ad libitum-fed controls. After zinc supplementation on day 14, plasma zinc was rapidly restored to the normal concentration.[40] This is further evidence of the importance of adequate and continuous supplies of dietary zinc throughout pregnancy.

ZINC DEFICIENCY IN LACTATION

The effects of a maternal dietary deficiency of zinc were also studied during lactation in rats. Normal pregnant rats were fed a stock ration until after parturition, then were given either a zinc-deficient (0.5 ppm

_____
Commercial rat chow, ad libitum, and crystalline vitamins.

zinc) or a zinc-supplemented diet. A third group served as restricted-intake controls. The zinc-deficient diet caused a marked reduction in zinc concentration of the milk, and of maternal blood plasma. Pups suckling deficient mothers showed poor survival, retarded growth, gross external signs of zinc deficiency, and reduced plasma zinc. Maternal dietary zinc deficiency during lactation thus results in zinc deficiency in the suckling rats.[41]

REFERENCES

1. Raulin, J.: Études cliniques sur la végétation. *Ann Sci Nat Botan Biol Végétale, 11*:93, 1969.
2. Todd, W. R., Elvehjem, C. A., and Hart, E. B.: Zinc in the nutrition of the rat. *Am J Physiol, 107*:146, 1934.
3. Hurley, L. S.: Studies on zinc deficiency in the developing rat. In Symposium on Zinc Metabolism. *Am J Clin Nutr, 22*:1332, 1969.
4. Swenerton, H., and Hurley, L. S.: Severe zinc deficiency in male and female rats. *J Nutr, 95*:8, 1968.
5. Davis, P. N., Norris, L. C., and Kratzer, F. H.: Iron deficiency studies in chicks using treated isolated soybean protein diets. *J Nutr, 78*:445, 1962.
6. Hurley, L. S.: Studies on nutritional factors in mammalian development. *J Nutr, 91*:2:II:27, 1967.
7. Dreosti, I. E., Tao, S., and Hurley, L. S.: Plasma zinc and leukocyte changes in weanling and pregnant rats during zinc deficiency. *Proc Soc Exp Biol Med, 127*:169, 1968.
8. Shrader, R. E., and Hurley, L. S.: Enzyme histochemistry of peripheral blood and bone marrow in zinc-deficient rats. *Lab Invest, 26*:566, 1972.
9. Tao, S., and Hurley, L. S.: Changes in plasma proteins in zinc-deficient rats. *Proc Soc Exp Biol Med, 136*:165, 1971.
10. Follis, R. H.: *Deficiency Disease.* Springfield, Thomas, 1958.
11. Millar, M. J., Fischer, J. I., Elchoate, P. V., and Mawson, C. A.: The effects of dietary zinc deficiency on the reproductive system of male rats. *Can J Biochem Physiol, 36*:557, 1958.
12. Barney, G. H., Orgebin-Crist, M. C., and Macapinlac, M. P.: Genesis of esophageal parakeratosis and histologic changes in the testes of the zinc-deficient rat and their reversal by zinc repletion. *J Nutr, 95*:526, 1968.
13. Diamond, I., Swenerton, H., and Hurley, L. S.: Testicular and esophageal lesions in zinc-deficient rats and their reversibility. *J Nutr, 101*:77, 1971.
14. Turk, D. E., Sunde, M. L., and Hoekstra, W. G.: Zinc deficiency experiments with poultry. *Poultry Sci, 38*:1256, 1959.
15. Blamberg, D. L., Blackwood, U. B., Supplee, W. C., and Combs, C. F.: Effect of zinc deficiency in hens on hatchability and embryonic development. *Proc Soc Exp Biol Med, 104*:217, 1960.
16. Keinholz, E. W., Turk, D. E., Sunde, M. L., and Hoekstra, W. G.: Effects of zinc deficiency in the diets of hens. *J Nutr, 75*:211, 1961.
17. Hurley, L. S., and Swenerton, H.: Congenital malformations resulting from zinc deficiency in rats. *Proc Soc Exp Biol Med, 123*:692, 1966.
18. Hurley, L. S., Gowan, J., and Swenerton, H.: Teratogenic effects of short-term and transitory zinc deficiency in rats. *Teratology, 4*:199, 1971.

19. Mills, C. F., Quarterman, J., Chester, J. K., Williams, R. B., and Dalgarno, A. C.: Metabolic role of zinc. In Symposium on Zinc Metabolism. *Am J Clin Nutr,* 22:1240, 1969.

20. Warkany, J., and Petering, H. G.: Congenital malformations of the central nervous system in rats produced by maternal zinc deficiency. *Teratology,* 5:319, 1972.

21. Dreosti, I. E., Grey, P. C., and Wilkins, P. J.: Deoxyribonucleic acid synthesis, protein synthesis and teratogenesis in zinc-deficient rats. *S Afr Med J, 46:*1585, 1972.

22. Diamond, I., and Hurley, L. S.: Histopathology of zinc-deficient fetal rats. *J Nutr, 100:*325, 1970.

23. Swenerton, H., Shrader, R., and Hurley, L. S.: Zinc-deficient embryos: Reduced thymidine incorporation. *Science, 166:*1014, 1969.

24. Hurley, L. S., Shrader, R. E.: Congenital malformations of the nervous system in zinc-deficient rats. In: Pfeiffer, C. C. (Ed.): *Neurobiology of the Trace Metals Zinc and Copper. International Rev of Neurobiol,* Suppl. 1, p. 7, New York, Acad Pr, 1972.

25. Fujioka, M., and Lieberman, I.: A Zn^{++} requirement for synthesis of deoxyribonucleic acid by rat liver. *J Biol Chem, 239:*1164, 1964.

26. Swenerton, H., and Hurley, L. S.: Teratogenic effects of a chelating agent and their prevention by zinc. *Science, 173:*62, 1971.

27. Hurley, L. S., Dreosti, I. E., and Swenerton, H.: Studies on zinc enzymes and nucleic acid synthesis in relation to congenital malformations in zinc-deficient rats. Proc Western Hemisphere Nutrition Congress II, August 1968, San Juan, Puerto Rico, p. 39.

28. Swenerton, H., Shrader, R. E., and Hurley, L. S.: Lactic and malic dehydrogenases in testes of zinc-deficient rats. *Proc Soc Exp Biol Med, 141:*283, 1972.

29. Prasad, A. S., Oberleas, D., Wolf, P., and Horwitz, J. P.: Studies on zinc deficiency: Changes in trace elements and enzyme activities in tissues of zinc-deficient rats. *J. Clin Invest, 46:* 549, 1967.

30. Weser, U., Seeber, S., and Warneke, P.: Reactivity of Zn^{++} on nuclear DNA and RNA biosynthesis of regenerating rat liver. *Biochem Biophys Acta, 179:*422, 1969.

31. Sandstead, H. H., and Rinaldi, R. A.: Impairment of deoxyribonucleic acid synthesis by dietary zinc deficiency in the rat. *J Cell Physiol,* 73:81, 1969.

32. Hurley, L. S., and Swenerton, H.: Lack of mobilization of bone and liver zinc under teratogenic conditions of zinc deficiency in rats. *J Nutr, 101:*597, 1971.

33. Hove, E., Elvehjem, C. A., and Hart, E. B.: Further studies on zinc deficiency in rats. *Am J Physiol, 124:*750, 1938.

34. Asling, C. W., and Hurley, L. S.: The influence of trace elements on the skeleton. *Clin Orthopaed, 27:*213, 1963.

35. Underwood, E. J.: *Trace Elements in Human and Animal Nutrition,* 3rd Ed. New York, Acad Pr, 1971.

36. Bronner, F.: Dynamics and function of calcium. In Comar, C. L., and Bronner, F. (Eds.): *Mineral Metabolism.* New York, Acad Pr, 1964, vol. II, part A, p. 341.

37. Hurley, L. S., and Tao, S.: Alleviation of teratogenic effects of zinc deficiency by simultaneous lack of calcium. *Am J Physiol, 222:*322, 1972.

38. Hurley, L. S., and Cosens, G.: Reproduction and prenatal development in relation to dietary zinc level. *Second International Symposium on Trace Element Metabolism in Animals,* June 18-22, 1973, Madison, Wisconsin, In press.

39. Swenerton, H. S., and Hurley, L. S.: Unpublished.

40. Hurley, L. S., and Mutch, P. B.: Prenatal and postnatal development after transitory gestational zinc deficiency in rats. *J Nutr, 103*:649, 1973.

41. Mutch, P., and Hurley, L. S.: Zinc deficiency in suckling rats. *Fed Proc, 30*:643, 1971.

DISCUSSION

Dr. Ruessner: I wonder if you know of any data that might be available on the incidence of fetal abnormalities in humans in the areas where Doctor Prasad worked, where there could be a zinc deficiency.

Dr. Hurley: I think that some of the other people here are more qualified to answer that question than I.

Dr. Ronaghy: In the cases that Doctor Prasad has already reported, we notice several bone abnormalities and that was in the first few cases. Actually, we saw this bone abnormality in two brothers which led us to believe that this could be some kind of genetic abnormality factor so there we started drawing some pedigrees to study all of the families. But we could not finally trace down any familial tendency because that was the only isolated case that we could find. However, in view of the fact that we have so many congenital anomalies in that area of the world, we are trying to find out if all the village mothers are zinc deficient. This is the study that we are working on at this time.

Dr. O'Dell: I thought your interaction between magnesium and zinc was very interesting, but what was the base line for your zinc? You said the zinc and the ash were low. Do you mean total zinc or zinc concentration in the ash or what was the actual measurement made?

Dr. Hurley: This was the total body ash and the zinc content was expressed as the zinc per milligram of total body ash.

Dr. Odell: The other question then was what was the total ash change? Was there less ash in the magnesium deficient fetus?

Dr. Hurley: I think the answer to that is no.

Dr. Chvapil: You said that in zinc and calcium deficient animals that you found less malformation. Still the changes in the zinc and calcium levels in the tissue, plasma, and bone were much less. In Doctor Hsu's experiment he showed in zinc deficiency, no changes in zinc level in the skin. Still there was quite a pronounced inhibition in protein synthesis be it collagenous or noncollagenous or be it DNA. I still wonder whether we are not losing something. Namely, just to correlate the level of the zinc with the malformation or the rate of protein synthesis doesn't seem to be proper. This is because such a relationship doesn't obviously exist.

Dr. Hurley: We did not correlate the level of zinc with the malformations. What we were doing is measuring the zinc in the maternal femur as an indication of whether or not zinc was removed from the bone in the zinc deficient animals. There was no change in the zinc in the maternal bone. But when the diet was lacking, both in calcium and zinc then the zinc concentration decreased.

Dr. Chvapil: This I understand, but it is still not quite clear whether you are able to make a correlation between the zinc level in a tissue and the decreased protein synthesis.

Dr. Hurley: We were not concerned with this at all. We were interested in learning about the movement of zinc in the body because the mothers don't show any effects. The fetuses are very much disturbed and deranged, but the mothers are quite normal. I hope that we may be able to pursue some of these questions in a more general session.

Chapter 5

NEW CONCEPT ON THE MECHANISM(S) OF THE BIOLOGICAL EFFECT OF ZINC*

Milos Chvapil

AND

Charles F. Zukoski

~~~~~~

THE BENEFICIAL EFFECT OF ZINC on various tissue injuries is usually explained by its effect on several zinc-dependent or zinc-containing enzymes. However, our experiments show that zinc markedly increases the stability of biomembranes in general by a mechanism(s) which is (are) restricted to the surface of the membrane. The evidence supporting this statement is outlined below.

Using the lysosomal membrane as a model, we have established the following facts on the control of membrane integrity:

When lysosomes isolated from rat liver are incubated in 0.25 M sucrose-acetate buffer, pH 5.0, at 37° (*in vitro* fragility test), there is a decrease in lysosomal integrity and an increase in the release of enzymes contained within the vacuole. The amount of the released enzyme (i.e. β-glucuronidase) is therefore proportional to the degree of membrane disintegration (labilization, lysis, or distortion) and serves as a handy assay for determining the stability of the membrane under various conditions. We found[1] that over a wide range of concentrations (0.05-2.5 mM), temperatures (20-37°), and pH's (4.5-7.0) zinc stabilizes lysosomal membranes, as shown in Figure 5-1. The fact that complexes of Zn:8-HQ (1:1 or 1:2) which do not permeate the cell membrane[2] are even more effective than Zn^{2+} alone indicates that this is a phenomenon occurring at the surface of the membrane. Furthermore, although the fully saturated complex (1:3) can pass through membranes, it, as well as 8-HQ itself, labilizes lysosomes in a concentration related fashion.[3]

This distribution of the zinc between the membrane and interior of lysosomes and mitochondria isolated from rat liver ranges from 2:1 to 3:1. When the vacuoles are incubated in 1 mM Zn^{2+}, this distribution remains essentially unchanged, while in particles incubated with the unsaturated Zn:8-HQ complexes (1:1 or 1:2) the zinc content of the membrane fraction but not the interest is increased (Table 5-I). These are just the complexes which cause the greatest stabilization of the lysosomal membrane.

*Experiments reported in this lecture were supported from Public Health Service grants ES 00790, AM AI 1648901, AM 15460-02, and National Science Foundation grant GB 33928.

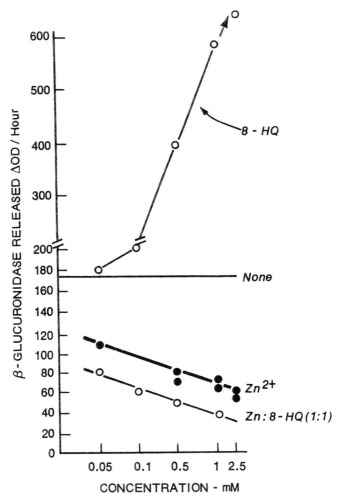

FIGURE 5-1. Effect of different concentrations of zinc, 8-hydroxyquinoline and of zinc + 8-hydroxyquinoline of the stability of isolated liver lysosomes.

Aliquots of the lysosomal suspension containing 10 to 15 mg. protein were incubated at 37° in 0.25 M sucrose, 0.1 M acetate buffer pH 5.0, and the substances being tested. The total volume was 3.0 ml. After 30 minutes the samples were centrifuged at 15,000 g and the supernatants assayed for released β-glucuronidase. Results are presented as released enzyme activity, as increased absorption at 550 nm x 1,000.[27]

Zinc is certainly not the only metal affecting the lysosomal membrane. Labilization by mercury[4] or copper ions[1,3] has been shown to be related to the formation of labile mercaptides with thiol groups of membrane constituents. We found that in addition to zinc and its nonsaturated complexes with 8-HQ, cadmium and lead ions at 1 mM final concentration stabilize the lysosomal membrane. In our system (see methodological de-

TABLE 5-I

DISTRIBUTION OF ZN²⁺ BETWEEN MEMBRANE AND INTERIOR OF CONTROL,
ZN²⁺ AND ZN:8-HQ TREATED LIVER MITOCHONDRIAL FRACTION

Sample	Total Zinc μg/mg Protein	Membrane Bound (in % of Total)	Free
Control	0.47 ± 0.071	61	39
Zn²⁺ (1 mM, pH 6.0)	3.32 ± 0.42	65	35
Zn²⁺ (1 mM, pH 7.4)	3.31 ± 0.07	65	35
Zn:8-HQ 1:1	3.66 ± 0.24	95	5
1:2	3.11 ± 0.18	97	3

A lysosome-rich fraction was prepared from rat liver and aliquots were incubated for 15 minutes at room temperature in the presence of two volumes of saline or the above substances (final conc. = 1×10^{-3} M). The lysosomes were washed 7 x with sucrose, then resuspended. A portion of this suspension was removed, hydrolyzed, and assayed for total protein and zinc. The remainder was treated with Triton X-100 and centrifuged. The pellet was hydrolyzed with redistilled HNO_3. Both pellet and supernatant were assayed for zinc (bound and free). Results are the average of three separate incubations. Source: Chvapil, Ryan and Zukoski.[3]

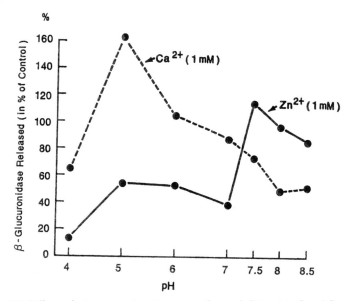

FIGURE 5-2. Effect of zinc and of calcium on the stability of isolated liver lysosomes at different pH values.

The conditions of incubation are the same as for Figure 1 except that the buffer contained 0.1 M acetate and 0.05 M PO_4 adjusted to the appropriate pH. The results are presented as the activity of released β-glucuronidase calculated as the percent of enzyme released in the control sample at each pH.[27]

tails in Fig. 5-2) manganese and nickel are inactive. The fact that neither zinc, cadmium nor lead ions interfere with the assay of pure β-glucuronidase led us to the conclusion that stabilization by these metals is related to an effect on the macromolecular components of the membrane.

The stabilizing effect of zinc is not restricted to lysosomal membranes but extends to biomembranes in general. There is quite a bit of experimental evidence supporting this view.

We found that low amplitude mitochondrial swelling is completely prevented in the presence of 1 mM zinc. Some other metals were also inhibitory, as shown in Table 5-II. This effect is very probably related to inhibition of the mitochondrial respiratory chain by zinc ions, as demonstrated by Chistyakov and Hendel.[5] These authors suggest that zinc successfully competes with iron for a ligand in a nonheme iron protein which takes part in electron transport in the respiratory chain. It has to be mentioned, however, that thyroxin-stimulated mitochondrial swelling (high amplitude) is enhanced by 10 to 100 μM Zn^{2+}.[6] The distinction between

TABLE 5-II

EFFECT OF SOME METALS AND CHELATING AGENTS ON
LOW-AMPLITUDE MITOCHONDRIAL SWELLING

Substance	Swelling (520 nm) ΔOD/sample/10 min.
Control	−0.163
Sodium EDTA	+0.125
Calcium EDTA	−0.217
2,2'-dipyridyl	−0.266
1,10-phenanthroline	−0.183
8-hydroxyquinoline	−0.300
Sodium diethyldithiocarbamate	−0.310
Zn^{2+}	+0.105
Cd^{2+}	−0.158
Fe^{2+}	+0.142
Ni^{2+}	+0.125
Au^{3+}	+0.057
Ca^{2+}	−0.163

Mitochondria isolated from rat liver were suspended in 0.25 M sucrose in final concentration 120 mcg protein/ml. All substances were tested at 1 mM final concentration. A change in O.D. at 520 nm was continuously recorded on Beckman DBG spectrophotometer with potenciometric recorder. Source: Chvapil and Ryan, unpublished results.

low and high amplitude changes is not entirely clear; the different effects of zinc, however, correspond to this distinction.

Our finding that lymphocytes purified from dog lymph by several washes have a significantly higher viability index when kept in the presence of 10 μM zinc agrees with a common experience of cytologists, who use zinc to isolate intact plasma-cell membranes.[7] It has also been shown that divalent metal ions, specifically Zn^{2+} and Ni^{2+}, present in natural ribosomes play an important role in preserving the compact structure of ribosomes.[8] On the contrary, in zinc deficiency polysomes disintegrate to oligo- and monosomes.[9]

These findings led us to the conclusion that zinc stabilizes a variety of biological membranes by some mechanism(s) which appears (appear) to be related directly to the membrane surface.

To better understand the proper meaning of the word "mechanisms" we tested several hypotheses on the possible mode of action of zinc:

Zinc Affects the Activity of Enzymes Controlling the Properties of Biological Membranes

Several phospholipases different in their pH optima and metal dependence have been reported to be present either within the lysosome or in the membrane fraction.[10,11] We thought it possible that zinc might affect lysosomal stability by altering the activity of such enzymes. We incubated lysosomes at various conditions of pH between 4 and 8.5 in the presence of sucrose or sucrose plus either Ca^{2+} or Zn^{2+}. In the presence of 1 mM Zn^{2+} the release of β-glucuronidase was decreased at acid pH yet increased at neutral pH relative to the controls (Fig. 5-3). In contrast, 1 mM Ca^{2+} stabilized lysosomes at neutral pH and labilized them under acid conditions. On the basis of these results it is certainly not possible to conclude whether or not zinc is acting to alter membrane stability via an effect on enzymes. However, these results do not reflect the metal and pH dependences of the known phospholipases[10,11] (M. A. Wells, personal communication). In this connection let us mention that a number of divalent metal ions, including zinc, exert an inhibitory effect on the ATPase activity of pulmonary alveolar macrophages.[12] This enzyme is located at the cellular plasma membrane and possibly constitutes an integral part of the plasma membrane structure.[13] It is felt that cell membrane functions such as chemotaxis, phagocytosis, and pinocytosis are governed by ATPase activity. On the other hand, it was found that complete cell disruption paralleled a 1.5-fold to 2-fold increase in ATPase activity.[13] Inhibition of the activity of this enzyme by zinc would therefore result in stabilization of plasma membranes, at least in pulmonary alveolar macrophages. Zinc may interact with certain reactive groups of the macromolecular constituents of the membrane, such as PO_4^{-3} or sialic acid, and as a result change the affinity of some as yet unknown enzymes to the modified substrate. An evaluation of this hypothesis is under study.

Zinc Acts by Decreasing Lipid Peroxidation in Biomembranes

A close relation between the lipid peroxidation and damage of biomembranes has been found repeatedly.[14,15] Since lipid peroxidation can be catalyzed by metals such as Fe^{2+}/Fe^{3+} and Cu^+/Cu^{2+}, we tested the hypothesis that zinc interferes with the metal-redox systems which initiate this oxidation. Lipid peroxidation was induced by administration of CCl_4 to rats for a period of three weeks. A group of control as well as CCl_4-

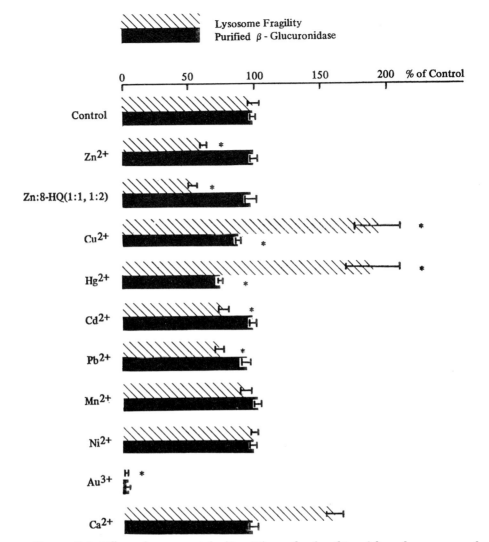

FIGURE 5-3. Effect of some metals (1 mM) on the fragility of liver lysosomes and activity of pure β-glucuronidase.

Method used was the same as described in Figure 1. All substances were tested in 1 mM final concentration. Results are the average of three to six determinations and are presented as Mean ± S.E. of % of control. Asterisk refers to results significantly different from controls ($P<0.01$ — <0.001). The specifity of the effect on lysosomal membrane was checked by direct assay of pure β-glucuronidase (Type B-1, bovine liver, Sigma) in the presence of 1 mM of each agent.

treated rats was administered zinc intragastrically (10 mg zinc acetate/day/rat) during this period. As shown in Table 5-III, simultaneous treatment with zinc caused a significant decrease in the level of lipid peroxides in the liver of rats injured by CCl_4, whereas in animals not exposed to

TABLE 5-III

EFFECT OF ZINC ON SOME PARAMETERS OF LIVER INJURY
INDUCED BY CCl₄

Group	Malonaldehyde (mitochondrial) μmoles/mg Protein	t/p	Collagen μmoles Hyp/g	Significance t/p
1. Control	21.27 ± 0.81		0.511 ± 0.016	
2. Control + Zn²⁺	21.11 ± 3.09		0.488 ± 0.057	
		3.8°°		2.31°
3. CCl₄—3 weeks	76.25 ± 14.45		0.778 ± 0.115	
		2.4°		2.8°
4. CCl₄ + Zn²⁺	40.04 ± 4.66		0.446 ± 0.033	

CCl₄ administered s.c. twice weekly 0.1 ml/100 g body weight for three weeks.
Zinc administered as 10 mg zinc acetate/day/rat by gavage.
There were four rats in each group. Results are presented as mean ± S.E.
Significance is given as student's t-test for the values being compared.
°P<0.05, °°P<0.01.
Source: Chvapil, Ryan, Elias and Peng.[27]

CCl₄ zinc treatment had no effect on lipid peroxidation in the liver.[29] A parallel change in the concentration of collagen proteins in the liver (see Table 5-III) is presented in this connection as evidence that the entire picture of liver injury induced by CCl₄ was improved by zinc treatment.°

Further evidence for such an effect of zinc on the formation of lipid peroxides in injured tissue was obtained in a model of lung edema produced by exposing mice to 35 ppm NO₂.[16] It has been shown that NO₂ as well as ozone or hyperbaric oxygen enhances lipid peroxidation[17] although it is not known whether this is the mechanism leading to edema. Pretreatment of mice with a low dose of zinc (4 μM/kg body weight by gavage for three days prior to NO₂ exposure) prevents the development of lung edema induced by NO₂ (Table 5-IV, unpublished results in collaboration with G. Gillette). Our studies on the control of lipid peroxidation in the liver or in the lung by zinc were done in highly complicated systems; we also used some simpler models. Lipid peroxidation was studied in isolated liver mitochondrial fractions stimulated by Fe²⁺-ascorbic acid-O₂ as well as in microsomal fractions in which lipid peroxidation was induced by CCl₄ *in vitro*. A representative example of such an experiment is presented in Table 5-V showing that lipid peroxidation in liver microsomes stimulated by CCl₄ was substantially decreased by zinc within a large range of concentrations. Addition of zinc (0.01-1 mM) to control microsomes also decreased lipid peroxidation.[28] This very probably is a result of the interference of this metal with electron transport in drug-oxidizing enzyme systems.[18]

°Later we found that the dose of zinc used in this experiment was too high; the optimal effective dose for rats is rather 1-2 mg ZnCl₂/100 g body weight, twice daily.

TABLE 5-IV

THE EFFECT OF ZINC PRETREATMENT ON LUNG EDEMA INDUCED IN
THE MOUSE BY NO₂ EXPOSURE

Group	N	Lung Wet Weight mg/g Body Weight	t-test	Lung Dry Weight mg/mg Lung Wet Weight	t-test
Control	7	6.98 ± 0.48		23.53 ± 0.46	
			3.15°		5.09°°
NO₂ (1.00 ppm)	6	10.03 ± 0.84		17.91 ± 1.00	
			3.79°		5.41°°
Zinc + NO₂	6	6.79 ± 0.14		23.42 ± 0.19	

Female mice, Cd-1 strain (Ch. Rivers), body weight 31.25 ± 1.20, were exposed for 30 minutes to a homogenous atmosphere of NO_2; 35 ppm. Zinc-treated mice received 0.6 ml of 0.2 mM zinc acetate solution by gavage, once a day for three days, prior to the NO_2 exposure. The animals were sacrificed three hours after removing from the chamber. The lung was dissected, cleaned from all extra pulmonary structures, and weighed. After the tissue was dried to constant weight, the dry substance was determined. The variability is given by standard error of the mean. Student's t-test was employed to test the significance ($P<0.01°$ or $P<0.005°°$). Source: Chvapil and Gillette, unpublished results.

TABLE 5-V

EFFECT OF ZINC ON LIPID PEROXIDATION IN LIVER MICROSOMES
IN VITRO

Sample	Lipid Peroxides μmoles/ml
Control	0.469
Zn²⁺, 1 mM	0.326
0.1 mM	0.360
0.01 mM	0.340
CCl₄ 5 μl/ml	0.680
Zn²⁺, 1 mM + CCl₄ 5 μl/ml	0.521
0.1 mM + CCl₄ 5 μl/ml	0.551
0.01 mM + CCl₄ 5 μl/ml	0.545

A microsomal fraction was prepared by a standard differential centrifugation procedure from dog liver and resuspended 1:1 (w/v) in Tris-KCl buffer (0.05 M, pH 7.4). Samples containing 2 ml of suspension (18 mg protein/ml), 1 ml of cofactors of microsomal oxidizing enzymes at the following final concentration: NADPH 0.2 mM, glucose-6-phosphate 2 mM, $MgSO_4$ 5 mM and nicotinamide 2 mM, plus 1 ml of the tested substance dissolved in Tris-KCl buffer at the concentration given in the Table, were incubated at 37° for 30 min. Samples containing both zinc and CCl₄ were pretreated with Zn^{2+} for 10 minutes at 20° before the addition of CCl₄. Source: Chvapil, Ryan, and Zukoski.[28]

CONCLUSIONS

We have presented data supporting our concept that zinc stabilizes biomembranes by some as yet unknown mechanism which is related to the surface of the membrane. More experimental data are needed in order to gain a deeper insight into the actual mechanisms involved. Our contemporary concept on the biological effect of zinc is illustrated in Figure 5-4. It postulates an interaction with macromolecules located at the membrane with resulting stabilization of the whole biostructure. Although it

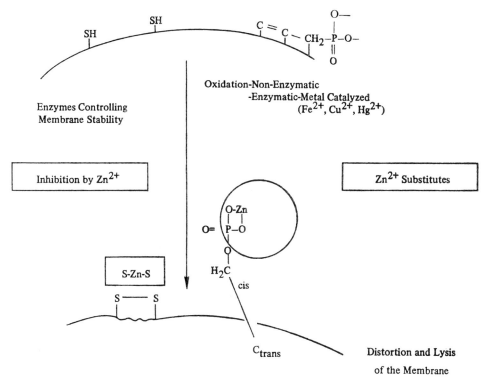

FIGURE 5-4. Schematic representation of the concept on biological effect of zinc. The following possible mechanisms are presented:
1) interaction with enzymes controlling the integrity of the membrane
2) interference with macromolecular components of the membrane, changing their conformation or enzyme-substrate specifity
3) Interference with metal catalyzed lipid peroxidation.

is possible that this effect may be mediated by enzymes, we favor a nonenzymatic mechanism. For example, zinc as a metal having only one oxidation state would not serve the redox function required for lipid peroxidation and thus might stabilize membranes by interfering with peroxidative damage. Such a reaction assumes that zinc successfully competes with iron or copper in biological systems. There exists quite a lot of evidence in favor of this assumption. Displacement of copper from SH-binding sites on metallothionein by zinc has been shown recently by Evans et al.[19] Zinc and cadmium antagonize copper absorption by displacing copper from the duodenal protein.[20] Zinc shows a marked preference for sulfur or nitrogenous ligand groups in the formation of its complexes[21] following the order of stabilities: $Hg^{2+} \gg Cd^{2+} > Zn^{2+} > Cu^{2+} > Ni^{2+} > Co^{2+} > Mn^{2+}$. We have found that Zn^{2+} (1 mM) will prevent labilization of lysosomes in the presence of an equimolar amount of Cu^{2+}. Thus, displacement of metals catalyzing lipid peroxidation by zinc seems theoretically feasible.

Even in the present version, the biological implications of this concept are multifold and in many respects offer a new aspect in the understanding of the tissue reactivity during injury. The beneficial effect of zinc in wound healing[22,29] revokes the question if uncontrolled process of phagocytosis, the extent of lysosomal rupture and cell necrosis in the dynamics of the inflammatory lesion are in accord with optimal rate of healing. Because of zinc administration the labilization of lysosomes in injured liver is decreased (unpublished results). In accordance, less collagen was deposited in the liver (See Table 5-III and Ref. 23), which agrees with the fact that collagen content in liver cirrhosis correlates with the extent of cell necrosis.[24,30]

Finally, one may speculate that the protection by zinc against carcinogenesis induced by dimethylbenzanthracene[25] is related to an effect on the characteristics of cell membrane or lysomal stability.[26]

SUMMARY

A new concept on the mechanism(s) of the biological effect of zinc is presented, showing that zinc interacts with macromolecules of various biomembranes by a mechanism which is restricted to the surface of the membrane.[31,32] The experimental evidence available so far favors the non-enzymatic mechanism. Interference with lipid peroxidation was demonstrated. This effect parallels an increased stability of lysosomal membrane and improvement of the entire picture of tissue injury.

REFERENCES

1. Chvapil, M., and Ryan, J. N.: Effect of selected chelating agents and metals on the stability of liver lysosomes. *Biochem Pharmacol, 21*:1097, 1972.
2. Albert, A.: *Selective Toxicity.* London, Methuen, 1965.
3. Chvapil, M., Ryan, J. N., and Zukoski, C. F.: Effect of zinc and other metals on the stability of lysosomes. *Proc Soc Exp Biol Med, 140*:642, 1972.
4. Verity, M., and Reith, A.: Effect of mercurial compounds on structure-linked latency of lysosomal hydrolases. *Biochem J, 105*:685, 1967.
5. Chistyakov, V. V., and Hendel, L. Ya: Mechanism of inhibition of mitochondrial respiratory chain by zinc ions. *Biokhimiia, 33*:1200, 1968.
6. Buchanan, J., Primack, M., and Tapley, D.: Relationship of mitochondrial swelling to thyroxine-stimulated mitochondrial protein synthesis. *Endocrinology, 87*:993, 1970.
7. Perdue, J. F., and Sneider, J.: The isolation and characterization of the plasma membrane from chick embryo fibroblasts. *Biochim Biophys Acta, 196*:125, 1970.
8. Tal, Moshe: Metal ions and ribosomal conformation. *Biochim Biophys Acta, 195*:76, 1969.

9. Sandstead, H. H., Hollaway, W. L., and Baum, V.: Zinc deficiency: Effect on polysomes. *Fed Proc, 30*:517, 1971 (Abstract).

10. Rahman, Y. E., and Verhagen, J.: Evidence of a membrane-bound phospholipase A in rat liver lysosomes. *Biochem Biophys Res Comm, 38*:670, 1970.

11. Franson, R., Waite, M., and LaVia, M.: Identification of phospholipase A_1 and A_2 in the soluble fraction of rat liver lysosomes. *Biochemistry, 10*:1942, 1971.

12. Mustafa, M., Cross, C. E., Munn, R. J., and Hardie, J. A.: Effects of divalent metal ions on alveolar macrophage membrane adenosine triphosphatase activity. *J Lab Clin Med, 77*:563, 1971.

13. Cross, C. E., Mustafa, M., Peterson, P., and Hardie, J. A.: Pulmonary alveolar macrophage. *Arch Intern Med, 127*:1069, 1971.

14. Wills, E. D.: Mechanisms of lipid peroxide formation in animal tissues. *Biochem J, 99*:667, 1966.

15. Witting, L. A.: The effect of antioxidant deficiency on tissue lipid composition in the rat. IV. Peroxidation and inter-conversion of polyunsaturated fatty acids in muscle phospholipids. *Lipids, 2*:109, 1967.

16. Thomas, H., Mueller, P., and Lyman, R.: Lipoperoxidation of lung lipids in rats exposed to NO_2. *Science, 159*:532, 1967.

17. Roehm, J. N., Hadley, J. G., and Menzel, D. B.: Oxidation of unsaturated fatty acids by ozone and nitrogen dioxide. *Arch Environ Health, 23*:142, 1971.

18. Peters, M. A.: The influence of magnesium and some other divalent cations on hepatic microsomal drug metabolism in vitro. *Biochem Pharmacol, 19*:533, 1970.

19. Evans, G. W., Majors, P., and Cornatzer, W. E.: Mechanism for cadmium and zinc antagonism of copper metabolism. *Biochem Biophys Res Comm, 40*:1142, 1970.

20. Starcher, B. C.: Studies on the mechanisms of copper absorption in the chick. *J Nutr, 97*:321, 1969.

21. Vallee, B. L.: The "active catalytic site", an approach through metalloenzymes. *Fed Proc, 20*:71, 1961 (Abstract).

22. Pories, W. J. and Strain, W. H.: Zinc and wound healing. In Prasad, A. S. (Ed.): *Zinc Metabolism.* Springfield, Thomas, 1966.

23. Saldeen, T.: On the protective action of zinc against experimental liver damage due to choline free diet or carbon tetrachloride. *Z Gesampte Exp Med, 150*:251, 1969.

24. Aterman, K.: Studies in fibrosis of the liver induced by carbon tetrachloride. I. Relation between hepatocellular injury and new formation of fibrous tissue. *Arch Pathol, 57*:1, 1954.

25. Poswillo, D. E., and Cohen, B.: Inhibition of carcinogenesis by dietary zinc. *Nature, 231*:447, 1971.

26. Allison, A. C.: Lysosomes and diseases. *Sci Am, 217*:62, 1967.

27. Chvapil, M., Ryan, J. N., Elias, S. L., and Peng, Y. M.: Protective effect of zinc on carbon tetrachloride-induced liver injury in rats. *Exp Mol Pathol, 19*:186, 1973.

28. Chvapil, M., Ryan, J. N., and Zukoski, C. F.: The effect of zinc on lipid peroxidation in liver microsomes and mitochondria. *Proc Soc Exp Biol Med, 141*:150, 1972.

29. Elias, S., and Chvapil, M.: Zinc and wound healing in normal and chronically ill rats. *J Surg Res, 15*:59, 1973.

30. Karl, L., Chvapil, M., and Zukoski, C. F.: Effect of zinc on the viability and phago-

cytic capacity of peritoneal macrophages. *Proc Soc Exp Biol Med, 142*:1123, 1973.

31. Chvapil, M., Elias, S. L., Ryan, J. N., and Zukoski, C. F.: Pathophysiology of zinc. In Pfeiffer, C. C. (Ed.): *International Review of Neurobiology*, New York, Academic Press, 1972, Supplement 1, p. 105.

32. Chvapil, M.: New aspects in the biological role of zinc: A stabilizer of macromolecules and biological membranes. *Life Sci, 13*:1041, 1973.

Chapter 7

THE EFFECTS OF ZINC IN MAN: NUTRITIONAL CONSIDERATIONS

WALTER MERTZ

T HE FINDINGS PRESENTED in this symposium are of eminent interest to the nutritionist. Zinc is one of the essential elements of the first transition series; it has been extensively studied in experimental animals. Zinc deficiency, severe enough to cause growth retardation and hypogonadism is known to occur in man in countries of the Middle East.[1] Is zinc nutrition a public health problem in the U.S. as well? It has been known for several years that the consumption of the average American diet does not always guarantee an optimal or even sufficient intake of certain trace elements. Iodization of table salt as well as iron enrichment of flour and bread were the first consequences of the recognition of this fact. In spite of these programs, iron deficiency as well as iodide deficiency continue to exist in certain age groups or geographic areas.[2,3] More recently, evidence began to emerge that the intake of the essential element chromium may be marginal as well.[4] The beneficial effects of zinc supplementation described by many authors point out the possibility that zinc may belong in this group of trace elements that are of nutritional concern.

ZINC DEFICIENCY

In evaluating the available results in a nutritional sense, it is necessary to distinguish between a physiological effect of a micronutrient and a pharmacological one. The first is essentially the correction of a prior deficiency, whereas the second is independent of the nutritional state.

In a study of 17 patients with delayed wound healing, Pories and others found that all subjects with serum zinc levels of less than 110 μg per 100 ml responded to zinc supplementation with a positive response of wound healing, whereas the remaining subjects who had zinc levels above 110 μg per 100 ml did not.[5] Similarly, in another study measuring the effect of zinc supplementation on atherosclerosis in 36 patients, those who improved upon supplementation had significantly lower initial serum zinc levels than the subjects who did not (85 versus 140 μg per 100 ml, $p <$ 0.005).[6] Similarly, in a third study 5 out of 6 atherosclerotic subjects who responded to zinc supplementation had initially subnormal serum zinc levels. In spite of the difficulties of interpreting serum zinc levels as a diagnostic means, it appears from these data that zinc supplementation is effective only in these cases who demonstrate some indication of a subnormal zinc state. Even though this concept is not entirely without contradiction,[7] the bulk of the available evidence strongly suggests that the effectiveness of zinc is dependent on the existence of a suboptimal zinc status; and therefore is not a drug effect.

The second problem is that of the etiology of the observed low zinc states. Are these exclusively a consequence of the disease that brought the subjects to the hospital or does the prior nutritional history of the subjects play a role and to what degree? It is well known that many diseases, infections, hormonal imbalances, and even exercise can alter zinc metabolism and decrease or increase circulating zinc levels.[8] However, one can assume on the basis of well controlled animal experiments that the influence of the disease or stress situation is not the overriding factor and that it is the previous dietary history that determines the performance of the animals. The zinc-sufficient rat does not benefit from additional zinc supplementation with improved wound healing.[9] If the zinc-responsive conditions as discussed in this symposium are indeed correlated with previous suboptimal zinc nutrition, the problem of zinc requirement and actual zinc intake in the U.S. becomes one of the highest urgency.

The third question is concerned with the incidence of marginal zinc nutritional states in the U.S. population. Zinc was not included in any of the large-scale nutritional surveys; therefore, exact data are not yet available. However, it is possible to make an approximate assessment of zinc nutrition from a variety of available data.

Henkin has shown that there is a large group of people who suffer from hypogeusia, dysgeusia, hyposmia, and dysosmia.[10] Even though these subjects did not exhibit any marked abnormalities of zinc metabolism, their taste acuity was significantly improved by zinc supplementation. Half of the subjects tested responded to as little as 25 mg of zinc per day in addition to their normal dietary intake. The condition also responds to other transition elements, such as copper or nickel. Therefore, it is difficult to interpret these findings as proof for widespread zinc deficiency. It can be said, however, that there is a large number of people in the U.S.A. who would benefit from an increased zinc intake.

Direct evidence for the existence of marginal zinc nutrition states has been obtained more recently by Hambidge.[11] Using hair as an indicator of the zinc nutritional status, this investigator found 9 children out of a total of 132 sampled who had abnormally low hair zinc levels. Upon individual examination, he was able to detect a marked impairment of taste acuity together with poor appetite and poor growth as compared with the Iowa standard. Increasing the zinc intake of these children by supplementing 2 mg of Zn per kilogram body weight per day resulted in improvement of taste acuity and increased appetite. The growth response is being evaluated. The combination of analytical, physiological and growth performance data, as well as the response to increased zinc intake presents proof for the existence of marginal zinc deficiency in children.

ZINC REQUIREMENT

The requirement of preadolescent children for equilibrium or positive balance has been estimated at approximately 6 mg per day.[12,13] Young college women were in positive balance on self-selected diets that furnished from 9.8 to 14.4 mg of zinc per day, with an average retention of 6.6 mg per day.[14] An average intake of 11.5 mg of zinc in balance studies with young college women resulted in near equilibrium. However, four of the nine subjects were in negative balance.[15] The studies of Spencer[8] conducted under strict control in a metabolic ward indicate that intakes of less than 9 mg per day in adults result in negative balance and that amounts of 10 to 12 mg are needed to obtain equilibrium or a slightly positive balance. On this basis, the Workshop on Zinc in Human Nutrition of the Food and Nutrition Board, National Academy of Sciences, tentatively recommended a dietary zinc intake of 15 to 20 mg per day for adults.[8] This recommendation is based on a safety factor of 1.5 to take into account the variation of availability of zinc in different foods as well as the individual variation of requirement. It can be assumed that with this range of intake the majority of the subjects would be in slightly positive zinc balance.

ACTUAL ZINC INTAKE

Values reported by different investigators are presented in Table 7-I. From these data it appears that the overall average zinc intake is somewhere between 12 and 13 mg per day. It must be realized that these

TABLE 7-I

DAILY ZINC INTAKE FROM MIXED DIETS

Author	Intake (mg)	Range (mg)
Tipton	14	11-18
Schroeder (Institutional)	16	
(Hospital)	8	
Engel (children)		5-9
White	12	
White (self-selected diets)	13	
Spencer	13	
Spencer (Hospital)	11	

values were obtained from good and balanced diets, such as given in hospitals, metabolic wards, or self-selected by well educated college women. It is likely that the daily intake would be considerably lower than the figures cited here if a less balanced diet were eaten or when the intake of calories were markedly reduced. It is obvious, therefore, that the recommended intake of 15 mg per day is not easily reached and that the actual consumption under adverse conditions may be considerably less than this figure.

Table 7-II gives a rough estimate of zinc concentrations in various groups of foods. With an average caloric density of 2 kcal per gram wet

TABLE 7-II

ZINC CONTENT OF FOODS (PPM)
(APPROXIMATE REQUIREMENT: 15 PPM IN 1 KG DIET)

Herring, Oysters		700-1600
Meats		30-50
Whole grains, lima beans, peas		20-30
Other seafoods		20-30
Bread, white	1-10	
Fruits, vegetables	1-4	
Butter, margarine, oils	1-3	
Sugar	<1-1	

weight of the daily diet, an intake of 1000 grams would furnish 2000 calories. In order to meet the estimated zinc requirement of 15 mg per day, the average zinc concentration would have to be 15 ppm, wet weight. This concentration is exceeded by meats, seafoods, and certain whole grains, peas, and beans. It is not known whether the availability of zinc in the latter three is comparable to that in meats. The rest of the major foods contains much less than the theoretical 15 ppm. This is particularly true for such important sources of food energy as bread, fat, and sugar. It is obvious from these data that a suboptimal zinc intake can easily result from a diet which does not contain sufficient animal proteins. With the outstanding position of the latter as a source of available zinc, any trend toward replacing meat with synthetic products, such as "textured meat" from soy protein is cause for considerable concern. This was expressed in the summary of the Workshop on Zinc in Human Nutrition: "The participants expressed strongly a recommendation that the 'textured meats' from plant proteins must be enriched with zinc to furnish the concentration of available zinc at least equal to that found in the meats that the substitutes are intended to replace."[8]

According to Schroeder's studies,[16] the low zinc content of vegetables is further reduced by canning. Losses due to this process were 40 percent for spinach, 60 percent for beans, and 83 percent in tomatoes. On the other hand, canned beets contained 60 percent more zinc than the raw product.[16]

Considerable losses of zinc and other essential trace elements occur whenever a food product is refined or separated into different fractions. The distribution of essential trace elements in milling fractions has been thoroughly studied.[17] Table 7-III, based on Schroeder's analyses,[16] shows

TABLE 7-III

ZINC IN PARTITIONED FOODS (PPM)

Wheat	32
Patent flour	9
Rice, whole	7
Rice, polished	2
Corn, whole	18
Cornstarch	1
Corn oil	2
Sugar, raw	9
Sugar, white	<1
Egg, whole	21
Egg, yolk	36
Egg, white	<1
Pork, whole	19
Pork, lard	2

Source: Schroeder, *Am J Clin Nutr,* 24:562, 1971.

that this is also true for other partitioning processes. The differences between whole wheat and flour, whole corn and cornstarch, raw sugar and white sugar, whole egg and egg white are of a sufficient magnitude to be nutritionally important.

ZINC BALANCE

The interpretation of the data discussed here with regard to nutritional sufficiency of dietary zinc intake has to be made with great caution. Too little is known about the availability of zinc in different foods, in the foods used for the balance studies as well as in the products analyzed for zinc content, and too little is known about other factors that govern absorption mechanisms. On the other hand, the reasonable agreement of analytical data from various laboratories as well as of the balance studies suggest that the estimated minimum requirement of approximately 10 mg per day for adults may be valid for a variety of circumstances. The presently available nutritional data then can be interpreted to mean that the average zinc intake from a well balanced diet is just slightly above the amount required to maintain zinc equilibrium. It is apparent that many diets, particularly when derived mainly from refined carbohdyrate and fat do not furnish enough zinc. The known rapid turnover of zinc in experimental animals and the rapid appearance of zinc deficiency symptoms suggest that the body stores of available zinc are not sufficient to compensate for any prolonged time of low zinc intake. The present average zinc intake of the adults in the U.S.A. does not appear to offer a desirable margin over the minimum requirement.

The negative zinc balance in the newborn and the subsequent sharp decline of zinc in hair of young infants may or may not be a physiological phenomenon.[11] Tissue levels of several trace elements are known to decline after birth. Hair zinc levels usually return to the concentration present at birth by the time the age of four years is reached. However, there are children whose hair zinc levels decline to extremely low levels and those whose hair level does not return to normal until much later in life. Milk, even mother's milk, is a poor source of zinc and many baby cereals may not contain enough zinc in an available form. The exact zinc requirement for the growing child is unknown. In analogy to iron nutrition, the zinc requirement of the growing child expressed on the basis of body weight or caloric intake may be higher than that of the adult. In this case the zinc nutrition of children would be an even greater problem than that of the adult.

SUMMARY

The average zinc intake in the adult population derived from a well balanced diet is only 2 to 3 mg above the estimated minimum requirement to maintain balance; it falls short of the intake of 15 mg recommended by the Workshop on Zinc in Human Nutrition. Deviations from the consumption of a well balanced diet containing sufficient animal proteins can be expected to result in negative zinc balance. On this basis, it is likely that marginal zinc nutrition states do exist in the population of the U.S.A. The incidence of marginal zinc deficiency is unknown.

REFERENCES

1. Prasad, A. S.: Metabolism of zinc and its deficiency in human subjects. In Prasad, A. S. (Ed): *Zinc Metabolism*. Springfield, Thomas, 1966, p. 250.

2. *Measures to Increase Iron in Foods and Diets*. Proceedings of a Workshop, January 1970. Food and Nutrition Board, National Academy of Sciences, Washington, D.C.

3. *Iodine Nutriture in the United States*. Summary of a Conference. October 1970. Food and Nutrition Board, National Academy of Sciences, Washington, D.C.

4. Mertz, W.: Chromium: Occurrence and function in biological systems. *Physiol Rev, 49*:163, 1969.

5. Pories, W. J., Strain, W. H., and Rob, C. G.: Zinc Deficiency in Delayed Healing and Chronic Disease. *Environmental Geochemistry in Health and Disease.* Memoir 123, Geological Society of America, 1971, p. 72.
6. Henzel, J. H., Holtman, B., Keitzer, F. W., DeWeese, M. S., and Lichti E.: Trace Elements in Atherosclerosis, Efficacy of Zinc Medication as a Therapeutic Modality. In: *Trace Substances in Environmental Health,* Columbia, 1969, p. 83.
7. Canning, E., and Fell, G. S.: Zinc in human health and disease. *Proc Nutr Soc 30:* 40A, September 1971.
8. *Zinc in Human Nutrition.* Summary of Proceedings of a Workshop. December, 1970. Food and Nutrition Board, National Academy of Sciences, Washington, D.C.
9. Sandstead, H. H., Lanier, Jr., V. C., Shephard, G. H., and Gillespie, D. D.: Zinc and wound healing. Effects of zinc deficiency and zinc supplementation. *Am J Clin Nutr,* 23:514, 1970.
10. Henkin, R. I.: Newer aspects of copper and zinc metabolism. In: Mertz, W. and Cornatzer, W. E. (Eds.): *Newer Trace Elements in Nutrition.* Dekker, New York, 1971, p. 255.
11. Hambidge, K. M., Hambidge, C., Jacobs, M., and Baum, J. D.: Low levels of zinc in hair, anorexia, poor growth, and hypogeusia in children. *Pediat Res,* 6:868, 1972.
12. Engel, R. W., Miller, R. F., and Price N. O.: Metabolic pattern in preadolescent children: XII. Zinc balance. In Prasad, A. S. (Ed.): *Zinc Metabolism,* Springfield, Thomas, 1966, p. 326.
13. Scoular, F. I.: A quantitative study, by means of spectrographic analysis, of zinc in nutrition. *J Nutr,* 17:103, 1939.
14. Tribble, H. M., and Scoular, F. I.: Zinc metabolism of young college women on self selected diets, *J Nutr,* 52:209, 1954.
15. White, H. S., and Gynne, P. N.: Utilization of inorganic elements by young women eating iron-fortified foods. *J Am Diet Assoc,* 59:27, 1971.
16. Schroeder, H. A.: Losses of vitamins and trace minerals resulting from processing and preservation of foods. *Am J Clin Nutr,* 24:562, 1971.
17. Czerniejewski, C. P., Shank, C. W., Bechtel, G. W., and Bradley, W. B.: The minerals of wheat flour, and bread. *Cereal Chem,* 41:65, 1964.

DISCUSSION

Dr. Henkin: I think the mystery of what happens in zinc metabolism during the first three years of life is even greater than you will lead us to believe when you consider how much zinc is in milk during the first week to two weeks of life. Mother's milk contains approximately 1000 mcg per hundred mls or certainly the amount that you would find in oysters or lobster or fresh calf's liver, which is about the highest that one can find. This then drops off, very markedly over time, probably under the control of prolactin. As time goes on, you end up with milk containing about 50 mcgs per 100 mls which is about what you might find in meat. Therefore, if a child gets only milk, and surprisingly enough there are many children in the United States who are getting primarily milk as their major source of food, you find a fairly large amount of zinc being ingested in comparison, say, to oil or fat in that population.

However, of course, you know you can supplement it with other foods so it is a much stranger problem than you might expect.

Dr. Pfeiffer: One of the factors not mentioned by Dr. Mertz has occupied our thoughts. We have grown peas in the backyard and run the zinc and manganese content and compared that with frozen peas from the chain store. The peas in the backyard have 100 percent zinc and manganese, while the frozen peas from the chain store have 20 percent of the zinc and manganese. They are a ghastly green when they are cooked. The reason for removing the trace metals is so they appear more wholesome when served, but they certainly are less nutritious. We did the same thing with carrots and apparently EDTA is not used to process carrots because the garden grown carrots are equal to frozen carrots.

Chapter 8

STUDIES OF ZINC METABOLISM IN NORMAL MAN AND IN PATIENTS WITH NEOPLASIA*

HERTA SPENCER, DACE OSIS,
LOIS KRAMER, AND
EMILIE WIATROWSKI

≈≈≈

INTRODUCTION

ALTHOUGH STUDIES OF ZINC METABOLISM and zinc balances in man have been reported many years ago[1], the analytical methods available for the analysis of zinc at that time were not only very tedious but also not very reliable. In recent years further zinc balance studies in man have been reported in which newer methods of zinc analysis, such as spectrographic techniques as well as atomic absorption spectroscopy have been utilized.[2,3] The studies of Tipton were carried out for a prolonged period of time in two adults on a self-selected diet[3] and the study of Engel was carried out in preadolescent girls in a summer camp.[2] In the present study, zinc balances were determined in adult males under strictly controlled dietary conditions in a Metabolic Research Ward.

MATERIALS AND METHODS

All patients were fully ambulatory and in good physical condition and had normal kidney and gastrointestinal functions. All clinical and laboratory tests were normal. The diet was kept constant throughout the studies and was analyzed for zinc, nitrogen, calcium, phosphorus, sodium, and potassium in each 6 day metabolic period. The basal diet contained an average of 2200 calories, 286 gm carbohydrate, 75 gm protein, 87 gm fat, 220 mg calcium, 770 mg phosphorus, and 12.7 mg zinc. The daily fluid intake was kept constant. When zinc balances were determined during high calcium intake, calcium gluconate tablets were added to the constant low calcium diet, raising the calcium intake about 10 fold. All other dietary constituents were kept constant. In studies of the effect of different intake levels of zinc on zinc metabolism, the changes in dietary zinc intake were achieved by increasing or decreasing the protein intake. In studies of starvation the "diet" chiefly consisted of water and beverages, such as tea or coffee without sugar. In all studies, all urine and stool specimens were collected from the start of the study. The body weight, the 24 hour urine

*Supported in part by Contract AT(11-1)-1231-92 from the U. S. Atomic Energy Commission and in part by the National Dairy Council.

volume, and the urinary excretions of creatinine, zinc, calcium, and phosphorus were determined daily.

Metabolic balances of zinc, calcium, phosphorus, and nitrogen were determined in each 6 day metabolic period on aliquots of the diet and on aliquots of 6 day pools of urine and stool. During starvation only urine collections were available as stools are usually not passed under these conditions. Zinc and calcium in the diet, plasma, urine, and stool were determined by atomic absorption spectroscopy,[4-6] nitrogen by the Kjeldahl method,[8] and phosphorus by the method of Fiske and SubbaRow.[7]

RESULTS

Table 8-I shows the analyzed values of the zinc content of the constant metabolic diet used in this Research Unit. The zinc content of the two

TABLE 8-I

ZINC CONTENT OF A METABOLIC DIET

Meal		Zinc, mg/meal	
		Diet I°	Diet II°
Breakfast		1.1	1.8
Lunch		6.8	7.1
Supper		3.2	5.6
	TOTAL	11.1	14.5

Average total calories = 2220 calories/day.
°Diets I and II are given on alternate days.

menus used on alternate days differed by about 3 mg per day due to the fact that these menus contained different types of meat.

Figure 8-1 shows that the main pathway of zinc excretion is via the intestine, the fecal zinc excretion approximated the zinc intake while the urinary zinc excretion was about 0.5 mg per day or 1/30th of the fecal zinc excretion.

Table 8-II shows the reproducibility of the zinc balances determined in the same subject for four consecutive 6 day periods. These data show again that the fecal zinc excretions reflected the zinc intake while the urinary

TABLE 8-II

ZINC BALANCES IN MAN

Period	Days	Zinc, mg/day°			
		Intake	Urine	Stool	Balance
1	6	14.08	0.87	12.66	+0.55
2	6	13.01	0.86	11.75	+0.40
3	6	14.11	0.97	12.42	+0.72
4	6	14.40	0.93	12.73	+0.74

°Values are averages for each 6-day period.

URINARY AND FECAL ZINC EXCRETION
IN MAN

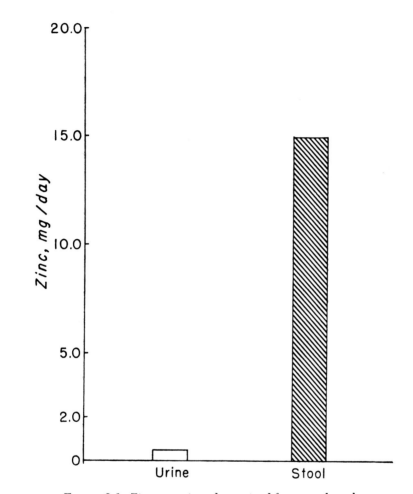

FIGURE 8-1. Zinc excretions determined for several weeks.

zinc was less than 1 mg per day. The zinc balances were in equilibrium and were similar in the four study periods.

Figure 8-2 shows that there was no correlation between the excretion of [65]Zn and urinary calcium: a similar lack of correlation between the urinary zinc and urinary calcium excretion was previously reported.[8]

Table 8-III shows data on zinc balances during different intake levels of calcium. The zinc intake was about 2 mg greater on the two high calcium intake levels than on the low calcium intake. The urinary zinc remained unchanged on increasing the calcium intake 8 to 10 fold. The fecal zinc in-

URINARY CALCIUM AND Zn65 EXCRETION

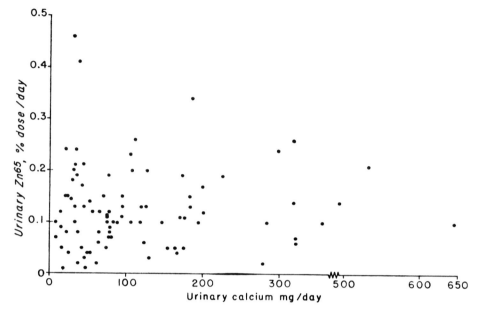

FIGURE 8-2. A single dose of ^{65}Zn was given orally to patients in various states of calcium metabolism.

TABLE 8-III

ZINC BALANCES DURING THE INTAKE OF
DIFFERENT AMOUNTS OF CALCIUM

Days	Calcium Intake mg/day	Zinc, mg/day*			
		Intake	Urine	Stool	Balance
20	212	12.60	0.75	11.33	+0.52
20	1658	14.67	0.85	13.87	−0.05
36	2168	14.45	0.74	14.12	−0.41

*Values are averages for the number of days indicated.

creased with increasing zinc intake and the zinc balances changed from slightly positive values during low calcium intake to slightly negative values in the two high calcium studies.

A 10-20 fold increase in urinary calcium induced by infusing calcium, resulted in only a very slight increase in urinary zinc excretion.[8] When stable strontium was infused in amounts equivalent to the amounts of calcium infused, similar changes in urinary zinc excretions were noted. When ammonium chloride was administered orally (9 gm/day for 6 days), the urinary zinc excretion increased slightly while the increase in urinary calcium was considerably greater (Table 8-IV).

TABLE 8-IV

EFFECT OF ACIDOSIS ON URINARY ZINC AND CALCIUM EXCRETIONS

Treatment	Urinary Excretions, mg/day[a]			
	Zinc	Calcium	Zinc	Calcium
Control	0.47	41	0.46	29
NH₄Cl[b]	0.60	105	0.72	132
Control	0.52	63	0.55	82
	Patient 1		Patient 2	

[a] Average values for six days.
[b] 9 gm NH₄Cl/day for 6 days.

Table 8-V shows that the urinary zinc excretion is independent of the urine volume. This is shown by the excretions of Patient 1 in whom the urine volume differed by 50 percent as well as by the zinc excretions of Patient 2 in whom the urine volume differed by 1100 cc per day while the urinary zinc excretions remained constant in the two patients.

Numerous plasma levels determined in the same patients on a constant dietary intake over time periods ranging from 1½ to 3 years varied by 20 to 30 mcg percent. For instance in one patient the plasma levels ranged from 84 to 112 mcg percent with an average of 96 mcg percent ± 7.6 and

TABLE 8-V

RELATIONSHIP BETWEEN URINARY ZINC EXCRETION
AND URINE VOLUME

Patient	Urine Volume ml/day	Urinary Zinc mg/day
1	3660	1.34
	2600	1.34
	1800	1.33
2	2900	0.24
	1800	0.22

in another the values were 96 to 116 mcg percent with an average of 105 mcg percent ± 8.1 in these time periods, respectively.

When the zinc intake was changed in the same subject from a low intake level of 6.5 mg/day to 16.7 mg/day, the zinc balances changed from negative to positive values. On a zinc intake of 9.5 mg/day, the zinc balance was only slightly negative. This zinc balance was similar to that determined during a higher zinc intake of 12.5 mg/day.

In malnutrition the zinc balance was found to be very positive on an adequate zinc intake of 15 mg per day. These zinc balances ranged from +5 to +6 mg/day and remained in this high range for several months. The zinc balance returned to normal values once the patient was nutritionally repleted.

Total calorie restriction resulting in marked weight loss led to a marked and sustained increase in urinary zinc excretion. These excretions reached a maximum of 6.5 mg per day and represented an approximate 10-fold increase in zinc excretion. Despite this marked loss of zinc, the plasma level of zinc did not decrease and in fact, these levels increased in the majority of patients during fasting (Fig. 8-3). This loss of zinc was independent of

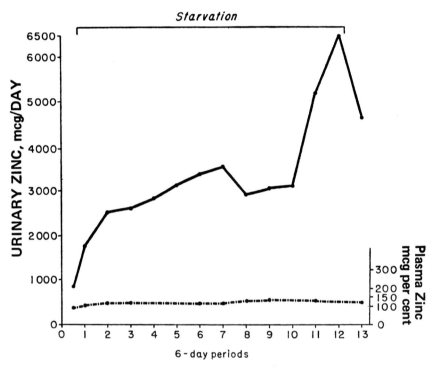

FIGURE 8-3. Each point of the urinary zinc excretion represents a 6-day average.

the addition of calcium during starvation. A similar loss of zinc via the kidney, however at a slower rate, was observed on a low protein-low calorie diet containing about 2 mg zinc per day which led to a gradual but continuous weight loss. During this dietary intake, the fecal zinc excretion averaged 4 mg per day and the urinary zinc excretion averaged 2 mg per day. Under these dietary conditions the plasma level of zinc increased also. The total loss of zinc during starvation and during prolonged low protein-low zinc intake was similar. In two cases studied for comparable periods of time, for 60 and 64 days, respectively, the total zinc loss was 276 mg during starvation and 250 mg on low protein intake.

In view of the reported changes in plasma zinc and urinary zinc in infectious diseases, the effect of tetracycline on zinc plasma levels and urinary zinc excretions has been studied in a patient with a urinary tract infection (E. coli). Figure 8-4 shows that prior to the administration of tetracycline the zinc plasma levels were low ranging from 71 to 77 mcg percent. During the administration of tetracycline for 24 days the plasma levels increased in the first 12 days to 89 and 91 μg percent and decreased

EFFECT OF TETRACYCLINE ON PLASMA ZINC AND URINARY ZINC LEVELS

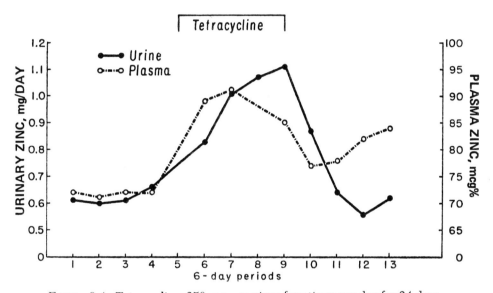

FIGURE 8-4. Tetracycline, 250 mg was given four times per day for 24 days.

in the next 6 days to 80 μg percent. In the 24 days following the discontinuation of this antibiotic, the plasma level remained in this range. The urinary zinc excretion averaged 0.6 mg/day prior to the administration of tetracycline. During tetracycline administration the urinary zinc excretion rose and reached 1.1 mg/day in the 4th 6 day period. Thereafter, the urinary zinc excretion decreased to control levels.

In patients with metastatic carcinoma of the prostate the observation was made that the intestinal absorption of ^{65}Zn was extremely low in the active stage of the disease. When a clinical and biochemical remission was induced by the administration of estrogen, the absorption of ^{65}Zn was markedly increased. This effect was not a result of estrogen therapy as the administration of estrogen to patients free of cancer did not increase the absorption of ^{65}Zn.

DISCUSSION

As has been pointed out previously, the dietary intake of zinc depends greatly on the dietary intake of protein.[8] Even the otherwise constant metabolic diet differed somewhat in zinc intake on alternate days due to the fact that a different type of meat was used in one of the meals of the two menus on these two days. The substitution of the portion of beef by a portion of chicken in this meal resulted in a 3 mg difference in the zinc intake per day. Assuming that the normal total zinc intake would be 12 mg per day, a 3 mg difference in zinc intake constitutes a considerable change. Despite this fluctuation, the zinc content of the metabolic diet was found to be very constant over a number of years.[8]

The zinc deficiency associated with endocrine changes in man[9] may be a result of an inadequate dietary intake including the intake of zinc. On the other hand, zinc deficiency in man may also develop despite an adequate zinc intake if the diet contains substances which complex zinc and make it unavailable for absorption.[10,11] The beneficial effects of zinc therapy for wound healing in surgical patients[12] and in patients with peripheral vascular disease[13] may indicate that these patients are actually zinc deficient. Since these patients were able to utilize the supplemental zinc and the main source of the zinc intake is the diet, one must assume that these patients may have had an inadequate dietary zinc intake for a prolonged period of time. Altered wound healing has also been demonstrated in zinc deficiency in experimental animals.[14] In diseases, such as myocardial infarction, which predominantly occur in the older age group, the zinc plasma level and the zinc tissue levels have been found to be low.[15,16] As peripheral vascular disease also occurs with great frequency in persons of the older age group, it is conceivable that changes in zinc metabolism may occur with age. However, this aspect has not been investigated.

In previous studies using ^{65}Zn as the tracer, it was shown that the urinary excretions of this radioisotope were extremely low after the oral or intravenous administration of ^{65}Zn.[17-19] The analyses of stable zinc as determined in zinc balance studies in man carried out in this Research Unit have also shown that the urinary zinc excretion is very low while the main pathway of excretion is via the intestine. The reason for this high intestinal excretion of zinc is not clear. The present studies have shown that the urinary zinc excretion in man is remarkably constant in a given individual despite marked changes in urine volume. The zinc balance data presented here have again demonstrated the constancy and reproducibility of these balances in subjects maintained under constant dietary conditions.

Little is known on the zinc requirement in man. In studies carried out in this Research Unit the zinc balance was about −4 mg per day when the zinc intake was at the extremely low level of 2 mg per day. On a zinc intake of 6.5 mg/day the zinc balance was less negative, −1.3 mg/day. In general, the zinc balance in man appears to be in equilibrium on a zinc intake of about 12 mg/day, although the requirement to attain equilibrium may vary greatly from person to person.

The factors which regulate the plasma zinc level and zinc homeostasis in man have not been delineated with certainty. Marked differences in the zinc plasma levels have been reported in different disease states.[20,21] The reasons for these changes may be many fold. The zinc plasma level as well as the urinary excretion of zinc have been reported to be decreased in man in acute infections.[22] Studies performed in this Research Unit have shown that, under normal conditions, the zinc plasma level was constant over periods of time extending from 1½ to 3 years. A study of the effect of the antibiotic tetracycline on the plasma level of zinc and on urinary zinc excretion carried out in a patient with an E. coli urinary tract infection has shown interesting results. Shortly after the institution of the antibiotic therapy both the plasma zinc level and the urinary zinc excretion increased. Although these changes may be a result of abolishing the infectious process, the mechanism of these changes is not clear. The low serum zinc values during infection have been attributed to redistribution of zinc in the body.[23]

In states of malnutrition the urinary zinc excretion has been found to be elevated[24] although not to the same extent as in total calorie restriction in obese man.[25,26] Despite this loss of zinc and the lack of zinc intake, the zinc plasma level did not decrease but, in fact, increased. The high urinary zinc excretions in both of these conditions may be a reflection of tissue breakdown associated with weight loss while the elevated zinc plasma level may result from dissociation of the zinc-protein complex secondary to tissue breakdown and circulation of increased amounts of ionic zinc in plasma prior to its clearance via the kidney. The increase in the zinc plasma level and the high urinary zinc excretion during starvation may also be related to the metabolic acidosis which may contribute to the dissociation of the zinc-protein complex. However, when acidosis was induced by ammonium chloride in normals, the urinary zinc excretion increased only by 20 to 30 percent. If the increase in urinary zinc during acidosis is a true increase, the reason for this excess excretion is not clear. It may be due to release of small amounts of zinc from bone as metabolic acidosis is invariably associated with loss of calcium and phosphorus. However, little correlation has been found between the urinary zinc and urinary calcium excretion.[8,17] Another explanation for the effect of acidosis on the slight increase in urinary zinc excretion may be a direct effect of acidosis on the kidney resulting either in a release of zinc from the kidney or in decreased tubular reabsorption of zinc. Whether the lower rate of zinc loss via the kidney during a low protein-low zinc intake is a result of the slower rate of weight loss and of the slower rate of tissue breakdown or of the absence of acidosis during a low calorie intake is not clear. The endogenous fecal zinc loss during a low calorie intake appears to be considerable and has been estimated to be 2 mg/day.[24] The total zinc loss during either starvation or during prolonged low calorie intake in time periods of about 2 months is considerable and has been calculated to amount to 10 to 15 percent of the total body zinc store.[27] Also, the total loss of zinc was similar in both conditions in this period of time.

The studies indicate that the plasma level of zinc does not reflect the zinc intake. An example of the lack of the correlation between the zinc status and the plasma level is the increase in the zinc plasma level despite a deficiency of zinc intake for several months during low calorie and low zinc intake. Another example is the increase in the zinc plasma level despite a marked loss of zinc during starvation. On the other hand, when large amounts of zinc were administered orally following protein and zinc depletion, the zinc plasma level did not increase but actually decreased, again indicating that the zinc plasma level did not reflect the dietary zinc intake.

The observation of a decrease in ^{65}Zn absorption in patients in the active stage of carcinoma of the prostate and the increase in the ^{65}Zn absorption during remission induced by estrogen[28] is intriguing. These studies have shown that the increase in ^{65}Zn absorption during estrogen therapy was not a direct effect of the estrogen but rather a result of the change in the neoplastic status, thus indicating that differences in zinc metabolism may exist in normals and in patients with neoplasia. Differences in ^{65}Zn concentration in normal and tumor tissue have been demonstrated in patients with cancer[29] and the plasma levels of zinc have been reported to be lower in patients with bronchogenic carcinoma[30] and in patients with Hodgkin's disease[31] than in normals. Whether these lower plasma levels of zinc in neoplasia are due to a deficient intake of zinc or to decreased zinc absorption, as shown in the patients with carcinoma of the prostate,[28] or to interference of the absorption of zinc by substances similar to those reported by others[10,11,32] needs clarification. The effect of zinc deficiency and of zinc excess in transplanted Walker 256 carcino-sarcoma has been reported.[33]

SUMMARY

The zinc balance studies in man have indicated that the amount of zinc necessary to attain zinc equilibrium is about 12 mg per day under normal conditions. However, in malnutrition the zinc balance may be very positive on a normal zinc intake and remains strongly positive until nutritional repletion is attained. The studies have demonstrated that the loss of zinc during weight reduction induced by a low calorie intake is as great as the loss of zinc induced by total calorie restriction during total starvation. The studies have also shown that the plasma level of zinc does not reflect the zinc intake nor the loss of zinc, and finally, that the metabolism of zinc may differ greatly in normals and in patients with certain types of neoplasia.

REFERENCES

1. McCance, R. A., and Widdowson, E. M.: The absorption and excretion of zinc. *Biochem J, 36*:692, 1942.
2. Engel, R. W., Miller, R. F., and Price, N. O.: Metabolic patterns in preadolescent children. XIII. Zinc balance. In Prasad, A. S. (Ed.): *Zinc Metabolism,* Springfield, Thomas, 1966, pp. 326-338.
3. Tipton, I. H., Stewart, P. L., and Dickson, J.: Patterns of elemental excretion in long term balance studies. *Health Phys, 16*:455, 1969.
4. Osis, D., Royston, K., Samachson, J., and Spencer, H.: Atomic absorption spectrophotometry in mineral and trace element studies in man. *Dev Appld Spectroscopy, 7A*:227, 1969.
5. Willis, J. B.: Determination of calcium and magnesium in urine by atomic absorption spectroscopy. *Anal Chem, 33*:556, 1961.
6. Willis, J. B.: Determination of lead and other heavy metals in urine by atomic absorption spectroscopy. *Anal Chem, 34*:614, 1962.
7. Fiske, C. H., and SubbaRow, Y. T.: The colorimetric determination of phosphorus. *J Biol Chem, 66*:375, 1925.
8. Spencer, H., Osis, D., Kramer, L., and Norris, C.: Studies of zinc metabolism in man. In Hemphill, D. D. (Ed.) *Proc. Conference on Trace Substance in Environmental Health,* V. University of Missouri—Columbia, 1972, pp. 193-204.
9. Prasad, A. S.: Metabolism of zinc and its deficiency in human subjects. In Prasad, A. S. (Ed.): *Zinc Metabolism,* Springfield, Thomas, 1966, pp. 250-303.
10. O'Dell, B. L.: Effect of dietary components upon zinc availability. A review with original data. *Am J Clin Nutr, 22*:1315, 1969.
11. Oberleas, D., Muhrer, M. E., and O'Dell, B. L.: The availability of zinc from foodstuffs. In Prasad, A. S. (Ed.): *Zinc Metabolism,* Springfield, Thomas, 1966, pp. 225-238.
12. Pories, W. J., and Strain, W. H.: Zinc and wound healing. In Prasad, A. S. (Ed.): *Zinc Metabolism.* Springfield, Thomas, 1966, pp. 378-394.
13. Henzel, J. H., DeWeese, M. S., and Lichti, E. L.: Zinc concentrations within healing wounds. *Arch Surg,* (Chicago), *100*:349, 1970.
14. Sandstead, H. H., Lanier, V. C. Jr., Shephard, G. H., and Gillespie, D. D.: Zinc and wound healing. Effects of zinc deficiency and zinc supplementation. *Am J Clin Nutr, 23*:514, 1970.
15. Wacker, W. E. C., Ulmer, D. D., and Vallee, B. L.: Metalloenzymes and myocardial infarction. II. Malic and lactic dehydrogenase activities and zinc concentrations in serum. *New Engl J Med, 255*:449, 1956.

16. Volkov, N. F.: Cobalt, manganese and zinc content in blood of atherosclerosis patients. *Fed Proc Trans Suppl, 22*:897, 1963.

17. Spencer, H., Vankinscott, V., Lewin, I., and Samachson, J.: Zinc-65 metabolism during low and high calcium intake in man. *J Nutr, 86*:169, 1965.

18. Spencer, H., Rosoff, B., Feldstein, A., Cohn, S. H., and Gusmano, E.: Metabolism of zinc-65 in man. *Radiation Res, 24*:432, 1965.

19. Spencer, H., Rosoff, B., Lewin, I., and Samachson, J.: Studies of zinc-65 metabolism in man. In Prasad, A. S. (Ed.): *Zinc Metabolism.* Springfield, Thomas, 1966, pp. 339-362.

20. Halsted, J. A., and Smith, J. C. Jr.: Plasma-zinc in health and disease. *Lancet, i*:322, 1970.

21. Sullivan, J. F., and Lankford, H. G.: Urinary excretion of zinc in alcoholism and postalcoholic cirrhosis. *Am J Clin Nutr, 10*:153, 1962.

22. Pekarek, R. S., Burghen, G. A., Bartelloni, P. J., Calia, F. M., Bostian, K. A., and Beisel, W. R.: The effect of live attenuated Venezuelan equine encephalomyelitis virus vaccine on serum iron, zinc, and copper concentrations in man. *J Lab Clin Med, 76*:293, 1970.

23. Pekarek, R. S., and Beisel, W. R.: Metabolic losses of zinc and other trace elements during acute infection. *Western Hemisphere Nutrition Congress III,* Mt. Kisco, N. Y., Futura, 1972, p. 352.

24. Spencer, H.: Unpublished data.

25. Spencer, H., and Samachson, J.: Studies of zinc metabolism in man. In Mills, C. F. (Ed.): *Trace Element Metabolism in Animals.* Edinburgh, Livingstone, 1970, pp. 312-314.

26. Spencer, H., Osis, D., Wiatrowski, E., and Samachson, J.: Zinc metabolism during starvation in man. *Fed Proc, 30*:643, 1971.

27. Underwood, E. J.: *Trace Elements in Human and Animal Nutrition,* 3rd ed. New York, Acad. Pr, 1971.

28. Spencer, H., Lewin, I., and Samachson, J.: Intestinal absorption of zinc[65] in patients with carcinoma of the prostate. *Cancer Res, 7*:67, 1966.

29. Rosoff, B., and Spencer, H.: Tissue distribution of zinc-65 in tumor tissue and and normal tissue in man. *Nature, 207*:652, 1965.

30. Davies, I. J. T., Musa, M., and Dormandy, T. L.: Measurements of plasma zinc. Part II. In Malignant Disease. *J Clin Pathol, 21*:363, 1968.

31. Auerbach, S.: Zinc content of plasma, blood, and erythrocytes in normal subjects and in patients with Hodgkin's disease and various hematologic disorders. *J Lab Clin Med, 65*:628, 1965.

32. Halsted, J. A.: Geophagia in man: its nature and nutritional effects. *Am J Clin Nutr, 21*:1384, 1968.

33. McQuitty, J. T., DeWys, W. D., Monaco, L., Strain, W. H., Rob, C. G., Apgar, J., and Pories, W. J.: Inhibition of tumor growth by dietary zinc deficiency. *Cancer Res, 30*:1387, 1970.

Chapter 9

ZINC DEFICIENCY AND CHRONIC ALCOHOLISM

James F. Sullivan

THE STUDY OF ZINC DEFICIENCY in patients with chronic alcoholism presents several problems in terminology and in interpretation. As seen in our hospitals, alcoholic patients quite regularly have acute and chronic liver disease ranging from fatty liver with mild alcoholic hepatitis to far advanced cirrhosis usually of the Laennec's type. Subsequently noted changes in zinc metabolism may be the result of hepatic pathology as well as of repeated alcoholic intoxication. The very low serum zinc levels are found in the most severely ill cirrhotic patients suggesting that hepatic pathology and dysfunction are the most important factors determining the altered zinc metabolism.[1] It is characteristic of these cirrhotics that the decreased serum zinc level is associated with a significantly increased excretion of urinary zinc.[2] In other disease states with low serum zinc there is a concomitant decrease in urinary zinc excretion, except in patients with the nephrotic syndrome. In the other conditions in which the serum zinc is decreased there is frequently found a decrease in serum albumin. Considering the relatively large percentage of zinc which is bound to albumin in the serum it seems likely that relative lack of zinc carrier is responsible for the abnormalities noted.[3] Thus in cirrhosis it is difficult to determine to what extent the zinc deficiency noted is primarily due to alcoholism and to what extent it represents hepatic dysfunction.

An additional factor which has made the study of clinical zinc deficiency difficult is the inability to delineate the enzyme systems and/or metabolic pathways which are impaired as a result of the deficiency. Zinc is undoubtedly needed for growth,[4] probably for sexual development[5] and aids greatly in the healing of wounds.[6] These observed results suggest an anabolic effect by the incorporation of amino acids into protein. Presently, the particular mechanisms involved in these phenomena are not clear.

MATERIALS AND METHODS

In earlier work from this laboratory the zincuria and decreased serum zinc levels initially described by Vallee and Wacker[7] were confirmed.[8] Repeated attempts to correlate zinc abnormalities with liver and renal function could be interpreted only as indicating that the most severe zinc deficiency occurred in the patients who were the most ill as judged by clinical criteria.[9] A brief description of the information obtained in this laboratory concerning trace metals in alcoholism follows:

Ingestion of alcohol by normal adults did not result in abnormalities in urinary zinc excretion.[10]

When acutely intoxicated alcoholic patients were studied, excess urinary zinc excretion was noted during the first few days of hospitalization but this returned to normal within a short period of time.[11] In this particular study effort was made to exclude all alcoholics with evidence of hepatic disease as manifested by jaundice, ascites or abnormal liver function.

The actual zinc content of cirrhotic livers was determined after measurement of collagen and correction by subtraction in this factor from the total hepatic weight. The zinc content was uniformly low in these cirrhotic livers.[12]

Studies of zinc metabolism with use of ^{65}Zn were carried out in 8 cirrhotic patients. The mean values were determined by endogenous fecal zinc (mean .0292 mg/Kg/24 hr) zinc pool (2.79 mg/Kg), zinc turnover (0.173 mg/Kg/24 hr) and an internal loss of 0.132 mg/Kg/24 hr,[13] the urinary zinc excretion was not elevated in four of the eight patients studied. Unfortunately similar two compartment analysis of zinc metabolism has not been performed in normal adults and thus the significance of these figures cannot be evaluated by comparison. It may be noted, however, that the actual zinc loss was much greater via the fecal route than by the urinary. However, even in the cirrhotic subjects with normal serum zinc and/or normal 24 hr urinary zinc excretion, the renal clearance of zinc was significantly higher when compared with normal subjects.

One source of zinc excretion into the intestinal tract is through pancreatic secretion, a mean rate of 142 mcg/60 min occurring as measured by duodenal drainage after secretin stimulation in normal subjects. Patients with cirrhosis or chronic pancreatitis appear to excrete a lower concentration in the pancreatic juice.[14]

In summary, these observations seem to indicate the following: (1) abnormal ethanol ingestion in the alcoholic is associated with at least transient excess zincuria in the absence of demonstrable liver disease, (2) the alcoholic cirrhotic has a significant decrease in hepatic and serum zinc, which is consistent and persistent, is not correlated with renal function but correlates to some degree with a decrease in serum albumin and the general severity of the disease process, (3) enzymatic or metabolic dysfunction specifically related to zinc deficiency is possible but as yet unproven.

RESULTS

In an attempt to clarify some of these observations several further studies have been performed in our laboratory.

Eighteen cirrhotic patients having a long history of alcoholism, hepatic cirrhosis on liver biopsy, normal renal function and decreased serum zinc values were studied. Normal serum zinc is 94 ± 11 mcg/100 ml (S.D.) in our laboratory. The patients studied had a mean value of 45 mcg/100 ml and a range of 22 to 66 mcg/100 ml. The serum content of copper, magnesium, calcium and iron was also measured to evaluate the possible changes in other divalent cations. Normal values for serum copper, iron and calcium are 70 to 140 mcg/100 ml, 75 to 175 mcg/100 ml and 9 to 11 mg/100 ml respectively in this laboratory. The normal plasma magnesium is 1.92 ± 0.16 mg/100 ml (S.D.). The data regarding zinc, calcium and magnesium appear in Table 9-I. These cations were decreased 100 percent, 76 percent and 28 percent respectively in the serum of the 18 patients

TABLE 9-I

DECREASE IN SERUM ZINC, CALCIUM AND
MAGNESIUM IN 18 CIRRHOTIC PATIENTS

	% Decrease	
Zinc	*Calcium*	*Magnesium*
100	76	28

studied. The decreased serum zinc was significant; however, it should be pointed out that selection of subjects was biased since low serum zinc was necessary for inclusion in this study. Copper and iron were abnormal in 11 and 22 percent of the patients but with each cation the abnormalities were equally divided between those greater than normal and those less than normal. Serum cholesterol, triglycerides and free fatty acid were also measured, wide variations were noted in each without a positive correlation with any of the other determinations. The urinary cation excretion in these patients is shown in Table 9-II. As expected the majority of the cirrhotics

TABLE 9-II

PERCENT URINARY ZINC, CALCIUM AND MAGNESIUM
IN 18 CIRRHOTIC PATIENTS

Variation	*Zinc*	*Calcium*	*Magnesium*
% elevated	76	28	17
% decreased	0	0	17

had urinary zinc excretion greater than 700 mcg/24 hr, the upper limit of normality in this laboratory. Urinary magnesium excretion (normal 30-140 mg/24 hr) was decreased in 3 patients and elevated in 3 patients. The calcium excretion was greater than 150 mg/24 hr in 6 patients.

In Table 9-III the serum protein values in this group of patients are

TABLE 9-III

PERCENT NORMAL SERUM PROTEIN CONTENT
IN 18 CIRRHOTIC PATIENTS

Alb	α1	α2	β	γ
76	17	17	17	76

shown. Depression of serum albumin (less than 3.5 gm/100 ml occurred in 76 percent depression of alpha$_1$ (less than 0.2 g/100 ml), alpha$_2$ (less than 0.5 g/100 ml and beta globulin (less than 0.6) each occurred in 3 patients. The majority (76 percent) showed elevation of the gamma globulin (above 1.7 gm/100 ml). Low serum zinc and increased zincuria were more frequent in patients with low albumin and high gamma globulin. The low calcium values were more frequently encountered in patients with low serum albumin. Positive correlations between the other serum protein fractions and the trace metals measured were not evident.

To evaluate the efficacy of zinc sulfate as a therapeutic agent zinc sulfate in the dosage of 100 mg bid was given to five cirrhotic patients for a period of two weeks. There was an increase in serum zinc values in each case and a simultaneous diminution in urinary zinc in 3 of the 5 patients. Serum transferrin, which is purported to measure protein synthesis,[16] was increased in 3 of the 5 patients. These data are shown in Table 9-IV.

TABLE 9-IV

RESULTS OF 14 DAYS ZINC SULFATE THERAPY

(200 mg/day)

Patient	Serum Zinc mcg/100 ml	Serum Transferrin mg/100 ml	Urine Zinc mcg/24 hr
H	44	50	1660
H + ZnSO$_4$	70	200	2630
J	64	200	1740
J + ZnSO$_4$	109	200	800
Ho	48	80	2124
Ho + ZnSO$_4$	67	110	2270
B	81	200	620
B + ZnSO$_4$	95	200	320
R	76	110	4231
R + ZnSO$_4$	100	200	2800

A survey of 25 noncirrhotic patients studied for steatorrhea by means of a 72 hour stool collection was made to evaluate actual fecal loss of zinc in normal subjects and in patients with steatorrhea. These results appear in Table 9-V and they suggest that there is increased zinc excretion with steatorrhea (a mean of 7.08 mg zinc/24 hours in the stool of patients without steatorrhea as opposed to 10.9 mg zinc/24 hr in patients with steatorhea). The small number and wide variations noted preclude any statistical validation of this suggestion.

TABLE 9-V

RELATION OF FECAL ZINC EXCRETION TO STEATORRHEA
IN NON-CIRRHOTIC PATIENTS°

Patients without Steatorrhea	Fat Excretion gm/24 hr	Zinc Excretion mg/24 hr
13	5	7.08
		(1.80-15.75)
Patients with Steatorrhea		
12	19.6	10.9
	(10.5-32)	(3.8-29.9)

°Values shown are means. Values in parentheses represent the range of the values obtained.

DISCUSSION

During the course of measurements of serum cations and their urinary excretion in the cirrhotic patient, the abnormality of decreased serum zinc, calcium and magnesium were observed. Both calcium and zinc showed some relation to decreased serum albumin. Magnesium did not. It is noteworthy that the patient with decreased serum magnesium continued to excrete significant amounts of magnesium in the urine. As shown by Shils this is in distinct contrast to the decrease in magnesium excretion noted in experimental magnesium deficiency.[15] The same type of phenomenon appears true of zinc. In neither case is the mechanism clear. Excessive excretion of magnesium is not necessarily associated with excessive excretion of zinc and vice versa. The comparison of serum zinc levels with protein levels shows a fairly consistent association between low serum zinc and low serum albumin and high gamma globulin. The failure of uniform correlation, however, indicates the presence of other determinants, as yet unrecognized.

In the study of zinc sulfate as a therapeutic agent the measurement of transferrin was used as an indicator of protein synthesis since it has been described as a sensitive indicator of such anabolic activity in Kwashiorkor.[16]

In general, after 14 days of therapy, elevation of serum zinc levels occurred while a decrease of urine zinc excretion and an elevation of transferrin occurred in 3 of 5 cases. These findings suggest that zinc sulfate might be of value as a therapeutic agent. However, similar changes have been noted in cirrhotics eating a full diet without zinc supplementation. Whether this could be related to dietary content of zinc is a moot point. Since the fecal route accounts for the major amount of zinc excretion per day a positive relation was not unexpected in patients with steatorrhea. Although the data are inconclusive, they suggest that a positive relation with steatorrhea does exist.

SUMMARY

The new data presented indicate that again abnormalities of zinc occur in alcoholic cirrhotic patients. The association of low serum zinc values and increased urinary excretion occurs frequently. Serum protein factors, especially low serum albumin, appear to be an important, but not the sole, factor in the low serum zinc levels. Steatorrhea which is known to exist frequently in cirrhotics, may play a significant role in development of zinc deficiency. Treatment with zinc sulfate appears promising with regard to restoration of body stores of zinc.

REFERENCES

1. Sullivan, J. F., and Lankford, H. G.: Zinc metabolism and chronic alcoholism, *Am J Clin Nutr, 17:*57, 1965.
2. Sullivan, J. F.: Renal clearance of zinc in acute and chronic alcoholism. *J Lab Clin Med, 64:*1008, 1964.
3. Boyett, J. D., and Sullivan, J. F.: Distribution of protein-bound zinc in normal and cirrhotic serum. *Metabolism, 19:*148, 1970.
4. Stiles, W.: *Trace Elements in Plants and Animals.* New York, Macmillan, 1948.
5. Prasad, A. S., Oberleas, D., Wolf, P., and Horwitz, J. P.: Studies on zinc deficiency: Changes in trace elements and enzyme activities in tissues of zinc-deficient rats. *J Clin Invest, 46:*549, 1967.
6. Pories, W. J., Henzel, J. H., Rob, C. G., and Strain, W. H.: Acceleration of wound healing in man with zinc sulphate given by mouth. *Lancet, i:*121, 1967.
7. Vallee, B. L., Wacker, W. E. C., Bartholomay, A. F., and Robin, E. D.: Zinc metabolism in hepatic dysfunction. I. Serum zinc concentrations in Laennec's cirrhosis and their validation by sequential analysis. *N Engl J Med, 225:*403, 1956.
8. Sullivan, J. F., and Lankford, H. G.: Urinary excretion of zinc in alcoholism and postalcoholic cirrhosis. *Am J Clin Nutr, 10:*153, 1962.
9. Sullivan, J. F.: The relation of zincuria to water and electrolyte excretion in patients with hepatic cirrhosis. *Gastroenterology, 42:*439, 1962.
10. Sullivan, J. F.: Effect of alcohol on urinary zinc excretion. *Quart J Stud Alcohol, 23:*216, 1962.
11. Sullivan, J. F., and Lankford, H. G.: Incidence and duration of increased urinary zinc in chronic alcoholism. *Am J Clin Nutr, 17:*57, 1965.
12. Boyett, J. D., and Sullivan, J. F.: Zinc and collagen content of cirrhotic liver. *Am J Dig Dis, 15:*797, 1970.
13. Sullivan, J. F., and Heaney, R. P.: Zinc metabolism in alcoholic liver disease. *Am J Clin Nutr, 23:*170, 1970.
14. Sullivan, J. F., O'Grady, J., and Lankford, H. G.: The zinc content of pancreatic secretion. *Gastroenterology, 48:*438, 1965.
15. Shils, M. E.: Experimental human magnesium depletion. *Am J Clin Nutr, 15:*133, 1964.
16. McFarlane, H., Adcock, K. J., Cooke, A., Ogbeide, M. I., Adeslima, H., Taylor, G. O., Reddy, S., Gurney, J. M., and Mordie, J. A.: Biochemical assessment of protein-calorie malnutrition. *Lancet, i:*392, 1969.

Chapter 10

DWARFISM AND DELAYED SEXUAL MATURATION CAUSED BY ZINC DEFICIENCY*

HOSSAIN A. RONAGHY

∽∽

A BOUT TEN YEARS AGO the clinical features of nutritional dwarfism were reported from Iran.[1] The features were growth retardation, absent sexual development, iron deficiency anemia, and geophagia. Growth retardation is shown to be a feature of zinc deficiency in animals and this led Prasad et al.[1] to think that zinc deficiency may be the cause of growth failure in man. Two years later biochemical abnormalities of zinc metabolism in a group of dwarfs were demonstrated.[2] A zinc supplementation program was carried out in Egypt in 22 nutritional dwarfs during 1961 to 1963.[3] This data suggested a beneficial effect of zinc on growth and sexual development. The present study was undertaken to see the effect of zinc on a group of patients under careful controlled study.

MATERIALS AND METHODS

Nutritional dwarfism is fairly common in Iran's villages. With the cooperation of Iranian Army Induction Centers an excellent source of cases became available. Since all males are called up for the draft at ages 19 to 20 and since the nutritional dwarfs were always rejected, it has been possible to identify 186 male cases from the induction center in Shiraz, all of about the same age. Dwarfs representing the syndrome described above, who also had other chronic organic disease, were excluded from consideration for the study. Such diseases included liver cirrhosis, nephritis, heart disease, urolithiasis with pyelonephritis and malabsorption associated with diarrhea and steatorrhea. From the rest, those willing to undergo a long period of observation were admitted to the Nemazee Hospital research ward where they received a well balanced diet with ample animal protein. After a two or three week stay for clinical and laboratory examinations, they were transferred to a nearby house, or annex, where 12 could be accommodated at a time, receiving the same hospital diet. Although diets were not analyzed, similar diets have been reported to contain from 27 to 31 mg of zinc, of which about 10 percent is reported to be absorbed.[4,5] Suitable supervision, entertainment, and occupational therapy were provided. They stayed in the annex for

*Supported by Contract No. CCD-69-53 between the University of Pennsylvania and the Department of Health, Education and Welfare, Washington, D. C.

119

six months to one year. Twenty cases were studied. Of these, 8 were observed for 12 months, 3 for 9 months and 9 for 6 months.

Two of the 20 dwarfs so studied were females, 1 of whom was found in a village, the other having been admitted to the hospital for malnutrition. They were aged 19 and 20 respectively and were transferred, after hospital studies, to the home of the author where they lived during the study, one for six months, the other for one year.

The dwarfs were divided into three treatment groups. Group I received a well balanced hospital diet plus a placebo capsule from the start. Group II received the hospital diet plus one capsule daily of 120 mg zinc sulfate from the start. This was $ZnSO_4.7H_2O$, containing 27 mg of elemental zinc. Group III received hospital diet plus placebo capsule for six months at which time the zinc sulfate capsule was substituted for the placebo. Selection of subjects for Groups I and II was by the method of lottery with replacements. The three members of Group III were drawn from Group I at the end of six months. The capsules were given seven days a week between the noon and evening meals by an attendant who assured that they were swallowed. A physician or a senior medical student supervised the program.

Iron doses of 100 mg of ferrous fumarate was given once daily only to those dwarfs whose hemoglobin on admission was 7.0 gm percent or less (four in all). The iron used was found to contain a negligible amount of contaminating zinc. Each three months the subjects were transferred back to the hospital for a few days for clinical and laboratory tests.

RESULTS

Pertinent clinical findings on admission to the hospital are shown in Table 10-I. They were moderately anemic. Serum proteins were essentially normal.

Analysis of the growth increment (height increase) for the 20 patients studied is shown in Figure 10-1. Group I were given only a well-balanced diet for six months. Group II were given the same diet plus one capsule daily which contained 120 mg of zinc sulfate for the same six months. Those receiving diet alone increased by an average of 3.6 cm in height.

TABLE 10-I

TREATMENT GROUPS

Group I	Well-balanced (hospital) diet, plus placebo capsule daily.
Group II	Well-balanced (hospital) diet, plus 120 mg $ZnSO_4·7H_2O$ in capsule daily, from the start (27 mg elemental zinc).
Group III	Well-balanced (hospital) diet, plus placebo capsule daily for six months followed by diet plus zinc capsule daily.

TABLE 10-II

CLINICAL FINDINGS ON ADMISSION TO HOSPITAL OF
NUTRITIONAL DWARFS

	Height (cm)	Weight (kg)	Hemoglobin (gm%)	Serum Protein (gm%)	Serum Albumin (gm%)	Serum Iron mcg/100 ml	Plasma Zinc mcg/100 ml
Mean	141	35	10.3	7.06	3.53	45	48
S.D.	8	5	4.0	0.69	0.40	23	17
Range	130-150	24-44	4.3-16.2	5.8-8.2	2.8-4.1	12-13	29-83
Normal Values	174.5°	61°	13-16†	6.3-7.9†	3.2-7.9†	3.2-5.0†	95±12§

°W. E. Nelson, *Pediatrics*, 9th ed., Philadelphia (W. B. Saunders Co., 1969), page 47.
†Values obtained in control subjects by research laboratory, Nemazee Hospital.
‡C. A. Finch, et al. "Ferrokinetics in Man," *Medicine*, 49:17-53, 1970.
§J. A. Halsted and J. C. Smith, "Plasma Zinc in Health and Disease," *Lancet* i, 322, 1970.

TABLE 10-III

PLASMA ZINC CONCENTRATION ON ADMISSION AND AFTER
SIX MONTHS OF THERAPY

(mcg/100 ml)

	Group I		Group II	
	On Admission	Six Months	On Admission	Six Months
Mean ± S.D.	51 ± 18	75 ± 9	42 ± 15	77 ± 9
Range	29-83	65-93	29-70	72-90
No. of Subjects	11	8	6	4

(Normal concentration in Iranian medical students was 95 ± 12)

Those receiving zinc sulfate daily in addition to the diet grew an average of 11.8 cm. These differences are statistically significant ($p < 0.01$).

During the following six months cases 1, 2, 3, and 7 continued to receive the diet without supplementary zinc therapy. Cases 8, 9, and 10 had one zinc capsule (120 mg zinc sulfate) added to their regimen (these constituted Group III). During this second six month period those continuing on the diet alone increased 2.4 cm in height whereas cases 8, 9, and 10, who were given the zinc sulfate daily in addition, increased 8.7 cm. The differences in these two groups were also highly significant statistically ($p < 0.001$).

Sexual development was evaluated by noting the first sign of sexual function, i.e. nocturnal emission in the male and first menstrual period in the two females of the group. Using these end points in numbers of weeks following admission to the hospital the results are shown in Figure 10-2. It can be seen that there was a strikingly longer period of time among those subjects who received a well balanced diet alone, in comparison with those who received zinc sulfate daily in addition, before sexual function occurred. The time interval before emission or menstruation was 33 weeks

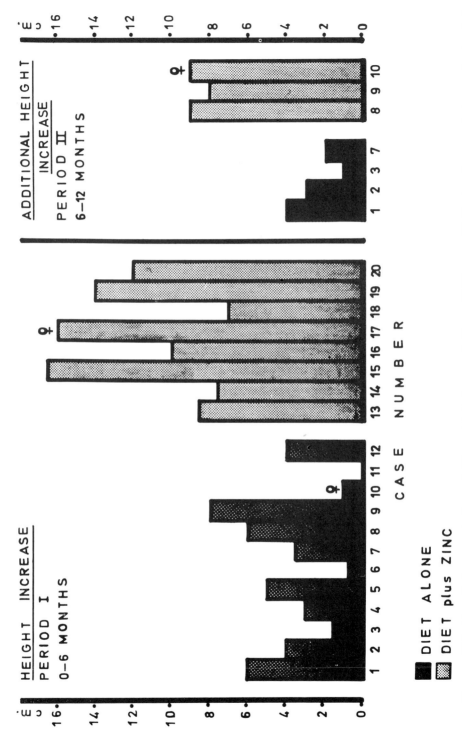

FIGURE 10-1. Growth Increment. Cases 1-12 constituted group I; Cases 13-20 group II. During the second six months (period II) Cases 1, 2, 3 and 7 remained in group I; Cases 4, 5, 6 and 11 having left the study and 8, 9 and 10 constituted group III.

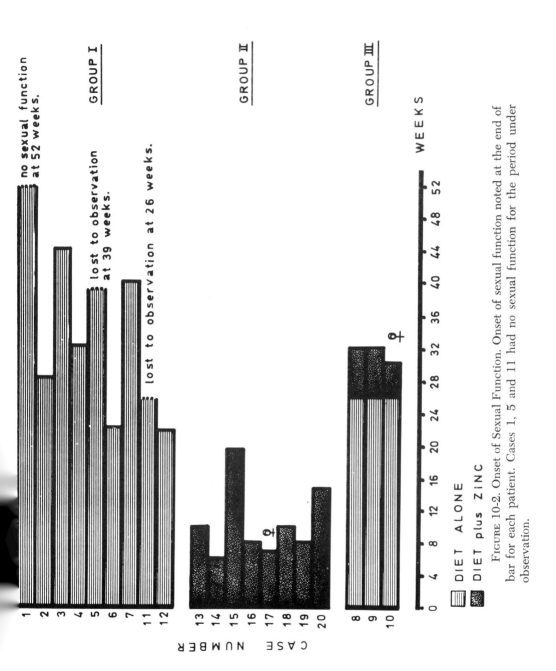

FIGURE 10-2. Onset of Sexual Function. Onset of sexual function noted at the end of bar for each patient. Cases 1, 5 and 11 had no sexual function for the period under observation.

in those receiving a well balanced diet alone, and 10.5 weeks in those who received zinc sulfate daily in addition. These differences are statistically highly significant ($p < 0.001$).

In case 1 no sexual function occurred after 52 weeks of treatment with diet alone. Case 5 was lost to observation at 39 weeks and case 11 at 26 weeks also with no sexual function occurring in either. If these three cases are included in the statistical analysis as if they had developed sexual function at or shortly after the times when they left the study the statistical differences are still highly significant ($p < 0.001$).

The three subjects in Group III who received the diet alone for six months had no evidence of sexual function up to that time. They were then given zinc sulfate daily and sexual function promptly occurred within 4, 6 and 6 weeks respectively.

It thus appears that a well balanced nutritious diet which contains from 25 to 30 mg of zinc resulted in slow but gradual growth, and eventual onset of sexual function. However, if 120 mg of zinc sulfate was given each day (27 mg of elemental zinc) growth was greatly enhanced and the onset of sexual function was greatly hastened.

Special attention was paid to the effect of therapy, i.e. either diet alone, or diet plus zinc sulfate, on appetite and food intake. It was noted that all subjects enjoyed the diet and had an ample intake of it. Although it was not possible under conditions of the study to make mathematical calculations of nutrient and caloric intake, observation indicated that those receiving zinc capsules had a better appetite and greater intake of food.

The subjects whose sexual development had not yet occurred were more cooperative and docile than after sexual function took place. Then they complained more, asked to be discharged and in a few cases (Nos. 4 and 6), left against advice.

The syndrome is entirely reversible with a good diet.[6] One subject upon attaining normal growth and sexual development was re-drafted and served in the army.

DISCUSSION

Evidence obtained from this study and that from the earlier Egyptian studies makes it clear that zinc may be a limiting essential nutrient in determining both growth and onset of puberty in man. In planning food supplementation programs in underdeveloped countries, such as adding lysine to wheat, this factor might profitably be considered.

The syndrome as described from Iran 10 years ago comprised eleven dwarfs, whose degree of anemia and thus weakness and other debilitating factors, were considerably more severe than the 20 subjects comprising the present report. The reason for this is probably not so much that rural conditions respecting food supplies may have improved but that the present subjects were selected from rejections of an army induction center (except the two females), whereas in the first group all had come to the hospital because they were too weak to survive without seeking medical attention. A follow-up study of the original 1960 group showed that the patients remained well, developing normally provided they avoided clay-eating and maintained a regular intake of animal protein. If they reverted to the old dietary pattern and practiced geophagia, relapse occurred.[6]

A study which was reported from Iran in 1968 indicated that zinc supplementation was effective in hastening sexual development in growth-retarded but outwardly healthy schoolboys with delayed puberty and low plasma zinc levels.[7] These observations indicate that a spectrum of zinc deficiency may occur, with "full-blown" dwarfism as defined by the features of this syndrome at one end, and but moderate growth retardation with late puberty at the other. The mild end of the spectrum may be very widespread in underdeveloped areas of the world where the chief food supplies are of cereal origin with high phytate content and thus probably lesser amounts of available zinc. One may rightly ask whether this is important from individual or public health viewpoints. Only further study can answer such a question but there are suggestions that zinc deficiency may lead to greater susceptibility to infection.[8] Doubtless other subtle signs of subnormal health may be traced to mild zinc deficiency when it is studied more extensively and when nutritionally-oriented physicians become more attuned to this possibility.

SUMMARY

Investigation in depth in man of the problem of mineral availability related to the role of complexants as well as to interrelationships of zinc with other metals is urgently called for. Obviously much of this research can be pursued most effectively where the clinical problems lie. Unfortunately, this is where facilities and adequate numbers of trained personnel for research are usually scarce. In addition to more detailed investigations of etiologic factors in zinc deficiency, knowledge of the results, especially endocrine dysfunction is needed.

A low plasma zinc concentration seems to be the rule among Iranian villagers.[8] The meaning of this is not entirely clear. A low plasma zinc level can only be considered suggestive and not diagnostic of zinc deficiency. The only certain criterion for zinc deficiency is a clinical response to administration of zinc under controlled conditions, as the author has attempted to accomplish in this investigation.

Geophagia must be considered as a possibly important factor in view of the fact that every subject in this investigation and all but one of the originally reported eleven Iranian dwarfs admitted to taking large amounts of clay. We believe that this may explain the fact that nutritional dwarfism is not clustered geographically and that with occasional exceptions only one member of the family was affected even though all ate the same diet. In Turkey the problem of geophagia has been studied by Minnich et al. who found that clay fed to both normal and iron deficient subjects inhibited the absorption of radioactive iron.[9] On the other hand Prasad and his co-workers did not mention that the Egyptian dwarfs admitted to the practice of geophagia.[3] The problem of geophagia obviously requires further careful investigation.

The patients with growth and sexual retardation caused by zinc deficiency approached normal growth and sexual development when they were provided with a nutritious, well balanced diet which included animal protein. The same revision toward normality occurs in nutritional iron deficiency when a well balanced diet is given. However, administration of an inorganic zinc salt in zinc deficiency and an iron salt in iron deficiency results in more rapid reversions toward normality in both conditions.

REFERENCES

1. Halsted, J. A., and Prasad, A. S.: Syndrome of iron deficiency anemia, hepato-splenomegaly, hypogonadism, dwarfism and geophagia. *Tr Am Climatol Assoc,* 72:130, 1960.

2. Prasad, A. S., Halsted, J. A., and Nadimi, M.: Syndrome of iron deficiency anemia, hepatosplenomegaly, hypogonadism, dwarfism, and geophagia. *Am J Med, 31:* 532, 1961.

3. Prasad, A. S., Miale, A., Farid, Z., Sandstead, H. H., Schulert, A. R., and Darby, W. J.: Biochemical studies on dwarfism, hypogonadism and anemia. *Arch Intern Med, 111:*407, 1963.

4. McCance, R. A., and Widdowson, H. M.: The absorption and excretion of zinc. *Biochem J,* 36:692, 1942.

5. Osis, D., Royston, K., Samachson, J., and Spencer, H.: Atomic-absorption spectrophotometry in mineral and trace-element studies in man. *Dev Appl Spectroscopy,* 7a:227, 1969.

6. Ronaghy, H. A., Moe, P. G., and Halsted, J. A.: A six-year follow-up of Iranian patients with dwarfism, hypogonadism, and iron-deficiency anemia. *Am J Clin Nutr, 21:*709, 1968.

7. Ronaghy, H. A., Fox, M. R. S., Garn, S. M., Israel, H., Harp, A., Moe, P. G., and Halsted, J. A.: Controlled zinc supplementation for malnourished school boys: a pilot experiment. *Am J Clin Nutr, 22:*1279-1289, 1969.

8. Halsted, J. A., and Smith, J. C., Jr.: Plasma-zinc in health and disease. *Lancet i,* 322, 1970.

9. Minnich, V., Okguoklu, A., Tarcon, Y., Arcasoy, A., Chin, S., Yorukoglu, O., Renda, F., and Demirag, B.: Pica in Turkey, II. Effect of clay upon iron absorption. *Am J Clin Nutr, 21:*78, 1968.

DISCUSSION

Dr. Sandstead: Did you determine the amount of zinc in the hospital diet?
Dr. Ronaghy: Yes, we did. Dr. Reinhold found that the diet of the so-called villager contained about 15 mg of available zinc.
Dr. Prasad: I would like to start with Dr. Sandstead. I understand he has some interesting slides to show that zinc deficiency of this severe type is not only present in Iran and Egypt, but also in the United States.
Dr. Sandstead: Thank you Dr. Prasad. I thought I might show you this patient, particularly in view of the interesting observations on the effect of steatorrhea on zinc losses and with Dr. Ronaghy's really beautiful presentation. We have, on occasion, been asked if the same thing could occur in the United States, and, if it doesn't occur in the United States, why should we be worried about it because it is obviously an Iranian or Egyptian problem.

This patient is presently a junior in pharmacy school at Auburn University and he was kind enough to come back to the clinic this summer so I could follow him up. He is now 21 years old. He has extensive regional enteritis with involvement of the small intestine from the mid jejunum by x-ray to the distal ilium. When we first saw him he did not appear this healthy. He was having seven to ten bowel movements a day, he had a serum albumin of 1.5, a very low serum carotene and low Vitamin A. He was having frequent night sweats and fever and abdominal pain.

Now, if I can have the next slide I will show you how he looked when we first saw him. Over on the left is this young man at age 20. He was a sophomore in college at that time, so you get a feeling that he is rather a remarkable person in the first place to get this far with his education. He had the appearance of about a ten year old boy and he didn't tell anybody how old he was at school because he was embarrassed and they thought he was a child prodigy. He lived with his mother and he had the behavior of a ten or twelve year old. So we were asked to see him and he appeared to us to be similar to the patients we had seen in Egypt. He had been seen at Vanderbilt at age 12 and there had been no change in his height or sexual maturation since age 12. He was age 20 when he came.

We admitted him to the Clinical Research Center and we did some studies and started him on what we thought was a lot of zinc. We gave him 100 mg of zinc a day and things happened slowly over the next year. You can see, from January to December he did increase body hair—a little appeared on his genitalia. His personality changed from being rather passive to somebody who has his own opinions of the time. He developed acne and began to go through puberty and he grew about an inch and one-half during that year.

We admitted him to the hospital in December and he had an attack of abdominal pain and we thought the regional enteritis was back. Incidentally, during this interval on zinc his symptoms of regional enteritis completely abated. He stopped having fever, night sweats, abdominal pain—he was having one to two stools a day which we didn't understand at all and his serum albumin rose into the normal range and his carotene and vitamin A came up. Anyway, in the hospital he then had an attack of abdominal pain. We thought he was having regional enteritis again, started him on intermittent steroids and sent him home because he wanted to get back to school. The steroids didn't help so we discontinued them. We increased the zinc to 300 mg of zinc a day in divided doses and dramatic things happened. You can see that from December, this is how he looks in May. There was a rapid change in his genitalia. We readmitted him to the hospital at this time because he was having recurrent abdominal pain and at laparotomy what he had was a whole series of partial intestinal obstructions and so his mid jejunum was resected. He went home, still on zinc, and you can see how he looked at me. He was rather pleased and doing quite well. At this time, the week prior to his clinical visit, he had his first erection and nocturnal emission and he couldn't wait to tell me about this.

Anyway, if I can have the next slide, you will see how he looked in August. I assure you, he was a bit short, but he is a perfectly normal man now and I have asked him if he is going to get a girlfriend and he said he is looking around.

Dr. Prasad: I would like to invite the audience to participate in the discussion. Has anybody any question about any of the papers that were presented?

Dr. O'Dell: I would like to ask Dr. Ronaghy a question that has bothered me about the people in these villages. In the first place there must be adults there that have children and so this thing that you have observed must have been going on for centuries. How did they develop and do you see any problems with the adults? Have you ever looked at the adults in these villages? Do they have any problems and do they have large families and how did they develop sexually in the first place?

Dr. Ronaghy: Actually, we are very interested in that part of the question because we have a very rapid rate of population growth. One of the highest in the world—3 percent. Once you get to higher altitudes there are no problems. The village people don't have anything else to do except make babies and they have a very large number of children—5, 6, 7, 8, 10 children in the family. But the fact is that those stricken with the syndrome unanimously admit eating large amounts of clay. One of the constant features of this syndrome is geophagia. Some patients said that they take one pound of clay every day and this is amazing. We have demonstrated by x-ray that you see the clay in the abdomen. Not all of them get it. In a family of 7 or 8 maybe one would be afflicted and this is because he eats large amounts of clay. We do not know why.

Dr. Henkin: I would like to make just one comment that would relate to Dr. Ronaghy's experience about geophagia in his patients in Iran. Because of his discussions with me some years ago at the V.A. Hospital in Washington, I went to a number of villages, if you want to call them villages, in Virginia where there are many poor people who practice a kind of geophagia. They eat various and sundry things that we wouldn't consider edible such as charcoal from fires or clay and they seem to prefer that to almost anything else. When one tests their taste acuity, one finds gross alterations. They have hypogeusia. When one looks at their zinc levels in the serum such as it is, they are also somewhat abnormal. These people are not necessarily hypogonadal. This is analagous to a very curious situation in rats. When a rat is made hypogeusic, he will accept food and fluids normally rejected. In other words, a solution of hydrochloric acid or sodium chloride which is normally rejected is now accepted. The hypogeusia is shown by an acceptance of material or food you would normally reject. This may relate to the kind of geophagsia that you describe, especially as you told the story that it is quite common for the people in the villages to take clay and eat it up to the age of two and then by habit, the parents tend to drive that out of the children and the acceptance of this kind of behavior then might very well persist because the sensory phenomena are such that they don't reject it.

Dr. Prasad: I might mention that there is some evidence in the literature to suggest that geophagia might effect the iron balance adversely, but to my knowledge there isn't any evidence in the literature that it affects the zinc balance adversely. As a matter of fact, Doctors Smith and Halsted reported that the rat at least, is able to get some zinc from the clay to survive on a zinc deficient regime. So this is quite an interesting phenomenon and I do not know what exactly is doing.

Dr. Woosley: One thing that concerned me about the study you mention by Doctors Smith and Halsted was the only time they could get those results was after they had extracted the calcium from the clay and it was not normal clay which they fed to the animals. The high calcium content of the normal clay could inhibit zinc absorption and cause the zinc deficiency state seen in geophagia.

Dr. Prasad: Now is there anyone who can elaborate on this? I do not know anybody from Washington. Dr. Smith is not here.

Dr. Hsu: It was acid extracted to remove the excess calcium.

Dr. Prasad: I see. Well, Dr. Woosley, your point is well taken.

Chapter 11

ZINC METABOLISM AND HOMEOSTASIS–
SOME NEWER CONCEPTS

W. Jack Miller
AND
Paul E. Stake

A SEVERE ZINC DEFICIENCY causes numerous pathological changes, reduction or cessation of growth, general debility, lethargy, and increased susceptibility to infection in animals. However, specific mechanisms which are responsible have not been elucidated. This information, along with conflicting observations on zinc requirements, led us to a series of zinc metabolism studies in ruminants. In this presentation we have integrated these results with other knowledge on zinc metabolism in animals, giving special emphasis to important, newly discovered principles. Since space is limited, reference is made to more complete reviews for additional details and original citations.[1,2]

ABSORPTION

Zinc is absorbed from the small intestine, especially the proximal portions, by a two-step process; uptake by intestinal mucosa and transport to blood. Even though transfer to blood apparently is the rate limiting step, this process is quite rapid. In calves, peak blood levels occur within one hour after zinc reaches the duodenum.[3] Zinc transfer from blood to biologically more active tissues, including liver, is relatively fast, indicating rapid accumulation and turnover. Even so, some zinc in these tissues appears tightly bound, with a slow turnover rate. Accumulation and turnover rates are very slow in tissues such as muscle and bone, with peaks occurring several weeks after absorption and fair quantities remaining for years. Evidence suggests that zinc often may be transported from one protein to another in different tissues (i.e. intestinal mucosa to blood) as metallo-ligand complexes, the same ligand being associated with complexes of both proteins. The ligand's nature influences zinc metabolism.[1]

EXCRETION

Feces are the main zinc excretion route, including much of the endogenous zinc. Animals have fairly effective, but far from complete, homeostatic zinc control mechanisms, which function through changes in zinc absorption and endogenous excretion via feces. The percentage of dietary zinc absorbed varies widely and is influenced by dietary zinc level, growth rate, age, and many other factors.

DIETARY ZINC CONTENT

With ruminants, and possibly all species, the most important factor influencing absorption is dietary zinc content. As dietary zinc is decreased, the percentage absorbed increases and endogenous losses are reduced. At high dietary zinc levels, the absorption percentage is reduced and endogenous losses increase, with the effect on absorption having more influence on homeostasis. However, when dietary zinc decreases, smaller absolute quantities are absorbed and vice versa when high zinc diets are fed, resulting in only partial homeostasis.

Animals fed severely deficient diets do not mobilize adequate body zinc to meet their needs for even short periods and are very dependent on absorbed zinc. However, they do reuse zinc normally released from various tissues at other sites. Since several weeks are required, after a single dose of ^{65}Zn to peak in tissues such as red muscle, considerable reuse is strongly indicated. With low zinc diets, tissue release rates decrease, indicating lower mobilization from body stores.

With severe zinc deficiencies, moderate reductions occur in zinc content of some tissues, including plasma, pancreas, liver, kidney, bone, and hair. But with high dietary zinc, content in several of these tissues increases sharply, indicating less efficient homeostatic control in high zinc diets. Even so, the zinc level required for any toxicity is many times the requirement. Zinc content of red muscle and heart tissue change very little with low or high zinc diets, suggesting a specific number of zinc binding sites which hold it with great affinity. In contrast to the apparent homeostatic breakdown in some tissues with high zinc diets, the reverse occurs in milk zinc content. As dietary zinc increases, milk zinc increases at a decelerating rate and plateaus. Plasma zinc does not decelerate, suggesting that the mammary gland regulates milk zinc content.

Until very recently, animals were believed to absorb only small and relatively fixed percentages of dietary zinc. This is incorrect: many factors affect zinc absorption and metabolism. Most naturally occurring zinc deficiencies observed in farm animals have been associated with other dietary factors, causing reduced availability and absorption. Several plant protein sources contain substances which interfere with zinc absorption for monogastric animals. Numerous other dietary components have been shown to materially affect zinc metabolism, including calcium, cadmium, copper, and chelating agents.

As animals become older the percentage of dietary zinc absorbed decreases. In many, or most, situations this is not due to a reduced absorption ability but to effects of other factors on the homeostatic control mechanisms. We recently observed 55 percent absorption of ^{65}Zn in lactating dairy cows fed a low zinc (16 ppm) diet (unpublished data). Since these was no indication of even a borderline deficiency, this probably does not represent maximum absorptive ability.

An unusual zinc deficiency occurs in a small percentage of Dutch-Fresian calves (personal communication, J. Kroneman and A. J. H. Schotman, Veterinary Faculty, State University of Utrecht, The Netherlands). This very characteristic zinc deficiency is temporarily correctable by very high zinc levels. Available data and observations lead to the speculation that a simple recessive inheritance pattern results in animals with serious impairments in zinc absorption or metabolism.

SUMMARY

Though sometimes helpful in diagnosing a zinc deficiency for a particular animal, tissue zinc often is an unreliable index. Many factors apparently influence tissue zinc. Obviously a zinc shortage must exist in some tissues for deficiency effects to occur. However, considering that the first deficiency effects can be corrected by feeding an amount of zinc which is less than 1 percent of that in the body, it appears that total tissue zinc may not be a good indicator. Rather, it seems that adequate labile zinc is crucial. Thus it appears important to study not only zinc metabolism in individual tissues, but also different fractions within tissues.

REFERENCES

1. Miller, W. J.: Zinc metabolism in farm animals. Proc. of a panel, *Mineral studies with isotopes in domestic animals,* International Atomic Energy Agency, Vienna. P. 23-41, 1971.
2. Miller, W. J.: Zinc nutrition of cattle: a review. *J Dairy Sci,* 53:1123, 1970.
3. Pate, F. M., Miller, W. J., Blackmon, D. M., and Gentry, R. P.: ^{65}Zn absorption rate following single duodenal dosing in calves fed zinc-deficient or control diets. *J Nutr, 100:*1259, 1970.

Chapter 12

PANEL DISCUSSION FOR SECTION B
HUMAN ZINC DEFICIENCY

Moderator: ANANDA S. PRASAD

Panelists: WALTER MERTZ, HOSSAIN RONAGHY, HERTA SPENCER, AND
JAMES F. SULLIVAN

Discussants: LUECKE, PETERING, KETTERING AND OTHERS.

Dr. Petering: Well, we have carried out a number of experiments with zinc being interested in what the environmental chemicals and other things that our changing environment may have on zinc metabolism and we had been attracted to Dr. Strain's work on the relationship of hair zinc and dwarfs and the effect of giving zinc to these patients as well as his work with medical students. But the problem we needed to know was what was the effect of age on hair zinc in the general population— whether there were any sex effects. Now, to follow Dr. Luecke's comments, we have also looked at hair zinc in rats fed approximately these same intakes and find that hair zinc actually does reflect the serum zinc and the intake of zinc.

The top regression lines are the ones we want. You see that the zinc concentration does vary with age, and I think this is of interest in view of the things that were mentioned previously about zinc in children. We do find that in the young, middle class children that there is a very low zinc level, approximately 100 ppm between the age of 1 and 2 years in the hair, these are parts per million and this goes up to a change at approximately 12 years of age and then there is a slow decrease. Now, this is of considerable interest because a few patients in the General Hospital—Cincinnati—who are indigent and obviously undernourished and have other problems all fell below 100 ppm, and some, as age advanced to 8 years, had dropped down to 60 ppm. We would consider that 100 ppm is a good place to begin to look for any changes that might be occurring or related to undernutrition. We didn't have the youngsters in the female group, but in the males in the age from 10 years on, the top line shows you the fact that the males and females in that age group were superimposable. There was no difference. So, in the age group beyond puberty, approximately, there is no sex effect in our studies with respect to hair zinc. I think this is a fortunate thing because you can see in copper, there is a difference in sex. However, our data would indicate that if you were to use hair, which I think should be used, and looked at in these surveys, particularly when you are looking for nutritional surveys and en-

vironmental surveys as we are, you must be careful to take a reasonably
narrow age group, because there can be changes which we don't understand. Whether this is nutritional, whether this is aging, or whether this is
the effect of the environment, these are some of the things that we are
interested in doing.

We have taken additional populations. We had a project with several
of our colleagues in Japan and some medical students from Tokyo University; a group of girls 17 and 18 from an academy in Cincinnati, medical
students and nurses, were all checked and these ages ran from 17 to 23
and they fell very closely to this general trend that we have, they were on
this side of this age group and they fell pretty closely into that line,
showing that again, that this may be an important relationship, to keep
in mind and that I do believe that hair offers a possibility of getting at
some surveys with respect to zinc in the population that isn't greatly
effected by sex in the post-puberty period, may not be in the below
either, because we don't have enough information on the girls, but that
there is an age relationship here. This age relationship may have considerable metabolic significance.

Dr. Spencer: Dr. Prasad, I would just like to make a remark to Dr. Luecke's
presentation. Dr. Luecke has shown very beautifully that the concentrations of zinc in the serum indirectly increased when zinc was given and
apparently in man we are faced with a much more complex situation
because the zinc plasma level in our own studies does not reflect the zinc
intake. One has to be careful in interpretation. When you give zinc to a
zinc depleted patient actually the plasma level decreases instead of increasing, which we interpret as the zinc being pulled into the tissues
and not circulating in the plasma. I wonder what sort of remark you
can make on this subject. Also, I would like to mention that we have
some preliminary indication that we get better retention of zinc if there
is protein in the diet, but if we add the zinc to just the low protein diet
alone, the retention is not so good.

Dr. Prasad: Where do you think the zinc is coming from in the plasma
and why is it that in other stress situations the plasma zinc drops so
quickly?

Dr. Spencer: I believe it has something to do with weight loss and with
tissue catabolism and the release of the zinc from the tissues.

Dr. Prasad: I would expect a similar phenomenon with a patient who has
severe pneumonia who drops his zinc level from 100 to 70.

Dr. Spencer: Well, there you have another complicating problem, the infection.

Dr. Luecke: Remember these are young growing rats and I think adults would probably be an entirely different situation. As to what happens in your case, I honestly don't know of an explanation.

Dr. Prasad: I would like to make a few comments about a subject which was brought up earlier. I know of a report from Turkey in which zinc-deficient dwarfs have been described similar to those Dr. Ronaghy presented. There have been reports from Portugal and from Morocco, and I was told by a good friend of mine from Brazil that ever since he saw our paper in the American Journal of Medicine, he sees them every day. But to our knowledge, no studies have been done in detail.

Dr. Petering: There is another factor here that I think needs to be considered. From our studies, we know that cadmium is accumulating in the population and when you starve a patient, I wonder what you do to the mobilization of any cadmium that is around in its relationship to the zinc. We know that in the rat, if you give cadmium, you alter the zinc metabolism rather strikingly. You could alter what is happening to the serum zinc as well as tissue levels of zinc by cadmium. On the contrary, if you are giving low levels of cadmium, you can protect the animal by giving zinc and sometimes you have to go beyond the physiologic range to do this.

Dr. Sandstead: Regarding your question of plasma levels of zinc in starvation versus infection. At the Western Hemisphere Congress on Nutrition, it was reported that in infection it appears that the zinc moves from the plasma to the liver and then during the period when the patient is recovering it leaves the liver and is excreted in the urine. So the situation with infection is entirely different than in starvation. There is some other undefined physiological phenomena happening to zinc distribution in infection.

Dr. Husain: We have been estimating the plasma zinc and skin zinc in dermatological conditions. We have found that in chronic debilitation, like pustular psoriasis, there is a marked decrease in plasma zinc. One particular patient I am going to discuss later was a case of chronic leg ulcers and we treated him with oral zinc sulfate. Later on, about three weeks after the treatment he went into a renal failure. It had nothing to do with the zinc therapy, but the plasma zinc fell down and the fecal zinc went up. He was excreting more zinc in the feces as compared to the urine, and I believe the zinc is most probably coming from the liver.

Dr. Sable: Dr. John Wood of the University of Illinois has been doing some beautiful work on still another metal, mercury. He's got some very lovely work on the formation of mono and dimethyl mercury in sludge, and I wonder if cadmium might somehow be exerting its effect because you get mono or dimethyl cadmium. Is that a possibility?

Dr. Petering: No. The stability of the methyl cadmiums is very, very low in an aqueous medium. So you have to have a nonaqueous medium in order to have stability. They can be made and they are used in chemical synthetic work, but they are highly unlikely to be of any importance in a biological system.

Concluding Remarks

Dr. Prasad: I would like to say just a couple of words about a few things, to which we have not addressed ourselves in this meeting and that is to ask "what is the effect of marginal deficiency on the maternal and fetal nutrition?" I think it is a very important point and about which we know so little at this time. The main difficulty is how do we make a diagnosis of marginal deficiency and one approach would be to find out some of the biochemical functions which we might determine under very carefully controlled conditions which we could relate to zinc.

To me, this is a crucial issue. There is no problem with the severe deficiency state, as you have seen in Iran and Egypt. It is particularly gratifying, however, that here are patients who have been deficient for 18 and 20 years and are completely reversible. Nothing is more gratifying to a physician than to see this situation.

SECTION C

Chapter 13

ZINC SULFATE THERAPY IN SURGICAL PATIENTS

WALTER J. PORIES

AND

WILLIAM H. STRAIN

Z INC IS AN ESSENTIAL FACTOR in wound healing. We[1] first suggested this essentiality in 1953 after observing that wounded and burned rats, which were maintained on diets accidentally enriched with zinc, healed more rapidly than animals fed control diets. Since this serendipitous result, the requirement of zinc for wound healing has been amply confirmed in many other animal and human studies. Zinc therapy now must be considered for zinc-deficient surgical patients, for burn patients, and for patients with other abnormal trace element levels. The mechanisms of the action of zinc are not known, but evidently the fundamental processes of protein synthesis are stimulated by this element.

INVESTIGATIONS IN ANIMALS

Rats

In addition to demonstrating the beneficial effects of dietary zinc on wound healing, our original investigations[1,2] showed that the effect of zinc medication is slow and is most evident during epithelization. Healing was studied in a series of eleven experiments using open standard wounds inflicted on young and old rats of both sexes. On standard commercial diets, young female rats healed within 30 days, young male and old female rats within 45 days, and old males required as many as 115 days. The addition of zinc salts to the diets accelerated the healing of old males as much as 40 percent, and of young males and old females up to 20 percent. Our studies also showed that the effect of the zinc supplement was to stimulate epithelization and that this stimulation was not evident before 15 days. In retrospect, it is probable that the diets used were slightly zinc deficient, and that with today's routinely enriched feeds, the observation would not have been made. Figure 13-1 illustrates our healing studies with rats.

Hamsters

Mesrobian and Shklar[3] extended these studies on epithelization by measuring the effect of zinc sulfate therapy on healing of gingival wounds in Syrian hamsters. The gingiva offered an excellent model because these

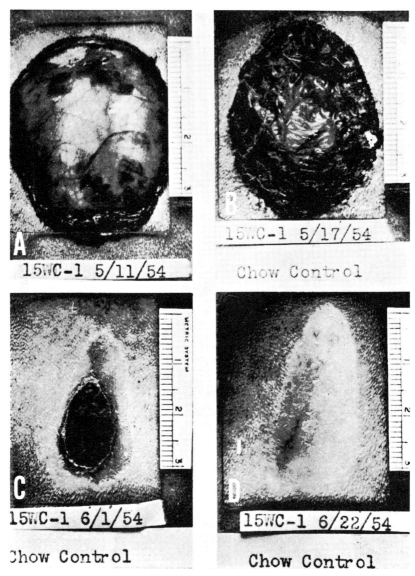

FIGURE 13-1. The healing of excised wounds of rats has characteristic phases as follows: (A) the original wound obtained by excising skin immediately dilates from the original area of 7.07 cm² to 10.5 cm²; (B) during the next six days, the wound contracts to the original size with the formation of a dark scab; (C) as healing continues, the scab peels off and a new one forms along with scar tissue; and (D) the wound is healed when no more scab forms. Healing is slower in male than in female rats, and the area of scar tissue is larger and more oval in the male. Healing time is much longer in old males than young males or old females. Young females heal very rapidly.

tissues have a much greater proportion of epithelium to collagen than skin and because they heal much more rapidly. They found that epithelization was better 3 days after wounding in the zinc supplemented hamsters, with greater tissue continuity and a less fragmented appearance. The difference between the medicated and control groups was less at one week, and both groups were fully healed at two weeks. Histologic examination confirmed that the zinc supplemented hamsters showed better epithelization with more mature granulation tissue, more regular connective tissue organization, less edema, less severe inflammatory infiltration, and fewer necrotic areas in the gingiva.

Domestic Animals

The epithelium is extremely sensitive to zinc deficiency. Miller's[4] enumeration of the cutaneous effects of zinc deficiency in cattle is classic: "Dry scaly skin . . . thickening of the skin around the nostrils . . . horny overgrowth of the mucosa . . . alopecia . . . red, scabby and wrinkled scrotal skin . . . tender, easily injured, and often raw and bleeding skin . . . wounds heal slowly, if at all." Similar symptoms have been observed in zinc deficient poultry and swine. When Tucker and Salmon[5] discovered that zinc deficiency was the cause of this troublesome skin disease of swine, they set the stage for the explosive growth of research on zinc metabolism. In addition, study of parakeratosis in swine furnished the impetus for zinc enrichment of commercial rations for monogastric domestic animals.

Miller[6] has confirmed that adequate zinc stores are needed for normal wound repair in animals. He demonstrated that zinc deficient cattle heal poorly and develop a halo of parakeratosis about the healing site, and that the addition of zinc to the feed produced rapid normal healing. As might be expected, the addition of excess zinc to a zinc-sufficient diet produced no acceleration of healing.

Failure to heal wounds is not the only defect in severely zinc-deficient calves. They are stunted, lethargic, and highly susceptible to nonspecific secondary infections which often result in death.[7,8,9,10] The oral mucosa of these calves is particulary liable to a rapid bacterial increase, but the condition is easily corrected by supplementary dietary zinc.[4,9,10] Whether the susceptibility is due to loss of epithelial continuity and bacterial invasion or to the production of ineffective white blood cells remains unknown.

Time Factors

Although zinc rapidly migrates into healing tissues, as shown by zinc-65 uptake studies in incised wounds of rats,[12] the effects of zinc medication

are slow and a difference in the rate of cutaneous healing between medicated and control animals is usually not apparent before 12 to 15 days.
Sandstead and Shepard[13,14] tested the effect of zinc deficiency on the
tensile strength of healing surgical incisions in the integument of rats
and found no difference at 6 days ($p < 0.2$), but did find a significant decrease at 12 days ($p < 0.001$).

Failure to appreciate the delayed effect of zinc deficiency or sufficiency
has misled several investigators. O'Riain, Copenhagen and Calnan[15] tested
the effect of zinc sulfate medication on the tensile strength of wounds
in rats at 7 days. They confirmed Sandstead's and Shepard's results that
there was no difference in wound strength at this time, but unfortunately
failed to continue the study into the critical period. Similarly, Groundwater and MacLeod[16] tested the bursting strength of abdominal wounds
in rats at 4, 7, and 10 days, and were unable to demonstrate any increase
in the strength of wounds in the zinc supplemented animals over controls.
In Kinnamon's[17] studies of zinc metabolism of irradiated wounds in rats,
no changes in collagen formation were found at 6 days, but radiozinc retention by the wounds was significantly elevated at that time, as we had
found earlier.[12] Figures 13-2A and 13-2B illustrate the type of measurements we made on radiozinc retention by wounds.

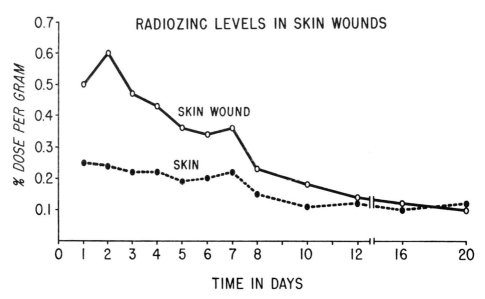

FIGURE 13-2A. Increased radiozinc retention in incised wounds of rats compared to
normal skin levels following intravenous injection of ca. 5 mcCi of zinc-65 chloride in
normal saline by tail vein at the time of wounding. The radioisotope accumulates
preferentially in the wound during the acute healing stage and demonstrates the
involvement of zinc with repair.

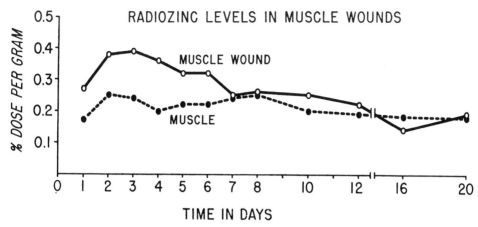

FIGURE 13-2B. Increased radiozinc retention in muscle wounds of rats compared to normal muscles following intravenous injection of ca. 5 mcCi of zinc-65 chloride in saline at the time of wounding. Radiozinc accumulates preferentially in the muscle wound during the acute healing stage, but the effect is not as pronounced as with the skin wound.

INVESTIGATIONS IN MAN

The empiric use of zinc to promote healing dates back to the early Egyptians who applied it topically in the form of calamine. Since then, zinc oxide, zinc sulfate, and zinc stearate in the form of powders, salves, solutions, and ointments have continued to be employed widely and effectively in the topical treatment of skin and eye lesions.

Evidence has rapidly accumulated that hospital patients are frequently zinc deficient, that poor healing is associated with low zinc levels, and that oral zinc therapy may stimulate previously indolent wounds to optimal repair. A good definition of zinc deficiency is sorely needed since current so-called "normal" are only "average" values, and vary among investigators.[18] All agree that plasma or serum values below 90 mcg percent indicate zinc deficiency. Two medications usually employed to treat zinc deficiency consist of zinc sulfate USP, 220 mg t.i.d., corresponding to the dosage of ferrous sulfate used in iron therapy, and 80 mg of zinc sulfate USP in combination with 300 mg of ascorbic acid.

Frequency of Zinc Deficiency in Hospital Patients

Zinc deficiency is common in hospital patients. This is well shown by the survey which Sullivan et al.[19] made of serum zinc concentrations in 225 consecutive hospital admissions. Zinc levels 3 standard deviations below their normal mean of 90 ± 10 mcg percent were found in 68 percent of cirrhotics and 21 percent of other patients. Hypozincemia has been well documented in patients with alcoholism;[20] atherosclerosis;[21] chronic cutaneous ulcers; [20,21,22,23] cirrhosis; [19,20] Down's syndrome; [20] dwarfism;[24,25] lung cancer;[20,26] leukemias;[19,20] malnutrition;[27] myocardial infarction;[20,27] pregnancy;[20] pulmonary infection, including tuberculosis;[19,20] and uremia.[20] Indeed, any patient presenting with chronic disease should be studied for zinc deficiency.

The high frequency of zinc deficiency in hospital populations is probably due to a combination of poor prior alimentation, inadequate parental nutrition, metabolic disorders, and excessive urinary and fecal losses of the metal. It is not surprising that a typical alcoholic patient with esophageal carcinoma and cirrhosis shows low serum zinc values because of poor nutrition, the metabolic and poorly understood effects of malignancy, and zincuria due to cirrhosis and other degenerative changes. Many similar common examples can be given.

Zinc Deficiency in Burns

Zinc deficits develop very rapidly in patients with major burns. Larsen et al.[28] have recently confirmed these observations by studies conducted on burned children at Shriners Burns Institute, Galveston. A total of 106 patients ranging in age from six months to 16 years were studied. They fell into three categories: (1) 68 acute burn patients with open wounds greater than 10 percent of the body surface; (2) 13 convalescent patients with burns over 12 weeks old, and wounds measuring less than 5 percent of body surface; and, (3) 25 patients admitted for reconstructive surgery who had no unhealed areas. The reconstructive surgery patients had normal plasma zinc levels, as did the majority of the convalescent burn patients. All of the acutely burned patients had persistent, low plasma zinc levels until near the 12th week when the majority of the wounds were epithelized. Nielsen and Jemec[29] also found hypozincemia with zincuria in their 7 patients with 16 to 53 percent body burns of partial or full thickness.

Association of Poor Healing and Low Zinc Levels

Patients with low zinc levels heal poorly and, conversely, poor healing is frequently associated with zinc deficiency. This relationship has been documented by measurements of zinc levels in serum, plasma, granulations, and skin.

In our first series of 17 patients referred to our study because of chronic, nonresponsive cutaneous ulcers, 11 had serum zinc levels below 100 mcg percent compared to our normal of 120 mcg and healed on zinc therapy, as shown in Figure 13-3.[27] Others have reported similar findings.

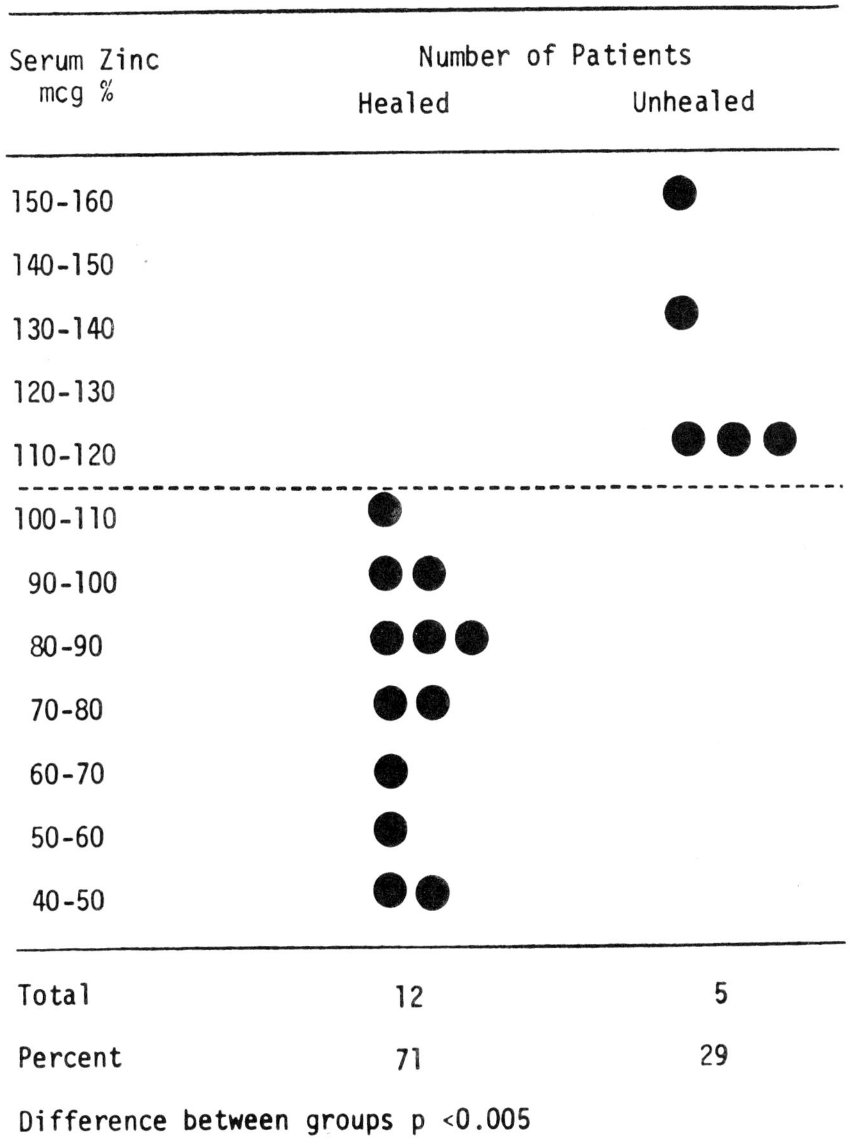

Serum Zinc mcg %	Number of Patients	
	Healed	Unhealed
150-160		●
140-150		
130-140		●
120-130		
110-120		● ● ●
100-110	●	
90-100	● ●	
80-90	● ● ●	
70-80	● ●	
60-70	●	
50-60	●	
40-50	● ●	
Total	12	5
Percent	71	29

Difference between groups p <0.005

FIGURE 13-3. Correlation of initial serum zinc levels with healing response of 17 patients to zinc sulfate therapy. As is evident, the patients with serum zinc levels below 120 mcg percent responded to zinc therapy, and those with zinc levels above 120 mcg percent did not respond. The difference in healing between the groups is highly significant (p<0.005).

Serjeant et al.[23] found serum zinc levels of 0.83 ± 0.12 µg per ml (83 ± 12 mcg percent) in a group of patients with leg ulcers associated with sickle cell anemia compared to their healthy control levels of 1.01 ± 0.08 mcg per ml. These serum zinc levels compare well with those reported by Husain[22] in his larger series of 104 patients. Halsted and Smith[20] reported 8 patients with indolent ulcers who had mean plasma zinc levels of 58 ± 15 mcg percent; only one patient had so-called normal levels over 96 ± 12 mcg percent. Greaves and Skillen[30] found that patients with chronic venous ulcers had significantly lower plasma zinc levels of 14.8 µmol in contrast with their controls of 18.1 µmol (p < 0.001). Sixteen patients who had wounds which had either failed to heal or were healing in abnormally slow fashion were measured by Henzel et al.[31] for cutaneous zinc concentrations. The patients with wound healing problems had zinc skin levels of 7.49 ppm versus two series of controls with levels of 16.84 and 16.63 ppm. Similarly, granulations of poorly healing ulcers contained 6.63 ppm of zinc compared to normally healing wounds which had concentrations of 11.66 and 11.17 ppm.

These observations on man are in accord with the animal data. In addition, it is common clinical experience that patients with malnutrition, cirrhosis, pulmonary infections, malignancies, and atherosclerosis heal poorly. The variations in techniques and manner of reporting zinc levels prevent easy comparisons between series, but the differences between the test groups and controls in each of the series are clearcut. Poor healing in man is frequently a consequence of zinc deficiency.

Zinc Therapy

Fortunately, healing problems due to zinc deficiency respond well to zinc sulfate therapy, and the medication is well tolerated. In 1965, we[32,33] began testing the effectiveness of zinc therapy in human healing. Twenty young men with operated pilonidal sinuses were randomly distributed into two groups prior to excision of the lesions. Ten of the patients were placed on zinc sulfate USP ($ZnSO_4 \cdot 7H_2O$), 220 mg t.i.d., while the ten in the control group were maintained on their usual diets without zinc supplementation. The methods of excision, dressing care, and activity were comparable in the two groups. Although the medicated patients had larger wounds than the controls (54.5 ml vs. 32.2 ml), the men treated with zinc healed 34.3 days faster (45.8 ± 2.6 days vs. 80.1 ± 13.7 days); (p < 0.02). Of great interest was the finding that healing curves of these patients resembled those seen in experimental animals; there was no difference in the rate of healing during the first 15 days after wounding and the major effect was apparent during the stage of epithelization. The technique of wound healing measurements is illustrated in Figure 13-4, and the data obtained are tabulated and analyzed in Table 13-I.

Many investigators have now confirmed the beneficial effects of zinc therapy, and three studies on venous leg ulcers are outstanding. Husain[22] reported a well controlled trial of zinc sulfate therapy in 104 patients with

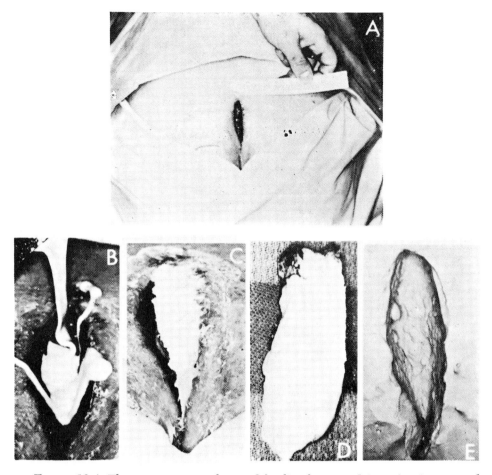

FIGURE 13-4. The measurement of wound healing by second intention in operated pilonidal sinus tracts is readily made by means of alginic acid casts, as shown: (A) the wound formed by operating a pilonidal sinus; (B) filling the wound with alginate hydrocolloid; (C) after one minute, the impression readily separates from the wound edges; (D) the finished impression is ready for volumetric measurement and casting in dental stone; and (E) the wound is easily reproduced in dental stone.

venous leg ulcers hospitalized during the entire study. The ulcers healed more rapidly in the treatment group; closing in 32 days on the average as against 77 days for the control group. In a group of 18 subjects with previously refractory venous ulcers, Greaves and Skillen[30] obtained re-epithelization after beginning zinc therapy. Some healing occurred in all patients and complete healing was evident in 13. Serjeant et al.[23] carried out a controlled trial on the effect of oral zinc sulfate in the healing of 34 patients with sickle cell leg ulcers and found the healing rate in the treatment group was three times faster than in the placebo group.

TABLE 13-I

WOUND HEALING IN CONTROLS AND TREATMENT GROUP

Patient No.	Age (yr.)	Wound Volume (ml.)	Days for Complete Healing	Healing Rate (ml. per day)
Controls:				
1	27	10.0	40	0.25
2	21	2.5	46	0.05
3	40	40.0	48	0.83
4	23	47.0	53	0.89
5	23	28.0	63	0.44
6	24	52.0	71	0.73
7	23	42.0	85	0.50
8	24	7.5	93	0.08
9	23	45.0	121	0.37
10	22	49.0	181	0.27
Mean ± S.E.	25.0	32.3	80.1 ± 13.7	0.44 ± 0.09
Treatment Group:				
1	19	100	33	3.03
2	24	28	34	0.82
3	22	30	43	0.70
4	18	44	44	1.00
5	28	35	46	0.76
6	40	140	46	3.04
7	28	30	48	0.63
8	23	50	51	0.98
9	22	49	52	0.94
10	22	39	61	0.64
Mean ± S.E.	24.6	54.5	45.8 ± 2.6	1.25 ± 0.30
Significance			$P < 0.02$	$P < 0.01$

Larsen et al.[28] reported that zinc therapy improved epithelization and graft acceptance in a series of 106 children with major burns. Henzel et al.[31] also identified 16 patients with impaired wound healing due to zinc deficiency. The addition of supplemental zinc to the diets of these subjects resulted in improved wound healing and occurred concomitantly with measurable increases in the concentration of zinc within the epithelium and granulation tissues of the wounds.

Zinc sulfate therapy promotes healing of chronic, indolent wounds in most cases. MacMahon et al.[34] described two bizarre cases, an elderly woman and an infant with advanced zinc deficiency due to malabsorption, both of whom had thin, glazed, and fragile skin. The woman's skin broke down repeatedly and failed to heal. Both patients cleared on zinc therapy. Pullen et al.[35] used zinc sulfate therapy successfully in the treatment of chronic respiratory tract granulations following laryngotracheal trauma. These lesions are particularly resistant to therapy and frequently occlude the airway. Seven of the eight patients treated with zinc healed rapidly and completely with no residual disease. In one of our controlled studies 13 out of 17 patients with chronic wounds responded rapidly to zinc sulfate;[27] all 13 were zinc deficient while the 4 who failed to respond had normal zinc levels.[27] In a limited double blind trial in a second group of patients with long term healing problems, we found that five of six treated with zinc healed, while three of four in the placebo group showed no change.

Several groups of investigators, using various methods, have failed to find any beneficial effects of zinc therapy on healing. In their initial study, Brewer et al.[36] treated the decubiti of 16 patients with oral zinc sulfate and found that 7 healed in an average of 8 weeks, 5 patients closed their wounds more than 50 percent in an average of 7 weeks, and 4 patients remained unchanged. In a second and double blind study involving a total group of 14 patients, they were unable to show any differences between the zinc medicated and control groups.[37] Myers and Cherry[38] failed to show any correlation of healing rates of chronic leg ulcers with serum zinc levels in 24 patients, nor did supplemental oral zinc therapy seem to accelerate healing.* Dr. Barcia,[39] also, reported lack of acceleration of healing with zinc sulfate therapy of pilonidal sinus tract incisions. Unfortunately, the zinc-deficient patients were not separated from the zinc-sufficient in these studies. In general, zinc medication is not beneficial to patients with high zinc stores.[40]

OTHER TRACE ELEMENTS AND HEALING

Healing is a complex biological process, and other trace elements are certainly involved, as well as a variety of organic moities. Although data are still incomplete on many of the interrelationships of trace elements, it is evident that healing is affected by deficiencies, and toxic excesses of the following: cadmium, cobalt, copper, iodine, manganese, molybdenum, and selenium.

Cadmium

Extensive studies[41] have been conducted on the toxic effects of cadmium since the discovery by Parizek and Zahor[42] that this metal produces chemical castration. It is only necessary to emphasize that cadmium damages the gonads of both sexes and that selenium and zinc protect against this damage. Anke et al.[43] have shown that cadmium is antagonistic to iron, as well

*Dr. Myers was good enough to allow us to analyze the raw data from this study on the healing of venous leg ulcers and the results appear to be consistent with a zinc effect. A nonparametric statistical Rank test was applied to the percent changes in ulcer area per week, the test is the Mann-Whitney U test which has a 95% confidence level compared to the parametric t-test. The difference in healing rate, although small, is significantly increased in the group with the higher zinc levels. Using Myers' data, a U of 30 was generated which for comparison of two groups of 11 each was significant at $p<0.05$. This significant difference is indicative of a zinc effect on the ulcer healing.

as to zinc, and drastically reduces the copper level of the fetus and milk. Cadmium thus becomes a significant cause of tissue damage since it is commonly present in commercial fertilizers, polluted air, and tobacco. Fortunately, zinc therapy and ascorbic acid[44] provide safe ways of offsetting cadmium toxicity.

Cobalt

An epidemic form of fulminating cobalt cardiomyopathy in man has focused attention on the tissue damage that can be produced by too much of this element.[45] Numerous deaths occurred in four localities during 1965 to 1966 from the addition of 1 ppm of cobalt to beer to enhance foaming qualities. The deceased were well nourished, but heavy beer drinkers. Polycythemia, pericardial effusions, and thyroid hyperplasia were some of the unusual features seen at autopsy, and were definitely different from alcoholic beri beri cardiomyopathies. Alcohol, cobalt, and protein-poor diets acted synergistically to produce the pathology.

Copper

The importance of copper to elastin formation in arteries has been reviewed by Hill.[46] Elastin is essential for arterial elasticity, and aortic aneurysms form and rupture as a consequence of this deficiency. Decreased formation of elastin results from a reduced synthesis of desmosine and isodesmosine, two amino acids which act as protein cross-links. The reduced formation of the desmosines in turn reflect lower activity of amine oxidase, an enzyme that appears to be copper dependent. Evidence that copper deficiency is involved in the production of human aneurysms has come from activation analysis of aneurysm tissue, which showed decreased copper content.[47] Copper therapy has not been developed for the prevention and treatment of aneurysms in man. Rather, the emphasis has been entirely on the removal of excess copper by penicillamine in Wilson's disease.[48]

Little work has been done on the effects of high copper levels on wound healing and the production of degenerative changes in man. This is in sharp contrast to the investigations on the very toxic effects of high copper levels in sheep.[49] Our preliminary observations suggest that blood and hair copper levels frequently are very high in patients with cancer, cardiovascular disease and other chronic illnesses.

Iodine

Hyperplastic changes develop in the thyroid as the iodine concentration falls below 0.1 percent of the dry weight of the gland.[50] The follicles of the gland distend with colloidal material and the cells lining the follicle become flattened and atrophied. Cellular necrosis, hemorrhage, and necrosis follow. The hyperplastic changes regress if iodine or thyroid hormones are supplied. As repetitive cycles of iodine deficiency and sufficiency occur, the metabolically active portions of the gland may hypertrophy excessively.

In this way, iodine deficiency may produce tissue damage and wounds, but the direct effect is to the thyroid gland. Prolonged iodine deficiency frequently leads to cretinism with permanent mental impairment and dwarfism due to the failure of the long bones to grow. In contrast to zinc deficiency, sexual development appears to be normal, but sexual drive seems to be absent.

Manganese

Although direct involvement of manganese in wound healing has not been demonstrated, we have studied two patients with healing problems who showed normal zinc and high manganese levels in their hair. In both patients, zinc therapy brought about healing without changing the zinc level, but with decrease in the manganese levels.

Molybdenum

Toxic effects of excess molybdenum in animals include joint deformities, growth impairment, anemia, diarrhea, and change of hair color, but not the production of wounds.[51] Cattle and sheep are more susceptible to excess molybdenum than other domestic animals. The element seems to act through reduction of liver sulfide oxidase activity, and this can be corrected by additional copper intake.

Selenium

Investigations on the biochemistry of selenium were summarized in a Selenium Symposium[52] in 1966. The element is present in liver factor 3 which protects against most of the symptoms of vitamin E deficiency. Traces of selenium are needed to prevent dietary liver necrosis in rats. Selenium deficiency appears to be very common, and has led to great losses in animal husbandry, since selenium-lack causes white muscle disease in cattle and sheep, hepatosis dietetica in swine, and exudative diathesis in poultry. Traces of selenium may be necessary to prevent peridontal disease in man, but excessive amounts seem to be cariogenic.[53]

Selenium is obviously involved in healing. It prevents the degenerative changes in cattle, poultry, sheep, and swine and protects against damage from cadmium. Direct application of selenium therapy to humans has not been made, other than treatment of seborrhea with selenium sulfide.

MECHANISMS

Although there is ample evidence that zinc is essential for healing in man and animals, the mechanisms remain poorly defined. There are probably multiple sites of action with local and systemic effects. Zinc moves rapidly into healing tissues.[12] We[54] have found the turnover to be high during the early stages of repair in skin, muscle, granulations, aorta, and bone.

Underwood[51] has reviewed the essentiality of zinc in processes which are basic in healing, e.g. protein synthesis, DNA and RNA production, and cellular growth and replication. More recent studies have demonstrated the need for zinc in amino acid metabolism and therefore the synthesis of collagen substrate.[55] We emphasize substrate because mature collagen contains little zinc in spite of the high zinc metabolism during the early stage of collagen formation.

The anti-infective action of zinc is of particular recent interest. Zinc sulfate (0.2 percent) drops have long been used effectively in the topical therapy of ophthalmic infections, and tons of zinc sulfate are used in chemical toilets. In one of our early healing experiments, respiratory disease ravaged our rat colony. All of our control animals died, while all the animals medicated with zinc survived. Mesrobian and Shklar[3] reported that in their studies postoperative deaths were four times fewer for zinc supplemented hamsters compared to the controls. Miller[4] has documented that zinc deficient calves are highly susceptible to nonspecific infections which often result in death. There are many possible reasons for the decreased resistance and stamina in zinc deficiency. Speculations include defective synthesis of proteins, white blood cells, interferons, and hormones.

ZINC MEDICATION

The usual form of oral zinc therapy is zinc sulfate heptahydrate (USP) capsules, 220 mg t.i.d. for adults, and half this level for children. The medication is well tolerated when taken after meals, but some patients do exhibit mild gastric distress. Oddly enough, oral zinc sulfate therapy was employed as 3 gr tablets in Great Britain in the early 1800's for the treatment of gleet and leukorrhea.[56] Perhaps this application should be reinvestigated in view of definite bactericidal properties of zinc salts.

Some vitamin-mineral preparations are available with a high zinc content. These are particularly satisfactory for maintenance since zinc-deficient patients seem to have permanently lost the ability to absorb the normal amount of zinc from the diet. Zinc-ascorbic acid preparations seem to be indicated if healing problems are involved, or if air pollution is a serious factor.

SUMMARY

Zinc is an essential factor for wound healing in animals. Compared to controls, zinc deficient animals heal poorly with characteristic epithelial defects and with decreased tensile strength. Although zinc migrates rapidly into healing tissues, the effects of zinc deficiency or supplementation on healing are slow to appear. Gross retardation or acceleration of cutaneous healing is not evident for 12 to 15 days, although rapidly healing tissues, such as gingiva, show the effects within three days.

Zinc deficiency in man is similarly associated with delayed wound healing. Because zinc deficiency is common in hospital patients and is characteristic of many chronic disease states, this deficit is probably a major factor in poor tissue repair and prolonged hospital stays. Fortunately, healing problems due to zinc deficiency respond well to zinc sulfate therapy, and the medication is well tolerated. Wider application of zinc therapy may be expected in the future as physicians become aware of the zinc deficiency syndrome. Insufficiency states are readily determined by atomic absorption spectroscopy, and inexpensive medication is now being evaluated.

Further advances are dependent on establishing optimal zinc levels for blood and other tissues of man, developing the interrelationships of the trace elements, and elucidating the mechanisms of zinc metabolism. Knowledge is especially needed on the availability of zinc from the diet and from the various body pools. Zinc deficiency is probably as common in man as iron and vitamin C deficiency, and appears to be of equal medical importance.

REFERENCES

1. Strain, W. H., Dutton, A. M., Heyer, H. B., and Ramsey, G. H.: *Experimental Studies on the Acceleration of Burn and Wound Healing*. Rochester, University of Rochester Reports, 1953.
2. Strain, W. H., Dutton, A. M., Heyer, H. B., Pories, W. J., and Ramsey, G. H.: *Acceleration of Burns and Wound Healing with Methionine Zinc*. Rochester, University of Rochester Reports, 1954.
3. Mesrobian, A. Z., and Shklar, G.: The effect of gingival wound healing of dietary supplements of zinc sulfate in the syrian hamster. *Periodontics*, 6:224, 1968.
4. Miller, W. J.: Zinc nutrition of cattle: A review. *J Dairy Sci*, 53:1123, 1970.
5. Tucker, H. F., and Salmon, W. D.: Parakeratosis or zinc deficiency disease in the pig. *Proc Soc Exp Biol Med*, 88:613, 1955.
6. Miller, W. J., Morton, J. D., Pitts, W. J., and Clifton, C. M.: Effect of zinc defi-

ciency and restricted feeding on wound healing in the bovine. *Proc Soc Exp Biol Med, 118*:427, 1965.

7. Miller, J. K., and Miller, W. J.: Experimental zinc deficiency and recovery of calves. *J Nutr, 76*:467, 1962.

8. Miller, W. J., Pitts, W. J., Clifton, C. M., and Morton, J. D.: Effects of zinc deficiency *per se* on feed efficiency, serum alkaline phosphatase, zinc in skin, behavior, greying other measurements in the Holstein calf. *J Dairy Sci, 48*: 1329, 1965.

9. Mills, C. F., Dalgarno, A. C., Williams, R. B., and Quarterman, J.: Zinc deficiency and the zinc requirements of calves and lambs. *Br J Nutr, 21*:751, 1967.

10. Ott, E. A., Smith, W. H., Stob, M., Parker, H. E., and Beeson, W. M.: Zinc deficiency syndrome in the young lamb. *J Nutr, 82*:41, 1964.

11. Mills, C. F., Quarterman, J., Chesters, J. K., Williams, R. B., and Dalgarno, A. C.: Metabolic role of zinc. *J Clin Nutr, 22*:1240, 1969.

12. Savlov, E. D., Strain, W. H., and Huegin, F.: Radiozinc studies in experimental wound healing. *J Surg Res, 2*:209, 1962.

13. Sandstead, H. H., and Shepard, G. H.: The effect of zinc deficiency on the tensile strength of healing surgical incisions in the integument of the rat. *Proc Soc Exp Biol Med, 128*:687, 1968.

14. Sandstead, H. H., Lanier, V. C., Jr., Shepard, G. H., and Gillespie, D. D.: Zinc and wound healing: effects of zinc deficiency and zinc supplementation. *Am J Clin Nutr, 23*:514, 1970.

15. O'Riain, S., Copenhagan, H. J., and Calnan, J. S.: The effect of zinc sulfate on the healing of incised wounds in rats. *Br J Plast Surg, 21*:240, 1968.

16. Groundwater, W., and Macleod, I. B.: The effects of systemic zinc supplements on the strength of healing incised wounds in normal rats. *Br J Surg, 57*:222, 1970.

17. Kinnamon, K. E.: Radiation and wound healing: influence of dietary methionine and zinc on zinc-65 distribution and excretion in the rat. *Rad Res, 29*:184, 1966.

18. Dawson, J. B., and Walker, B. E.: Direct determination of zinc in whole blood, plasma and urine by atomic absorption spectroscopy. *Clin Chim Acta, 26*:465, 1969.

19. Sullivan, J. F., Parker, M. M., and Boyett, J. D.: Incidence of low serum zinc in noncirrhotic patients. *Proc Soc Exp Biol Med., 130*:591, 1969.

20. Halsted, J. A., and Smith, J. C., Jr.: Plasma-zinc in health and disease. *Lancet, i*: 322, Feb. 14, 1970.

21. Pories, W. J., Strain, W. H., and Rob, C. G.: Zinc deficiency in delayed healing and chronic disease. In Cannon, H. L., and Hopps, H. C. (Eds.): *Environmental Geochemistry in Health and Disease*, Memoir 123. Boulder, Colorado, Geological Society of America, 1971.

22. Husain, S. L.: Oral zinc sulphate in leg ulcers. *Lancet, i*:1069, May 31, 1969.

23. Serjeant, G. R., Galloway, R. E., and Gueri, M. C.: Oral zinc sulphate in sickle-cell ulcers. *Lancet, ii*:891, Oct. 31, 1970.

24. Prasad, A. S., and Oberleas, D.: Zinc: Human nutrition and metabolic effects. *Ann Intern Med, 73*:631, 1970.

25. Caggiano, V., Schnitzler, R., Strauss, W., Baker, R. K., Carter, A. C., Josephson, A. S., and Wallach, S.: Zinc deficiency in a patient with retarded growth, hypogonadism, hypogamma globulinemia and chronic infection. *Am J Med Sci, 257*:305, 1969.

26. Davies, I. J. T., Musa, M., and Dormandy, T. L.: Measurements of plasma zinc. *J Clin Pathol*, *21*:359, 1968.
27. Pories, W. J., Strain, W. H., Peer, R. M., and Landew, M. H.: Zinc deficiency as a cause for delayed wound healing. In *Current Topics in Surgical Research*, *Vol. I*. New York, Acad Pr, 1970.
28. Larsen, D. L., Maxwell, R., Abston, S., and Dobrkovsky, M.: Zinc deficiency in burned children. *Plast Reconstr Surg*, *46*:13, 1970.
29. Nielsen, S. P., and Jemec, B.: Zinc metabolism in patients with severe burns. *Scand J Plast Reconstr Surg*, *2*:47, 1968.
30. Greaves, M. W., and Skillen, A. W.: Effects of long-continued ingestion of zinc sulphate in patients with venous leg ulceration. *Lancet*, *ii*:879, Oct. 31, 1970.
31. Henzel, J. H., DeWeese, M. S., and Lichti, E. L.: Zinc concentrations within healing wounds. *Arch Surg*, *100*:349, 1970.
32. Pories, W. J., Henzel, J. H., Rob, C. G., and Strain, W. H.: Promotion of wound healing in man with zinc sulfate given by mouth. *Lancet*, *i*:121, Jan. 21, 1967.
33. Pories, W. J., Henzel, J. H., Rob, C. G., and Strain, W. H.: Acceleration of healing with zinc sulfate. *Ann Surg*, *165*:432, 1967.
34. MacMahon, R. A., Parker, M. L., and McKinnon, M. C.: Zinc treatment in malabsorption. *Med J Aust*, *ii*:210, Aug. 3, 1968.
35. Pullen, F. W., II, Pories, W. J., and Strain, W. H.: Delayed healing: the rationale for zinc therapy. *Laryngoscope*, *81*:1638, 1971.
36. Brewer, R. D., Jr., Leaf, J. F., and Mihaldzic, N.: Preliminary observations on the effect of oral zinc sulfate on the healing of decubitus ulcers. *Proc Annu Clin Spinal Cord Inj Conf*, *15*:93, 1966.
37. Brewer, R. D., Jr., Mihaldzic, N., and Dietz, A.: The effect of oral zinc sulfate on the healing of decubitus ulcers in spinal cord injured patients. *Proc Annu Clin Spinal Cord Inj Conf*, *17*:70, 1967.
38. Myers, M. B., and Cherry, G.: Zinc and the healing of chronic leg ulcers. *Am J Surg*, *120*:77, 1970.
39. Barcia, P. J., Lack of acceleration of healing with zinc sulfate. *Ann Surg*, *172*:1048, 1970.
40. Pories, W. J., and Strain, W. H.: Zinc in wound healing. In Prasad, A. S. (Ed.): *Zinc Metabolism*. Springfield, Thomas, 1966.
41. Friberg, L. T., Piscator, M., and Nordberg, G. F.: *Cadmium in the Environment*. Cleveland, CRC Press, 1971.
42. Parizek, J., and Zahor, Z.: Effect of cadmium salts on testicular tissue. *Nature* (Lond.), *177*:1036, 1956.
43. Anke, M., Hennig, A., Schneider, H. J., Ludke, H., Von Gagern, W., and Schlegel, H.: The interrelations between cadmium, zinc, copper and iron in metabolism of hens, ruminants and man. In Mills, C. F. (Ed.): *Trace Element Metabolism in Animals*, Edinburgh, Livingstone, 1971, p. 317.
44. Spivey Fox, M. R., and Fry, B. E., Jr.: Cadmium toxicity decreased by dietary ascorbic acid supplements. *Science*, *169*:989, 1970.
45. Alexander, C. S.: Cobalt and the heart. *Ann Intern Med*, *70*:411, 1969.
46. Hill, C. H.: The role of copper in elastin formation. *Nutr Rev*, *27*:99, 1969.
47. Strain, W. H., Rob, C. G., Pories, W. J., Childers, R. C., Thompson, M. F., Jr., Hennessen, J. A., and Graber, F. M.: Element imbalances of atherosclerotic aortas. In Devoe, J. R. (Ed.): *Modern Trends in Activation Analysis*. Washington, National Bureau of Standards Special Publication 312, 1969, Vol. I, p. 128.

48. Walshe, J. M.: Wilson's disease—new oral therapy. *Lancet, i*:25, Jan. 7, 1956.
49. Thompson, R. H., and Todd, J. R.: Chronic copper poisoning in sheep—Biochemical studies of the haemolytic process. In Mills, C. F., (Ed.): *Trace Element Metabolism in Animals.* Edinburgh, Livingstone, 1970.
50. Anonymous. Goiter and iodine deficiency. *Nutr Rev, 22*:169, 1964.
51. Underwood, E. J.: *Trace Elements in Human and Animal Nutrition*, 3rd ed. New York, Acad Pr, 1971.
52. Muth, O. H. (Ed.): Symposium: *Selenium in Biomedicine: First International Symposium,* Oregon State University. Westport, Avi, 1966.
53. Hadjimarkos, D. M.: Effect of selenium on dental caries. *Arch Environ Health, 10*:893, 1965.
54. Strain, W. H., Pories, W. J., and Peer, R. M.: Unpublished results.
55. Hsu, J. M., and Anthony, W. L.: Zinc deficiency and urinary excretion of taurine-^{35}S and inorganic sulfate-^{35}S following cystine-^{35}S injection in rats. *J Nutr, 100*:1189, 1970.
56. Graham, C. W. M. S.: On the internal use of zinc in gleet and leucorrhea. *Edinburgh Med Surg J, 88*:107, 1826.

DISCUSSION

Comments

Chairman: Dr. J. H. Henzel: Are there any questions relative to Dr. Pories presentation? He has not only summarized beautifully, but also has added some new unpublished work. Most importantly of all, I waited to see if he would mention anything about Dr. Barcia's work. He's reviewed thoroughly the studies, that would seem to indicate that zinc is not as effective or as efficient as all of the original data. As he has pointed out, it is extremely important to find your parameter before you start the type of study as was done in the original work by Dr. Pories and Dr. Strain and also, to follow through quite thoroughly on it.

Dr. Chvapil: Let me just very briefly comment on this impressive work. The first comment is just a definition. I don't think that you are measuring tensile strength because according to the definition, tensile strength should be expressed as a factor of a homogenous material. Therefore, what you are measuring here is breaking strength and this is a common situation in all these measurements with very complicated material like skin or intestine or any other tissue. But what I would really like to ask Dr. Pories is the meaning of increased tensile strength. Is it because collagen is more accumulated, collagen is more cross-linked, the remodeling—that means the degradation of collagen—is less rapid, by the zinc effect? I really would like to understand better the meaning of the increased breaking strength which you find in your experiments. And, finally, it just occurred to me that the reason that you have the pronounced differences after zinc—the pronounced promotion of wound healing after 12-14 days—is very probably related to the technique that you have been using. Because, in my opinion, the wound healing is nothing less than a continuous dynamic process. which should start the first or second day. But if you are measuring, let's say, the polimetric area—I really need to know more about your technique to understand it better—or if you are just measuring the tensile strength, then very probably you will find these changes after 12-14 days. Howevery, if you focus on some activity of some enzymes related to healing— e.g., protocollagen hydroxylase—I am sure you should find a parameter of collagen synthesis faster than 12-14 days.

Dr. Pories: Well, firstly, I think your comment is well taken that we are talking about breaking strength, and not tensile strength. Secondly, our own experiments did not yield breaking strength. These were Dr. Sandstead's studies, and perhaps he would like to comment and elaborate on them. I don't think that healing is a continuous process and I am not sure that collagen is a measure of good healing. We talk about hydroxyproline, we talk about collagen as a measure of healing, and yet I am not sure that development of increasing amounts of collagen is necessarily what we want. A thick scar, a joint which is filled with collagen, an inelastic scar on the face—these are not things that we would like. In many ways, collagen is actually a bad by-product of healing. I would hope that when we heal vascular tissue that we could build elastin, and muscularis, and just a minimum of collagen. The questions you ask are very profound and the answers are not available. I wonder if Dr. Sandstead would comment.

Dr. Sandstead: Dr. Chvapil's question about the breaking strength is difficult to answer. If you examine the wounds histopathologically, the wound of the pair fed control animal is much more dense on histochemical staining for collagen than that of the zinc deficient animal. And it is obvious, you know!

Dr. Petering: I don't think you can measure tensile strength of a healing wound, but you certainly can measure tensile strength of skin. And this is the accepted parameter that the people working in leather use all the time. We are working with the Tanners Research Laboratory in Cincinnati, and this is exactly what they calculate for us—the tensile strength of skin. About the wound Dr. Chvapil may be correct, but I don't think that you are right about the point that you can't measure tensile strength of skin.

Chapter 14

ORAL ZINC SULFATE IN THE TREATMENT OF VENOUS LEG ULCERS

KNUT HAEGER, ERIK LANNER, AND
PER-OLOW MAGNUSSON

O UR INTEREST IN ZINC as a possible adjunct in wound healing was aroused by the paper of Pories et al.[17] in which they demonstrated the beneficial effect of oral zinc sulfate on the healing of operative wounds after removal of pilonidal cysts. We decided to test the effect of the drug on venous leg ulcers which were proven to show delayed healing.

We feel that we have to explain exactly what kind of ulcers we have dealt with. For this purpose it is necessary to know the background of the syndrome of chronic venous insufficiency. Our conception of this syndrome is shown in Figure 14-1. The immediate mechanisms of the

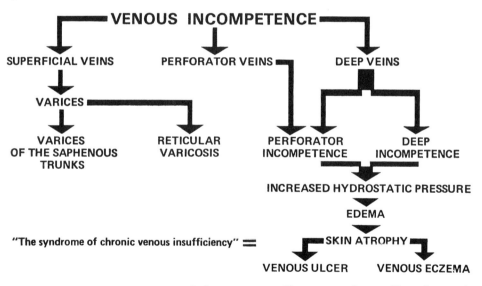

FIGURE 14-1. Our conception of the venous insufficiency syndrome. Note that varicosis does not cause leg ulcers, for which insufficient perforator veins are a prerequisite!

pathogenesis of a venous ulcer are not known in detail. It is quite clear, however, that perforator insufficiency is always present,[1] and that an increased hydrostatic pressure and an increased tissue pressure are prerequisites for ulceration. Possibly also locally produced toxic agents are at least partly responsible.

Healing of venous ulcers follows the same laws as that of any other ulcer with the addition that the healing mechanisms apparently do not work unless the increased pressure is eliminated. This can be done either by bed rest with elevation of the leg, or by compression with bandages so that the counterpressure equals the internal pressure of the leg. Even if bed rest usually results in a somewhat faster healing (compare the work by Husain in this symposium) it has been proved that ambulant therapy with the patient working also leads to desirable results. In our practice we have used the later method.

Hypostatic ulcers of the usual size and the typical location usually heal within 8 weeks after the beginning of compression therapy. Larger ulcers, and ulcers on certain locations, however, may stay unhealed for considerably longer periods. Properly treated they always heal, but in certain cases it may require a very long time. These longstanding ulcers appeared to be a very proper material for the study of the effects of a drug supposed to have a healing promoting action.

MATERIAL

Fifty-three patients of both sexes were treated. The average age of the patients treated with zinc was 63.3 years (range 49-83 years); the control group averaged 63.9 years (range 44-81 years). There were no statistically significant differences between ages and the distribution of sex between the two groups. In all cases, uncomplicated venous crural ulcer was diagnosed and verified by phlebography, which in all cases revealed perforator incompetence and/or deep venous incompetence. The rate of deep incompetence was the same in the treated series and the placebo series.

Naturally, in a series consisting of patients in this age group, there is some degree of arterial disease. However, patients with clinical symptoms of atherosclerotic disease were not included. Although not verified by arteriography or plethysmographic examination in all cases, it may be assumed that the incidence and degree of arterial disease is similar in both groups.

METHODS

Local Treatment

The local treatment was identical for all patients. The methods are previously reported and are summarized as follows: wound treatment with Katadyn® silver spray, compressive bandages with aluminium foil, rubber foam and elastic bandage with Lohmann Kräftig®. All patients were treated ambulantly and the ulcers were dressed two or three times a week, depending on the degree of seepage and size. All bandaging was made by the same specially trained nurse.

Medical Treatment

Patients with edema were given diuretics in the lowest possible dose to keep them at the lowest possible degree of swelling in the lower leg and ankle region. With the exception of two patients (one treated, one control) the diuretic treatment consisted of either clopamid (Brinaldix®, Sandoz) 20 mg p.d., or chlorthalidon (Hygroton®, Geigy) 100 mg three times weekly. The incidence of patients on diuretics and the relative distribution of the two preparations were similar in the treated group and control group.

Zinc Sulfate Treatment

The patients were given alternatively zinc sulfate capsules and placebo capsules according to a randomized double blind system. A third group was treated with zinc sulfate in the pharmaceutical form of effervescent tablets (Solvezink®, Draco*). The dose of zinc sulfate was in either case 200 mg three times daily.

Investigated Parameters

The ulcer area was measured according to the method of Fergusson and Logan.[4] The healing quotient, expressed as healed surface area in mm² divided by the number of days until complete healing, was calculated. The appraisal of complete healing was made by one and the same person in all cases. The progress of healing was checked at weekly intervals, and the ulcer area was registered.

Laboratory investigation, including all parameters listed in Table 14-IV, was made before treatment and after three weeks and six weeks of treatment. In patients requiring a prolonged treatment, checks of the haematological parameters were made as a matter of routine. By urinalysis, it was checked that patients on zinc really ingested the tablets.

After one week, three weeks, six weeks and when treatment was finished, the patient was interviewed about side effects. If present, a rough estimate of the duration and intensity of such effects was made.

RESULTS

Fifteen patients received zinc sulfate in gelatine capsules, 17 patients received zinc sulfate in effervescent tablets, and 21 patients received placebo. The healing quotients (HQ) for each series are given in Table 14-I for the patients who during the study were completely healed.

After three months of treatment, the number of patients with healed and nonhealed leg ulcers were counted in each group. The results of the double-blind study are given in Table 14-II. Student's t-test showed that

*AB Draco, Lund, Sweden, a subsidiary of AB Astra, Södertälje, Sweden.

the rate of healed patients in the zinc-treated group was significantly higher, t = 2.52 p < 0.05, than in the placebo group. In the third group,

TABLE 14-I

HEALING QUOTIENTS FOR CRURAL ULCERS

Mean Values

Medication	Initial Ulcer Surface Area (mm^2)	Healing Time (days)	HQ
Zinc sulfate (capsules)	557	85	5.94
Zinc sulfate (efferv. tablets)	573	59	8.26
Placebo	370	70	5.28

TABLE 14-II

HEALED AND NON-HEALED ULCERS IN DOUBLE BLIND TEST

Treatment	Total No. of Patients	No. of Healed Ulcers	No. of Non-healed Ulcers
Zinc sulfate (capsules)	12	11	1
Placebo	19	11	8

difference: t = 2.52; p<0.05

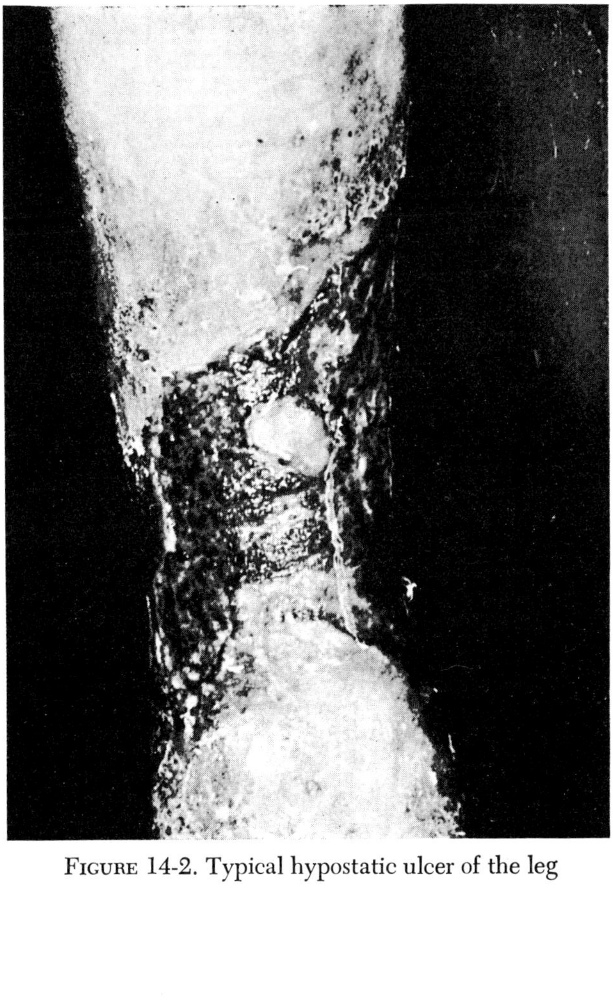

FIGURE 14-2. Typical hypostatic ulcer of the leg

TABLE 14-III

PERCENTAGE OF INITIAL ULCER AREA DURING PERIOD OF TREATMENT

Duration of Treatment (days)	Zinc Sulphate	Placebo	Significance
20	54 %	72.7%	N.S.
30	35.5%	53.8%	N.S.
40	20.0%	46.4%	$p < 0.05$
50	11.2%	40.2%	$p < 0.01$
60	5.6%	38.6%	$p < 0.01$
70	3.3%	37.4%	$p < 0.01$
80	1.9%	35.4%	$p < 0.01$
90	1.0%	35.7%	$p < 0.01$

TABLE 14-IV

MEAN VALUES OF HEMATOLOGICAL PARAMETERS BEFORE AND
AFTER ZINC TREATMENT

Hematological Parameter	Before Treatment	After Six Weeks of Treatment
Hemoglobin (gm/100 ml)	13.05 ± 0.38	13.49 ± 0.41
Red cell count ($\times 10^6$/cmm)	4.05 ± 0.12	4.24 ± 0.13
White cell count (per cmm)	5625 ± 402	5131 ± 641
Sedimentation rate (mm/hr)	20.38 ± 2.80	17.50 ± 2.44
Neutrophilic-myelocytes (percent)	1.20 ± 0.40	0.47 ± 0.19
Neutrophilic-granulocytes (percent)	70.60 ± 2.19	68.20 ± 2.92
Eosinophilic-granulocytes (percent)	2.33 ± 0.47	1.53 ± 0.35
Basophilic-granulocytes (percent)	0.40 ± 0.13	0.33 ± 0.13
Lymphocytes (percent)	21.07 ± 2.04	25.47 ± 2.71
Monocytes (percent)	4.33 ± 0.75	4.00 ± 0.50
Thrombocytes (per cmm)	212500 ± 1364	192500 ± 1142
Bilirubin/serum (mg/100 ml)	0.53 ± 0.06	0.53 ± 0.05
Alkaline phosphatase (units)	6.67 ± 0.65	6.67 ± 0.67
SGOT (units)	24.93 ± 3.01	22.73 ± 1.54
SGPT (units)	18.53 ± 4.88	15.33 ± 1.05

where the patients were treated with effervescent tablets, all 17 patients were completely healed.

Further, the progress of healing for each patient was shown on a diagram. The ulcer area after 20, 30, 40, 50, 60, 70, 80, and 90 days was interpolated on the ordinate and the means of these areas calculated for the placebo group and for the entire zinc-treated group. The results are given in Table 14-III. There were no statistically significant differences during the first 30 days of treatment. From 40 days on, however, the differences started to be increasingly greater and became significant. The healing curves for zinc sulfate and placebo, respectively, are diagramatically represented in Figure 14-3.

SIDE EFFECTS

All patients, except one with a hemoglobin value of 9.8 g percent (normal values in this laboratory 11.9-14.6 g percent), showed normal values of all investigated parameters. The results of the analysis before

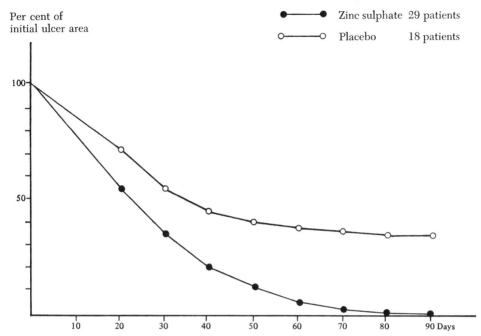

FIGURE 14-3. Diagrammatic representation of percentages of initial ulcer area throughout the period of observation in patients with and without oral zinc therapy.

treatment and after six weeks of treatment with zinc sulfate are given in Table 14-IV. From this table, it is clear that no parameter was significantly influenced. Individually, no pathological value was observed even in patients requiring prolonged treatment. It may be concluded that zinc sulphate 200 mg three times daily for six weeks has no toxic effect, either on liver function, as expressed by the declared haematological tests, or on other registered parameters.

Out of 15 patients on zinc sulfate in capsules, three discontinued the treatment. Their stated reasons were dizziness, itching, and nausea, respectively. No patients on effervescent tablets discontinued therapy. The percentage of undesirable effects after zinc treatment and leading to a discontinuation of therapy was 9.4 percent and after placebo treatment 9.6 percent. The stated reasons for discontinuation after placebo was dizziness in one case and exanthema in another.

Minor disturbances, usually rapidly disappearing, were noted in six patients on zinc (dizziness 2, itching 1, nausea 1, constipation 2), and in six patients on placebo (dizziness 1, itching 1, minor gastroenterologic inconvenience 4).

DISCUSSION

The average HQ was less in this series than in earlier reported series from this clinic.[7,8,9] The reason for this is threefold; an abundance of rather large ulcers, ulcers located near and below the malleoli, and a high rate of legs with both perforator and deep venous insufficiency. All three factors have been shown to markedly prolong the healing time for venous ulcers.[9] The average age of the patients in this series was approximately 7 years higher than in the collected material of more than 2000 leg ulcers from this clinic during the last eight years. In an earlier study, however, we were not able to prove that the age factor *per se* did influence healing time.

Comparing patients whose ulcers were healed within the period of the experiment, there were no significant differences in HQ between those given placebo and those given zinc sulfate in the double blind study.

It should be noted, however, that only 58 percent of patients in the placebo group were healed within this period compared with 91.7 percent in the zinc treated group. If the patients given effervescent tablets are included, the total healing rate is 96.5 percent in the treated group.

Because healing did not occur in a large part of the placebo-patients, the overall comparison between placebo treated and zinc treated patients showed significant differences regarding the progress of healing. These differences, however, did not appear until after 30 days of treatment (Figure 14-3).

It is tempting to speculate on the reasons for this pattern.

Halsted et al.[10] showed that patients with indolent ulcers often had low zinc-serum levels compared with normal individuals. One hypothesis is that the patients in the placebo-group who were completely healed had normal or almost normal zinc-serum levels already from the start whereas the 8 patients who received placebo without healing had subnormal levels at the start.

The results of our investigation are supported by an observation by the Henzel group. It appeared that zinc concentration in the tissues of the healing wound did not reach normal skin values until after about 30 days of medication. In fact, the curves shown in Figure 14-3 appear to be almost identical with those presented by Dr. Pories at this symposium. The delayed effect may also explain why some workers using a short period of observation failed to observe a beneficial action of zinc treatment.

Recently, Drs. Henzel, Holtmann, Keitzer, DeWeese and Lichti[12] published some evidence that the administration of zinc may act as a pharmacological agent permitting an improved local perfusion of ischaemic areas. Even in venous ulcers, particularly in the age group to which the majority of our patients belong, a certain amount of nutritional deficiency may be present.[6,14] In some pilot experiments on patients with ischaemic leg ulcers caused by atherosclerosis of the main vessels of the leg, we studied the influence of oral zinc therapy. As far as can be judged from these studies, oral zinc sulfate appears to be beneficial also in this type of leg ulcers. A full report will be published later.[*]

Drs. Husain[13] and Greaves and Skillen,[5] respectively, reported on beneficial results of zinc sulfate in leg ulcers. Their results were corroborated by case reports by Cohen[3] and Carruthers.[2] On the contrary, Myers and Cherry,[16] in a series of 40 ambulatory patients with chronic leg ulcers, did not find that the addition of oral zinc accelerated the healing rate. This, however, does not necessarily imply that their observations differ from ours. During the first weeks of treatment, we found no difference in the healing quotient, a term synonymous with the healing rate of these authors. It is also very plausible that there were cases of ischaemic ulcers in their series. It should be observed that the duration of the ulcers before treatment varied between 3 months and 25 years with a mean of 4.7 years. This indicates that it is not very likely that the main part of the ulcers were of venous origin, since even a large venous ulcer is usually healed within a considerably shorter time on proper bandaging treatment. On the contrary, ischaemic ulcers may require an extremely long time for healing: in our clinic, sometimes up to 24 months or even longer.

This interpretation of a controversial result is supported by the fact that Myers and Cherry[16] already from the beginning of their well-controlled experiment noted one particular group of cases showing rapid healing. Could this very group of patients possibly represent pure venous ulcers in a series of ischaemic or combined arterial and venous ulcers?

Another question of interest is whether locally applied zinc may have the same effect as ingested zinc sulfate. By tradition, zinc ointments have been widely used even for the treatment of leg ulcers. However, it seems that local zinc has been more or less abandoned in the modern ambulant compressive therapy of venous leg ulcers, and conclusive evidence on the role of local zinc has not been traced in the literature. Experimentally, Murray and Rosenthal[15] did not find any healing effect of local zinc in rat wounds.

The rate of side effects appears to be rather large after oral zinc sulfate. However, effects of the same type and severity were also found to a similar degree after placebo medication. Objective parameters were not influenced. The results are what can be expected in any double blind trial. It should be noted, however, that there was a significant difference between the pharmaceutical forms regarding side effects. Thus, the main part of side effects was caused by zinc in gelatin capsules, whereas the effervescent tablets gave very few such reactions (Table 14-V).

[*]Note added in proof: The report was published by Haeger, K., and Lanner, E.: Oral zinc sulphate and ischaemic leg ulcers. VASA 3:77, 1974.

TABLE 14-V

SIDE EFFECTS

Treatment	No. of Patients	No. of Pat:s with Side Effects	Discontinued Treatment Due to Side Effects	Gastric Side Effects
Zinc sulfate (capsules)	15	7	3	5
Zinc sulfate (effervescent tablets)	17	2	0	1
Placebo (capsules)	21	8	2	2

Difference between zinc sulfate and zinc sulfate effervescent tablets $t = 2.042$, $p < 0.05$.

SUMMARY

This investigation revealed (a) that the addition of oral zinc to the local treatment of long-standing venous leg ulcers improved the rate of healing (b) that this effect was obvious after 40 days of treatment (c) that haematological standard parameters remained normal throughout the period of observation (d) that no serious side effects were observed and that minor side effects apparently were modified by an improved pharmaceutical form.

Obviously, it would be extremely interesting to correlate the rate of healing in patients with or without zinc therapy with initial and running estimates of plasma and tissue zinc levels. Work along these lines is in progress in our laboratory.

REFERENCES

1. Arnoldi, C. C., and Haeger, K.: Ulcuscruris venosum—crux medicorum? *Lanartidningen 64*:2149, 1967.
2. Carruthers, R.: Zinc and wound healing. *Med J Aust, 1*:731, 1967.
3. Cohen, C.: Zinc sulphate and bedsores. *Br Med J, 2*:561, 1968.
4. Fergusson, A. G., and Logan, J. C. P.: Leg ulcers: assessment of response to certain topical medicaments. *Br. Med J, 1*:871, 1961.
5. Greaves, M. W., and Skillen, A. W.: Effects of long-continued ingestion of zinc sulphate in patients with venous leg ulceration. *Lancet, ii*.889, 1970.
6. Greither, A: Krampfaden und varikösen Symptomenkomplex. In: Grottron, H. A. (Ed.): *Dermatologie und Venerologie*, Stuttgart, Thieme, 1959, Vol. III, 212.
7. Haeger, K.: The treatment of venous ulcers of the leg. *Geriatrics, 19*:760, 1964.
8. Haeger, K.: *Venous and Lymphatic Disorders of the Leg.* Lund, Scandinavian University Books, 1966.
9. Haeger, K.: The influence of certain factors on the healing time of leg ulcers in ambulant patients. *Zbl Phlebolog, 9*:28, 1971.
10. Halsted, J. A., Hackley, B., Rudzki, C., and Smith, J. C. Jr.: Plasma zinc concentrations in liver diseases; comparison with normal control and certain other chronic diseases. *Gastroenterology, 54*:1098, 1968.
11. Henzel, J. H., DeWeese, M. S., and Lichti, E. L.: Zinc concentrations within

healing wounds. Significance of postoperative zincuria on availability and requirements during tissue repair. *Arch Surg, 100*:349, 1970.

12. Henzel, J. H., Holtmann, B., Keitzer, F. W., DeWeese, M. S., and Lichti, E.: Trace elements in atherosclerosis, efficacy of zinc medications as a therapeutic modality. In Hemphill, D. D. (Ed.): *Trace Substances in Environmental Health —II*, Columbia, Mo., University of Missouri, 1969, p. 83.
13. Husain, S. L.: Oral zinc sulphate in leg ulcers. *Lancet, i*:1069, 1969.
14. van der Molen, H. R.: Elastizitätsveränderungen der Haut und ihre Bedeutung für Entstehung der Phlebopathien. *Zbl Phlebolog, 5*:75, 1966.
15. Murray, J., and Rosenthal, S.: The effect of locally applied zinc and aluminium on healing incised wounds. *Surg Gyn Obstet, 126*:1298, 1968.
16. Myers, M. B., and Cherry, G.: Zinc and the healing of chronic leg ulcers. *Am J Surg, 120*:77, 1970.
17. Pories, W. J., Henzel, J. H., Rob, C. G., and Strain, W. H.: Acceleration of wound healing in man with zinc sulphate given by mouth. *Lancet, i*:121, 1967.

DISCUSSION

Chairman: John H. Henzel: Very beautiful piece of work, Dr. Haeger. Are there any questions with respect to this paper?

Dr. Larson: I was just curious to know how much do you think edema plays a part because one question that always comes in my mind is why don't we see the same amount of ulceration in lymph edema, and in Galveston they tend to gravitate in that direction. We have a large number of lymph-edematous patients and rarely do we see ulcerations until we have venous obstruction.

Dr. Haeger: I don't think you can heal a venous leg ulcer if you don't treat edema perfectly. All these patients were treated with compression therapy and it is a most important thing to get a real good compression. I think Dr. Husain will agree with that. And, also, we give diuretics in rather large doses, not as large as in hypertension, but fair doses. We have seen very good effects from that.

Chapter 15

ORAL ZINC SULFATE IN THE TREATMENT OF LEG ULCERS

S. Latafat Husain

AND

Rodney G. Bessant

~~~~~~

L EG ULCERS PRESENT a difficult therapeutic problem. Both patients and doctors tend to accept the presence of an ulcerated leg with a grim stoicism born of years of unsuccessful treatment. If this attitude prevails these chronically disabled patients may not seek treatment again unless given the stimulus of new hope.[12] Therapeutic agents recommended for topical use in the treatment of chronic leg ulcers are legion, and this itself suggests that none is entirely satisfactory. Most leg ulcers take an average eleven weeks to heal completely, irrespective of treatment.[7]

Zinc is an essential trace element in nutrition and is a constituent of most foods. Zinc salts are mainly used topically as mild astringents and disinfectants,[2] and several topical preparations containing zinc salts are used for the treatment of leg ulcers. In recent years there has been a renewed interest in this metal. This is due to the reports of rare cases of zinc deficiency disease in man. In condition of severe malnutrition, cases of anemia, with dwarfism and hypogonadism, were described which responded to zinc therapy when tissue zinc was low and its intake poor.[11] Great interest and much attention has been given to the role of zinc in the healing of wounds, suggesting that zinc may play here a fundamental role. Pories et al.[9] in a brilliant piece of work showed that, after excision of pilonidal sinus tracts, if zinc sulfate was given orally to young airmen during the period of healing, the healing rates were nearly three times greater in the treated group.

MATERIALS AND METHODS

It has been reported[5] that zinc sulfate given orally in a dose of 220 mg three times a day accelerated the healing of leg ulcers. In that study one hundred and four patients of various ages were included. All the

We thank the following: Drs. A. Lyell, J. O'D. Alexander, and J. Thomson, Consultant Dermatologists, Glasgow Royal Infirmary, for allowing study of their patients; the Nursing Staff, Glasgow Royal Infirmary, for their cooperation; Dr. G. S. Fell, Pathological Biochemistry, Glasgow University, for plasma zinc estimations Dr. W. R. Greig and staff, Nuclear Medicine, Glasgow Royal Infirmary, for use of their facilities; and Dr. F. C. Gillespie, Clinical Physics & Bio-Engineering, Western Regional Hospital Board, Glasgow, for helpful discussions.

patients were admitted to the dermatological wards and were on the normal hospital diet. Identical capsules containing 220 mg of lactose (placebo) or zinc sulfate were given three times a day to equal numbers of controls and treated patients. Ulcers healed more quickly in the treatment group. The ulcers of the treatment group healed in 32 days on average, as against 77 days for the control group. The ranges for the total number of days required for healing were 12 to 71 days for the treatment group and 35 to 232 days for the controls. Time to complete healing was independent of age and sex. There was no significant difference in the serum zinc estimations between the control and the treatment groups although some patients suffering from chronic leg ulcers did have low plasma zinc values, but statistically it was not significant.

In a later study 90 patients (62 females, 28 males) of various ages (34 to 82 years, average 62.8 years) with chronic ulcers of the lower limb were included. These patients were treated as out-patients, and most of them were ambulant. Only those patients who did not respond to the conventional topical therapy were included in this study. Zinc sulfate 220 mg B.P. in white gelatine capsules were prescribed. They were asked to take one capsule three times a day, half an hour after meal. Each patient received the same form of topical therapy depending upon the severity of the ulcer (i.e. Eusol dressing, 25.0 percent sodium sulfate soaks, or anaflex paste). The areas of the ulcers were measured by a planimeter.

Samples of venous blood were taken for the estimation of plasma zinc, full blood count and sedimentation rate, liver function tests, electrolytes and urea. The above mentioned investigations were carried out, before resuming the treatment, during the treatment (three weeks), and after stopping the treatment.

As shown in Table 15-I, 18 patients did not heal completely before the end of the trial (112 days) but 62 patients responded to the treatment. The average time required for complete healing was 63 days (as compared to the first study where the ulcers healed in 32.3 days). The average plasma zinc values were 93 ± 23 mcg/100ml before the therapy was commenced. Ten patients defaulted and were omitted from the trial.

As we have extended our series of patients, now, we feel all the cases of leg ulcers do not respond to the zinc sulfate therapy. Of course,

TABLE 15-I

Sex	Total No. of Patients	Failed to Respond	Healed Completely	Mean Plasma Zinc mcg/100 ml
Female:	56	10	46	93 ± 23
Male:	24	8	16	90 ± 19

one explanation could be the multifactorial etiology of the ulcers. Initially, we presumed that the zinc supplements corrected the deficiency states. Low plasma zinc values have been reported by some workers[1,3] and we also found low plasma values in some cases of leg ulcers,[6] but in our study it was not significantly demonstrated. In a series of several hundred plasma zinc values in patients with various diseases, we have found consistently low values only in severe and generalised illnesses such as cirrhosis of the liver and malignant diseases. The method of assay by atomic absorption spectrophotometry is essentially that described by Davies et al.[1] in 1968. Too much importance has been given to plasma zinc alone, since it represents less than 12 percent of whole blood zinc and like many other plasma values may remain at near normal levels until tissue reserves are greatly reduced. We are now looking at red cell and tissue zinc values in leg ulcer cases. Before zinc deficiency is postulated, two out of the three indices—plasma red cell, and tissue—zinc must be lowered.

The main role of oral zinc is probably to provide excess available zinc ions to cells at sites where extra demands are being made for nucleic acid and protein synthesis.[10] In postoperative patients, a fall in zinc stores in the early postoperative period has been shown.[8] In rats, radioactive zinc was mostly concentrated in healing tissue, the highest level being found immediately after injury.[14] The activity of zinc in wound healing is highest in the period of epithelization, which may also be related to the fact that 20 percent of the body zinc stores are in epithelial structures of skin.[9]

In many papers, uptake, absorption, and excretion of radioactive zinc have been studied in experimental animals to gain a better understanding of its metabolism under different conditions, but only limited data are available about the metabolism of ^{65}Zn in the human body. Some aspects of zinc metabolism have been studied by Ross et al.[13] and Craig and Siegel.[4] The most prominent studies were conducted by Spencer et al.[15] whose studies gave a full picture of the organ uptake and excretion of a single dose of radio zinc given intravenously or orally.

Radiozinc Studies

We have commenced a study to examine in more detail the metabolic pathway of zinc in the human body with special reference to any involvement in healing processes, using zinc-65 as a tracer. Six subjects with healing problems in the form of unilateral leg ulcers have been studied so far with a view primarily to determining whether there is an increased uptake of radiozinc in the ulcer and to find a possible explanation for the delayed response to treatment. Patients with unilateral ulceration were selected so that any concentration of radiozinc in the ulcer could be detected by external counting while using the clear leg as a control.

Each patient was given orally a single dose of two microcuries of zinc-65 (as chloride) in water, after fasting overnight. The physical half life is 245 days and measurements were made using the 1.11 MeV gamma radiation emitted in 45 percent of disintegrations. The total amount of zinc in the oral dose was well below one microgram so the radiozinc behaved as a true tracer of the dietary zinc.

Radiozinc was measured as follows:

(a) In separated plasma.

(b) In separated red blood cells.

(c) In urine samples collected separately for each voiding over the first 72 hours; thereafter in 24 hour urine collections.

(d) In 24 hour fecal collections.

(e) In the whole body, using a scanning bed whole-body monitor of the Warner-Oliver type.

(f) By external counting over the ulcer site, the corresponding region of the clear leg, forearms, thighs and liver, using a 5 inch diameter sodium iodide detector with cylindrical lead collimator.

This study is still in its preliminary stages so the results obtained to date should be regarded as qualitative indications only. Working from these results the study is continuing in order to examine a statistically

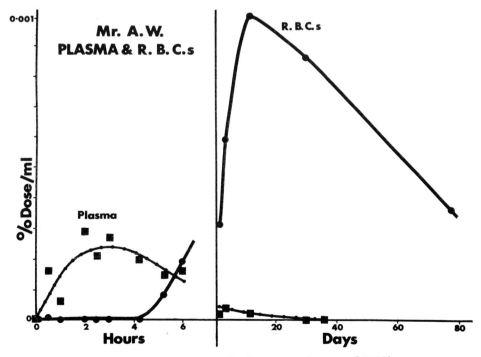

FIGURE 15-1. Appearance of radiozinc in plasma and RBC's.

significant number of subjects. The results obtained to date will be illustrated by reference to individual subjects. While in no sense representing any sort of quantitative mean the data illustrated are typical of the behaviour of five of the six subjects. The sixth is discussed later.

Figure 15-1 shows the appearance of radiozinc in plasma and RBC's of subject A. W. following the oral dose. The plasma activity in all five subjects is characterised by a rapid rise to a peak level between two and three hours, suggesting the probability of gastric absorption. Peak levels covered a wide range between 0.2 and 1 percent of dose per liter and activity fell to a low level again after 7 to 10 hours.

In the RBC's, activity remained low throughout the period of high plasma activity but rose slowly to reach a maximum at 5 to 20 days. Thereafter there was a slow decline at a rate similar to that of the whole-body activity. In two subjects measured to 80 days the fall was 60 percent at that time. In the subject followed the longest, RBC activity was still detectable after 120 days.

Figure 15-2 shows the rise of activity in early urine samples which were collected separately for each voiding for two subjects. It is noteworthy that the peak of 0.05—0.10 percent dose per liter, is reached after about 36

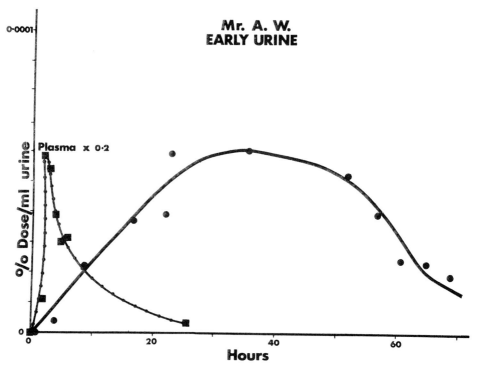

FIGURE 15-2. Rise of radiozinc activity in early separate urine samples.

hours whereas at the time of the peak in plasma activity the urine specific activity is still low. Thus newly absorbed zinc is in a form not cleared by the kidneys but after three days a steady daily loss is established. This probably is a result of newly entered zinc being fairly firmly bound to plasma transport proteins.

In two patients external counting over the liver region was performed from the time of administration of the radiozinc. Although the counter resolution did not permit exclusion of the spleen, pancreas or kidneys, the liver is regarded as the most likely site of the radio zinc. The results for subject R. S. in Figure 15-3 show a rapid rise in liver activity with the plasma, followed by a continued rise as the plasma activity falls. Liver activity starts to fall within one day. No doubt the early measurements are complicated by the passage of unabsorbed radiozinc through the stomach and intestines, but for subject R. S. a logarithmic plot of measure-

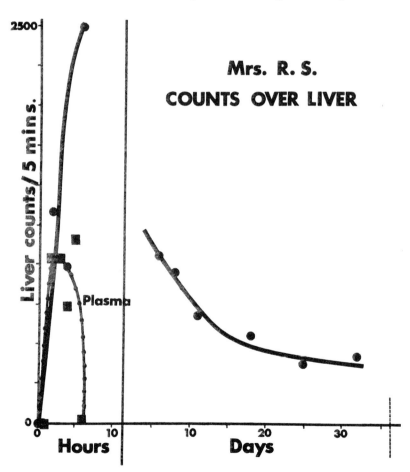

FIGURE 15-3. Radiozinc in liver.

ments over 40 days indicated a good fit to a single exponential with half life in liver for newly absorbed zinc of about 18 days.

As indicated in Figure 15-4 the study failed to detect any preferential uptake of radiozinc by the ulcer which might be expected if zinc were taking a direct part in the healing process. In none of the five subjects was any significant difference in activity between the clear and ulcerated legs detectable. It should be remembered that all the subjects had long-

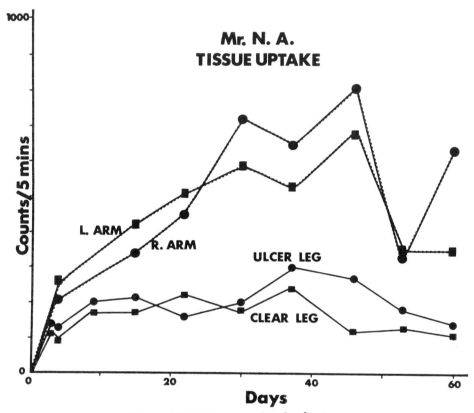

FIGURE 15-4. Tissue uptake of radiozinc.

standing healing problems so this result could simply be confirmation of the correlation between zinc and healing.

Figure 15-4 also shows that radiozinc uptake in the legs, which were measured near the ankles, is low compared with uptake by the muscular tissue of the forearm. Two patients were also measured over the thighs and this confirmed that uptake was concentrated in muscular regions. Calculation showed that the activity of circulating RBC's was far too low to produce the observed count rates. If the uptake was in bone the distribution would have to be very nonuniform to give these results.

It is perhaps significant that the concentration in tissue of radiozinc rises over the same order of time as that in the liver falls. After reaching a peak at 20 to 50 days the tissue activity falls at a similar rate to the whole-body activity.

Figure 15-5 shows the decline in whole-body activity for two subjects. After the initial rapid fall due to excretion of unabsorbed radiozinc the whole-body activity of subject A. W. between days 7 to 70 followed a single exponential with half-life of 54 days. Subject R. S. who was not on

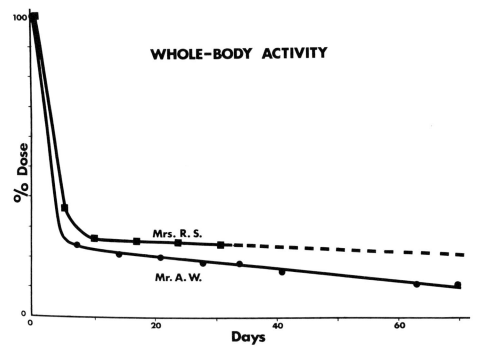

FIGURE 15-5. Decline in whole-body radiozinc activity.

zinc therapy indicated a whole-body half-life of about 200 days from the measurements which were possible. Subject A. W. commenced zinc therapy on day 11 and it is tempting and not unreasonable to ascribe the shorter whole-body half-life to this cause. Further subjects are, of course, needed to give statistically sound support for this conclusion. Extrapolating the exponentials back to zero time gives oral absorption factors for the radiozinc chloride of 25.1 percent and 26.2 percent for these two subjects.

From the foregoing preliminary results an outline of zinc metabolism may be suggested. Oral zinc in ionic form is rapidly absorbed into the bloodstream either from the stomach or duodenum. It is deposited in liver and there is little urinary loss. After one or two days the zinc, presumably in bound form, leaves the liver and accumulates in muscular tissue and

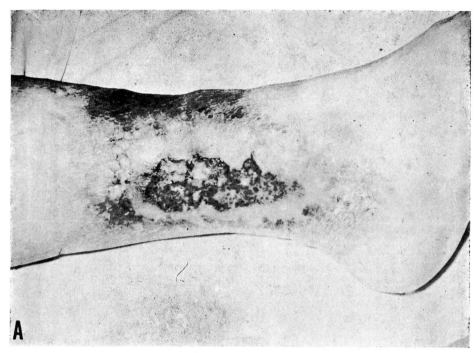

FIGURE 15-6a. Leg ulcer before oral zinc sulfate treatment.

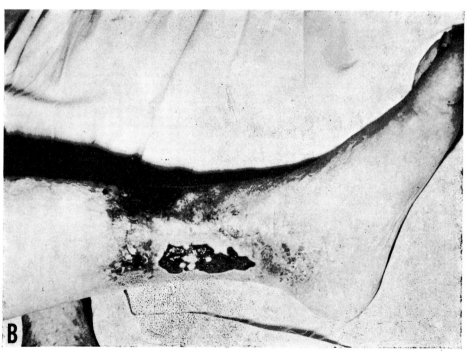

FIGURE 15-6b. Leg ulcer after three weeks treatment with oral zinc sulfate.

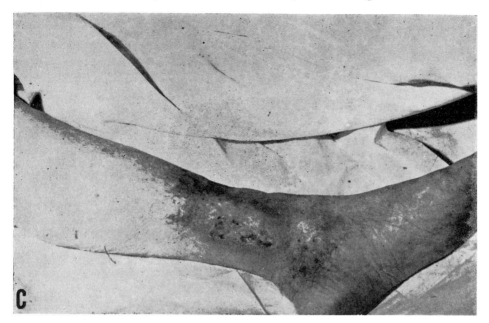

FIGURE 15-6c. Leg ulcer after six weeks treatment with oral zinc sulfate.

loss via urine and feces begins. By about 21 days a maximum concentration is reached in tissue and steady loss of whole body activity is occurring, divided between feces and urine in the ratio of about six to one.

This scheme is very consistent with the observation of Drs. Pories and Strain[8] that it was about 14 days before oral zinc therapy was effective in accelerating healing of surgical wounds. It suggests that where a healing need can be predicted, as in surgery, zinc therapy should be started 2 to 3 weeks beforehand for maximum benefit.

The sixth subject, M. B., who was on the therapy for four months and did not show any improvement was an interesting case. She was 69 years old, suffering from rheumatoid arthritis for fifteen years, had been treated with prednisolone systemically for ten years, and had a plasma zinc level 69 mcg/100ml. After administration of ^{65}Zn no radioactivity was detected in the plasma but 98 percent dose was excreted in the stool in the first 48 hours. Later on malabsorption studies were carried out, and this case was proved to be suffering from the malabsorption syndrome.

SUMMARY

We have now been using oral zinc sulfate in cases for leg ulcers for more than four years and most of the pharmacists in Glasgow are familiar with this type of therapy. We have been using zinc in inpatients and outpatients suffering from leg ulcers and we are quite convinced that the oral zinc sulfate therapy promotes their healing. Although the clinical appearance of the ulcers varied from patient to patient initially, it was quite clear that after 2 to 3 weeks treatment with local therapy combined with zinc sulfate systemically, the ulcers were cleaner and showed healthy granulation tissue. There was also a striking reduction in the purulent exudate. However, it is difficult to assess the effects of many forms of treatment on the healing rate of leg ulcers due to their multi-factorial etiology and the different in size and depth of these ulcers. Initially, in all patients the ulceration had been present for many months or years and failed to respond to conventional treatment. It seems unlikely that the incidence of healing would have been so high in the absence of the oral zinc.

REFERENCES

1. Davies, I. J. T., Musa, M., and Dormandy, T. L.: Measurements of plasma zinc. *J Clin Pathol, 21*:359, 1968.
2. *Extra Pharmacopaeia.* 25th Ed., London, The Pharmaceutical Press, 1968.
3. Greaves, M. W., and Boyde, T. R.: Plasma zinc concentrations in patients with psoriasis, other dermatoses and venous leg ulceration. *Lancet, ii*:1019, 1967.
4. Craig, F. A., and Siegel, E.: Distribution in blood and excretion of Zn^{65} in man. *Proc Soc Exp Biol Med, 104*:351, 1960.
5. Husain, S. L.: Oral zinc sulphate in leg ulcers. *Lancet, i*:1069, 1969.
6. Husain, S. L., Fell, G. S., and Scott, R.: Zinc and healing. *Lancet, ii*:1361, 1970.
7. Munro-Ashman, E. J. E., and Wells, R. S.: The treatment time for varicose ulcers. *Br J Clin Pract, 22*:129, 1968.
8. Pories, W. J., and Strain, W. H.: Zinc and wound healing. In Prasad, A. S.: *Zinc Metabolism.* Springfield, Thomas, 1966.
9. Pories, W. J., Henzel, J. H., Rob, C. G., and Strain, W. H.: Acceleration of healing with zinc sulphate. *Ann Surg, 165*:432, 1967.
10. Pories, W. J., and Strain, W. N.: The functional role of zinc in epidermal tissues. In Mills, C. F. (Ed.): *Trace Element Metabolism in Animals.* Edinburgh, Livingstone, 1970.
11. Prasad, A. S., Miale, A. Jr., Farid, Z., Sandstead, H. H., and Schulert, A. R.: Zinc metabolism in patients with syndrome of iron deficiency anaemia hepatosplenomegaly, hypogonadism, dwarfism. *J Lab Clin Med, 61*:537, 1963.
12. Rivlin, S.: Gravitational leg ulcers in the elderly. *Lancet, i*:1363, 1958.
13. Ross, J. F., Ebaugh, F. G. Jr., and Talbot, T. R. Jr.: Radioisotopic studies of zinc metabolism in human subjects. *Trans Assoc Am Phys, 71*:322, 1958.
14. Savlov, E. D., Strain, W. H., and Huegin, F.: Radiozinc studies in experimental wound healing. *J Surg Res, 2*:209, 1962.
15. Spencer, S., Rosoff, B., Lewin, I., and Samachson, J.: Studies of zinc-65 metabolism in man. In Prasad, A. S. (Ed.): *Zinc Metabolism.* Springfield, Thomas, 1966.

DISCUSSION

Dr. Ronaghy: I am a bit confused about the time which you mentioned. In 30 days your patients' ulcers healed while Dr. Haeger, in a previous

the placebo and the treated group was not significant at all. Now, I wonder what this contradiction is between these two presentations. The other thing is, that I am surprised that you didn't have any complication or any side effect of zinc while you are giving a large dose of zinc, something like 220 mg three times a day, you haven't got anything. While on the treatment of the school children which were put on zinc, we got some dermatitis, abdominal complaints, nausea or vomiting as side effects. We had quite a large number of side effects. I am surprised that you didn't get them.

Dr. Husain: As you have seen in the first study, that the average healing time was 33 days and the span was from 21 days to 71 days and one of the patients 104 days. Fifty-two controls and fifty-two on zinc. As far as the ambulant patients are concerned, the average healing time was 63 days. These are the patients who are hospitalized and who are observed there in the hospital. We were quite sure that they were taking zinc sulfate and those patients who are ambulant, we are not sure whether they were taking the zinc sulfate or not. This may be one explanation.

Now as far as toxic effects are concerned, we have been estimating the electrolytes, urea, liver functions tests and full blood count and ESR and we haven't noticed any toxic effects so far.

Dr. Ronaghy: Laboratory side effects you mean?

Dr. Husain: Yes, and, clinically, we have not noticed any toxic effects. Being a dermatologist, we are very particular to keep looking if there are signs of dermatitis.

Dr. Spencer: I just want to make a remark in regard to the side reactions. As long as one gives zinc sulfate, like any other medication, for instance fluoride, with food in the middle of the meal or half an hour after, we have no problem whatsoever. The gastric irritation and diarrhea or the gastrointestinal symptoms would come if you are not careful about giving it with the food.

Dr. Husain: I quite agree with you. Another point, if I could bring it into this discussion, that when these ulcers heal completely, I stop the treatment and the zinc sulfate was not given after that. And how long were your patients getting the zinc sulfate therapy?

Dr. Ronaghy: Two years. I should like to mention the answer to Dr. Spencer, that we gave this zinc with the help of Dr. Fox who made special cookies for us and these were given along with some food and we really didn't know who was getting what. As you say, it was double blind, but we fairly soon noticed that one group was complaining, while the iron group and placebo group enjoyed their medication.

Dr. Pories: I think there is a marked difference between the ability of people to tolerate zinc sulfate therapy and it depends on their age. I think young patients tolerate it much more poorly, they have many more side effects and complications of gastric irritation. Patients with a pilonidal sinus series had this as a complaint. Patients who we have treated who were much older did not have this problem. So I think age may express the difference between the two groups.

Dr. Prasad: I might like to urge at this point that zinc sulfate is not a very good choice. I think perhaps if you could use zinc carbonate or oxide you would have much less trouble. It looks like, that by tradition, everyone has started to use sulfate and it has become very much ingrained. The very unfortunate thing is that we cannot use any other salt at this time in the United States. We have to use zinc sulfate.

Dr. Spencer: I would like to say that in my work on animals, I found no toxicity either clinically or on autopsy. We used the same proportion per gram of body weight in animals as Pories and Strain used on humans, reducing it by proportion.

Dr. Ronaghy: This is highly individual as we have used the drug for a longer period of time. We have patients who are on six and eight capsules a day depending on the condition that is being treated. We have GI problems with women occasionally, much more so than with men. If your back is really put against the wall, 30 cc. of any of the mint-flavored antacids work marvelously.

Dr. Haeger: I was intrigued by the difference of zinc uptake in the arms and the legs. You had considerably less uptake in the legs. Couldn't that be due to atherosclerotic disease of the legs? In that case, we come to the question of diagnosis of the ulcer. Was that really a pure venous ulcer or was it combined arterial and venous ulcer. This might explain a very long healing time in some cases.

Dr. Husain: That is a very good question which I forgot to mention in my talk. The uptake was less in the legs as compared to the forearm and thighs. It may be due to decreased circulation of muscular in contrast to the bony areas of the leg. There is the other possibility that since these six patients did not respond to zinc sulfate therapy, they might have had lower concentration of zinc in the leg areas.

Regarding the second point of your question, these are chronic patients who had leg ulcers for more than 5 to 8 years. Therefore, any arterial ulcer may have begun as a venous ulcer, and now the arterial deficiency has a definite role in delaying healing.

Chapter 16

DESIGN OF LARGE SCALE CONTROLLED STUDIES OF ZINC THERAPY

JOHN B. HERRMANN

T HE CONCEPT OF A CONTROLLED CLINICAL TRIAL as an indispensable step
in the evaluation of a new therapeutic method has become firmly
established despite considerable reluctance, and even active opposition
on the part of the medical profession. This technique has proven to be
the most reliable and efficient method of evaluating new treatments and
comparing the relative efficacy of various modes of therapy in the management of human disease. The waste of human life and medical resources
due to the application of ineffective, or dangerous methods of treatment
is incalculable. Trial and error techniques and vague "clinical impressions"
are notoriously unreliable as a basis for making therapeutic decisions. Even
retrospective or prospective clinical studies utilizing historical or other
not truly comparable control groups may provide misleading information
leading to erroneous and even hazardous conclusions. All of these methods
may, however, provide information useful in the design of large properly
controlled clinical studies.

The design of an appropriate controlled clinical trial is often the most
difficult part of conducting such a study. There are a number of essential
features which are necessary for the formulation of a controlled clinical
trial. These are:

1. Justification of the need for the study.
2. Availability of sufficient preliminary data.
3. Proper definition of the problem to be solved.
4. Availability of precise methods to evaluate results.
5. Definition of the population to be studied.
6. Assurance of adequate numbers of patients.
7. Choice of an appropriate randomization technique.
8. Identification of primary determinant variables.
9. Formulation of a detailed experimental protocol.
10. Appropriate questionnaires and forms to ensure complete data
    recording.
11. Availability of proper coordination and statistical collaboration.
12. Adequate funding for conduct of the trial.
13. Proper attention to ethical considerations.

Recently we have begun a controlled clinical trial to test the effect
of oral zinc sulfate upon the healing of chronic decubitus ulcers in hu-

mans. This trial, being conducted by a group of Veteran's Administration Hospitals, could easily serve as a model for other large-scale clinical trials of zinc therapy and will be used to illustrate the essentials of a controlled clinical trial listed above.

Justification of the Need for the Study

Delayed wound healing continues to represent a significant clinical problem despite the voluminous research and knowledge which has accumulated concerning the mechanisms of wound repair. Failures and delays in healing still account for the majority of surgical complications and the associated morbidity constitutes a major economic factor both for individuals and for the entire health care system. The need for improvement in this sphere is obvious; and because of the complexity and variability of the repair mechanism, carefully controlled clinical studies are essential.

The trace element zinc has been implicated as an essential ingredient of the healing mechanism, and presumed deficiencies of zinc have been found in a wide number of chronic conditions. The application of zinc therapy to healing problems in humans under the conditions of a controlled clinical trial appears warranted.

Availability of Sufficient Preliminary Data

Prior to the design of a controlled clinical trial, sufficient preliminary information must be available in the form of both laboratory and preliminary clinical studies to determine the safety and the efficacy of the treatment under consideration. In the case of zinc, there is abundant experimental evidence in the literature that this trace element plays an important role in growth, development, and the repair of injured tissues. There is also abundant clinical evidence that oral zinc therapy in the form of zinc sulfate, 220 mg p.o. t.i.d. is both safe and undeniably efficacious in the treatment of disorders of growth and development associated with zinc deficiency. This dose also appears to be effective in the treatment of delayed wound healing due to a number of causes and also possibly effective in the treatment of other diseases such as atherosclerosis obliterans. Sufficient background information is therefore available upon which to formulate a number of controlled clinical trials of oral zinc therapy. Zinc sulfate is probably not the most effective form of zinc therapy but sufficient background information is not yet available to recommend a change at this time.

The background of this present controlled trial must include a preliminary study conducted by Dr. James Halsted and myself at the Veterans Administration Hospital in Washington, D.C. several years ago. This study was a random, double-blind, clinical study comparing the effects of oral zinc sulfate, 220 mg p.o. t.i.d. with a placebo upon the rate of healing of chronic cutaneous ulcers in humans. The study included patients with ulcers due to arterial insufficiency, venous insufficiency, other non-specific ulcers, and ulcers of the decubitus type. The results of this study, although not statistically significant because of insufficient numbers of patients, were striking. Patients who had received zinc showed improvement in their ulcers, while patients receiving a placebo showed progression of their lesions (Fig. 16-1). In addition, the majority of patients with

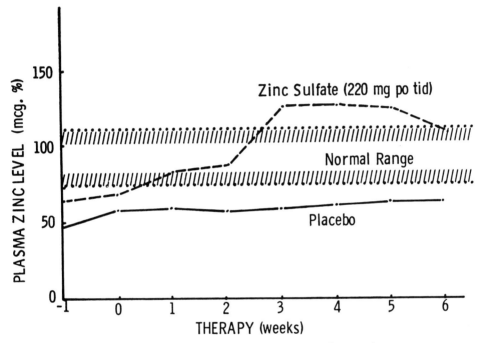

FIGURE 16-1. Average plasma zinc levels in treated and control patients in a preliminary study of the effects of oral zinc on the healing of chronic cutaneous ulcers.

these chronic ulcers were apparently zinc deficient at least upon the basis of plasma zinc levels (Fig. 16-2). We felt that this provided sufficient indication to conduct a large scale cooperative study of the effects of oral zinc therapy upon healing.

Proper Definition of the Problem to be Solved

Historically, some clinical trials, although properly conducted, have yielded results of no real benefit because the preliminary formulation of

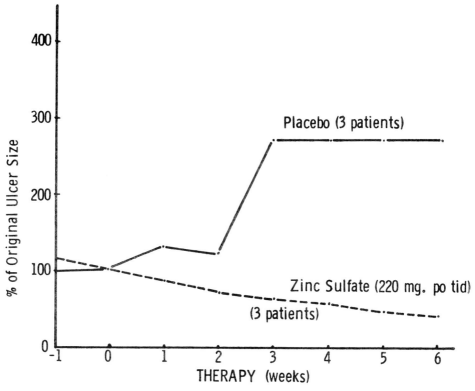

FIGURE 16-2. Changes in ulcer size of patients treated with oral zinc or a placebo in a preliminary trial of the effects of oral zinc sulfate on the healing of chronic cutaneous ulcers.

the problem was not correct. An appropriate formulation should ideally pose a basic question to which a yes or no answer can be given. A careful review of the literature and our own preliminary results indicated that two major questions in the area of zinc and wound healing needed to be answered: (1) Does oral zinc improve the rate of healing?; and (2) Does zinc deficiency play a determinant role in the vulnerary effects of zinc therapy? Our current study is designed to answer both of these questions.

Availability of Precise Methods to Evaluate Results

Objective methods of evaluating results are extremely important if useful information is to be derived from any clinical trial. The objective measurement of wound healing, however, presents certain problems. One of the reasons for using decubitus ulcers in our present study was that these lesions can be evaluated by nondestructive techniques rather than resorting to the biopsies and tensile strength measurements used for incised wounds. Perhaps the simplest criteria for the measurement of healing in open wounds of the decubitus type would be "time to complete healing". This method, despite its simplicity and ease of statistical analysis, was not considered applicable for this study because of the notoriously slow healing of ulcers of this type, and because of the difficulty in defining an appropriate end point. The length of time required in many cases would be an undue hardship on patient, professional staff and hospital and would deny the use of accepted plastic surgical procedures for these patients.

We therefore elected to perform serial measurements of ulcer area and volume which can be used to develop healing curves for each ulcer. These curves tend to follow a log-linear pattern with respect to time. The average rate of healing of control and experimental groups thus calculated over a 10 week interval can then be compared and correlated with many of the other variables documented on the report forms used in the study.

Uniformity and accuracy of measurements obtained is strengthened by using both direct and photographic measurement techniques with independent evaluation by impartial judges. This is extremely important to ensure uniformity when a number of investigators are involved in independent observations.

Definition of the Population to be Studied

Prior to the initiation of a clinical trial, the investigators must have a firm knowledge of the characteristics of the population from which the study sample will be drawn. The results of the study will theoretically only apply to this population and then only if the sample is truly representative of the entire population. A randomly chosen sample is ideal, but rarely possible in clinical investigations.

Confining our current investigation to patients in Veterans Hospitals poses certain well recognized limitations in interpretation and extrapolation of results. This has not, however, proven to be a serious problem in the many controlled clinical trials conducted within the Veterans Administration Hospital System.

In our initial phases of planning, it was necessary to make certain decisions regarding the population which we would be studying. Rather than including a wide variety of diseases with diverse etiologies, we felt that limitation to a certain lesion was of practical benefit. For a number of reasons, decubiti, or pressure sores, were chosen as an appropriate study lesion. One reason for choosing this entity was the difficult problem that patients with this type of lesion present in any hospital, particularly in a VA hospital. A review of recent VA statistics (Fig. 16-3) revealed that the incidence of decubitus ulcers was rising rapidly in the veteran population. The reasons for this were not clear but probably related to changing

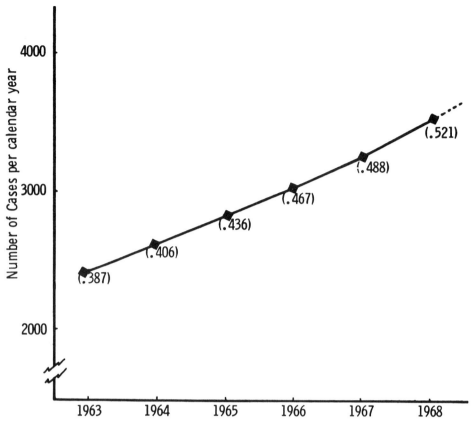

FIGURE 16-3. Incidence of decubitus ulcers in the V.A. Hospital System 1963 to 1968. Figures based upon hospital discharge diagnosis. Percentage of total VA discharges shown in parentheses.

factors in the veteran population rather than specific factors in treatment because the increase was limited to certain age groups (Fig. 16-4) and not an overall increase. Spinal cord injury is a very common denominator in the development of decubiti. We have carefully avoided limiting our study to this group, however, so that the results of the study will not be limited to this group and have more general application.

The design of an appropriate experimental protocol must include a specific list of criteria for eligibility of patients for the study; and another list of specific criteria for excluding some of these patients from the final study group. It is extremely valuable to collect data on patients who are excluded for one reason or another but were otherwise eligible. In our current study a screening log is kept to record such information for later analysis.

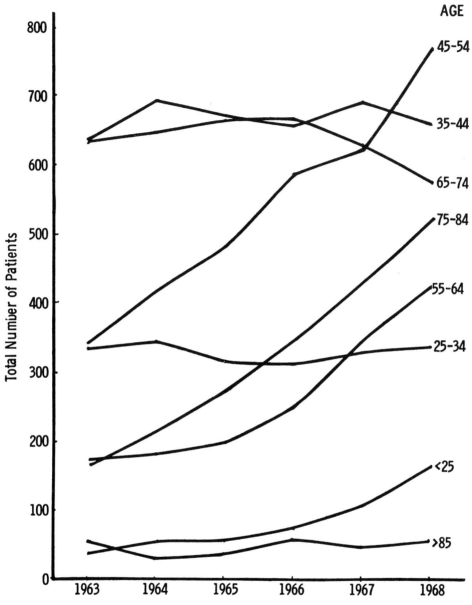

FIGURE 16-4. Age distribution of decubitus ulcers. V. A. Hospital System 1963 to 1968.

Assurance of Adequate Numbers of Patients

Although it is often impossible to accurately predict how many patients will be necessary to provide an adequate study, statistical methods are available which will provide reasonable estimates based upon preliminary studies and a careful estimation of the magnitude of difference which would be significant.[2] Close communication between the investigator and his consultant statistician at this point is necessary to arrive at some reasonable figure. In our study, we estimate that at least 100 patients will be necessary for meaningful interpretation.

Preliminary figures, however, have a tendency to escalate once the project is underway; and therefore, it is necessary to ensure that more than adequate numbers of patients will be available within a reasonable period of time. In many situations, including our study, sufficient patients are not available in any one area for this purpose, and therefore cooperative efforts among several or many investigators in a number of hospitals are necessary for conduct of the trial.

The cooperative clinical trial in which the resources of several hospitals and investigators are combined has become an increasingly important method of conducting controlled clinical studies. The first large study of this type was conducted by the Veterans Administration and the Armed Forces to evaluate the chemotherapy of tuberculosis.[1] Numerous other cooperative studies have been organized since then, primarily in the field of cancer chemotherapy; and many of these have involved the Veterans Administration hospital system. This organization is ideally suited to studies of this type. Because of this unique capability, the VA Research Service has been quite receptive to funding controlled studies of the cooperative type. Our current study has been reviewed and approved by the VA Research Service and has, within the past month, become fully operational. At present, a total of 5 hospitals with 2 investigators in each hospital are cooperating in this controlled study.

One problem which became obvious in attempting to study something as unexciting as decubitus ulcers was that very few physicians were interested in this problem. On the other hand, the prevention and treatment of decubitus ulcers has long been a vital part of nursing care and a considerable amount of interest in this problem was expressed by the VA Nursing Service. Accordingly, the study was organized as a combined project of nurses and physicians. To my knowledge, this is the first cooperative study in which nurses have played a key role as co-principal investigators.

Choice of An Appropriate Randomization Technique

Allocation of patients to treatment groups must be performed by strict randomization. Historical comparisons; comparisons between hospitals; alternating techniques; and assignment by birth date, social security number, day of week, etc., are not acceptable. Patients who refuse treatment or are not treated for other extraneous reasons are not suitable controls.

Groups chosen by any technique other than strict randomization are not likely to be truly comparable.

An even more insidious error can occur after randomization if the care of the patients differs from one group to another in aspects other than the specific treatment under study. This can be best avoided by utilizing a "double-blind" technique in which neither the patient nor the physician knows what treatment is being given. This technique is not always feasible, and other methods to assure uniformity of management and assessment must be considered. We have utilized the "double-blind" technique in both our preliminary and our current study.

Randomization in our study was performed so that equal numbers of patients will be assigned to treatment and control groups and sequencing at each participating hospital has been accomplished so that numerical equality of control and experimental groups will occur in steps of every 10 patients.

Identification of Primary Determinant Variables

All of the variables which may influence the course of treatment cannot, of course, be identified prior to the trial. Known, or highly suspected variables, should, however, be anticipated and the study designed to take these into account. Other variables which might influence the treatment should be identified for later analysis. Randomization of groups will theoretically evenly disperse these factors so that the validity of the study in terms of its primary purpose will not be impaired even if the suspected variable turns out to be highly significant. Further controlled studies will usually be necessary to fully resolve the effects if they appear of significant importance unless they were incorporated as a primary factor in the original study design.

The potential variables involved in a process as complex as healing are indeed legion. Age, underlying disease, nutrition, level of activity, infection, location, status of surrounding tissue, ancillary therapeutic endeavors and nursing care practices are but a few of the many variables which we have considered. We have attempted to control a few of these variables, such as ancillary therapeutic measures, by specific instructions in the protocol, but the remainder have been left as random variables. One additional important variable found in all cooperative studies is the variability between participating hospitals. Upon recommendation of various consultants and reviewers, we are attempting to control this undefined variable by stratification of the randomization scheme. This will ensure that equal numbers of control and treated patients will occur at each participating hospital. The problem of zinc deficiency was also recognized as a probable significant variable, but since this state is difficult to define, we felt that controlling this factor would be perilous and not worth the additional complexity of experimental design required.

Formulation of a Detailed Experimental Protocol

Considerable time and effort must be spent in developing a detailed protocol for the conduct of the trial. This protocol should be specific in regards to patient selection and exclusion, the randomization scheme to be used, the experimental design and the method of analysis to be used, the criteria of assessment of the effects of treatment, the number of subjects required, the details of the treatment under test, the ancillary therapeutic measures to be employed, the recording forms that will be used to document progress of the patient and possibly significant variables, and the general organization of the trial. In a collaborative study, all participants must agree to follow the specifics in the protocol.

There is often considerable pressure to change portions of the protocol after the study is underway, particularly in fields in which knowledge is being rapidly accumulated. Careful experimental design will minimize tendencies to change the protocol by anticipating problems which might occur. Occasionally, however, changes must be made. This occasionally can be accomplished without significant damage to the study, but often the study will have to be restarted.

Over a year was spent in designing the current trial of zinc therapy of decubitus ulcers including several meetings with consultants, reviewers and participating investigators. It is still too early to assess the results of our efforts to avoid pitfalls but we hope that the time and effort was worthwhile.

Appropriate Questionnaires and Forms to Ensure Complete Data Recording

The same careful planning must go into the design of appropriate recording forms that was used in the protocol design. Forms should be complete in regard to necessary information but not overburdened with extraneous matter. They should be in a form readily transcribed for computer processing. This usually means a check list type form rather than a narrative report. It often requires considerable effort to design forms which are specific without ambiguity and which incorporate all the necessary information.

At least two forms are necessary—an initial form to be completed when the patient enters the study and a follow up form to record the progress of the patient under treatment. Usually, the follow up form is completed periodically throughout the course of the study, and often a final form is necessary at the completion of the study to record any changes in the multiple variables detailed in the initial form.

Our current study employs an initial form, a weekly report form to be completed during the twelve weeks of the study period and a final report form. All are of the check list variety for expediency in data processing. Because of the many variables inherent in wound healing problems of this type, the forms are somewhat more detailed than ideal, but hopefully will not place too great a burden on the investigators.

Availability of Proper Coordination and Statistical Collaboration

A controlled clinical trial is an important piece of experimental work. As such, sufficient time and effort must be devoted to it to ensure that results will be meaningful. Proper administration of the study is a prime requisite, particularly in cooperative studies where the coordination of a number of investigators is necessary. It is necessary to ensure that forms are being completed properly, the protocol is being adhered to, and that patients are being properly entered into the study. It is also necessary to maintain close contact with investigators, to distribute information when it is available, and to check on the homogeniety of work from different centers.

The active collaboration and participation of a statistician is essential in the conduct of a controlled clinical trial. It is important that the statistician be involved in the preparation of the protocol and forms as well as the continued interpretation of results. It is extremely difficult for a statistician to make meaningful interpretations from data derived from a study which was not properly designed to yield such information. A competent statistician can be of extreme value in choosing the appropriate experimental design, designing appropriate forms, monitoring the data as it comes in, and analyzing the results of the study.

We are fortunate to have the services of Dr. Leonard Chiazzi from the Division of Biostatistics of the Georgetown University as an active consultant in our VA Cooperative Study on the Effect of Oral Zinc Sulphate on the Healing of Decubitus Ulcers.

Adequate Funding for the Conduct of the Trial

Controlled clinical trials of the type outlined here are expensive. Adequate funding for the proper conduct of such a trial is essential if meaningful results are to be obtained. Although the greatest single cost of conducting such a trial—the professional time and effort involved—is most commonly provided gratis by an interested investigator or group of investigators, funds are necessary for travel, the preparation of forms, obtaining appropriate equipment and supplies, laboratory studies, statistical support and computer time, and many other items.

Within recent years the Veterans Administration has recognized the need for controlled clinical trials and has encouraged such trials within the Veterans Administration System. The VA is uniquely suited to investigative work of this type, particularly when the collaborative efforts of a number of hospitals are required. We have, therefore, been able to obtain funding from the Veterans Administration for the conduct of this study.

In addition to providing funds, the VA has also provided us with a careful critical review of the protocol with a number of suggestions which were extremely helpful in strengthening the study.

Proper Attention to Ethical Considerations

Last, but not least, is the question of ethics. This is still an extremely controversial topic. Recent guidelines have emphasized the necessity for informed consent on the part of patients involved in clinical trials. Despite the furor created by the strict requirement of informed consent, in practice this has not been a serious stumbling block in the conduct of clinical trials. Perhaps a more important question involves the ethics of controlled clinical trials in general. The guidelines proposed by Mr. John Hayward of Guy's Hospital, London, at the Ninth International Cancer Congress,[4] perhaps most adequately express the current feeling on this problem:

1. It is unethical to attempt to analyse the effect of a treatment by the haphazard and uncontrolled administration of that treatment.

2. It is unethical not to carry out a clinical trial when there is doubt whether a new treatment is better than an established treatment.

3. It is unethical to conduct a clinical trial unless the clinical and statistical design of the trial is appropriate.

4. It is unethical to carry out a clinical trial without due responsibility for the patients' care and, if the procedures do not contribute to the benefit of the patients, without their understanding and permission.

5. It is unethical to terminate a clinical trial unless a meaningful result has been obtained.

We hope that this study will provide an incentive and guide for others in establishing additional properly controlled trials of zinc therapy in humans.

REFERENCES

1. Canada, R. O., Allison, S. T., and D'Esopo, N. D., Dunner, E., Moyer, R. E., Shamaskin, A., Tempel, C. W., and Charter, W. V.: Three-year follow-up study on 202 cases of pulmonary tuberculosis treated with streptomycin. *Am Rev Tuberculosis, 62*:563, 1950.

2. Gehan, E. A.: The determination of the number of patients required in a preliminary and a follow-up trial of a new chemotherapeutic agent. *J Chronic Dis*, 13:346, 1961.
3. Flamant, R. (Ed.): *Controlled Therapeutic Trials*, Geneva, Switzerland, International Union Against Cancer, Technical Report Series, vol. 7, 1970.
4. Hayward, J. L.: Ethics in Clinical Trials. UICC Monograph Series Vol. 10: Ninth International Cancer Congress, Springer-Verlag, Heidelberg, 1967.
5. Higgins, G. A.: Controlled therapeutic trials. *Arch Surg*, 102:160, 1971.

DISCUSSION

Dr. Herrmann: I have tried to outline some of the basic fundamentals for you, and I hope this will be a stimulus to members of the audience here to conduct such trials. I think they are sorely needed in this field and I hope that a number of them can be started in such fields such as peripheral vascular disease which you will hear about tomorrow, etc. I did not go into too much of the details of our own study. It is just underway and we have no results as yet, obviously. Those of you who may be interested in the protocol and experimental design, I will be glad to furnish with a copy of our protocol if you'll just give me your name and address. Thank you very much.

Dr. Henzel: John, I have one very rapid question concerning the patient population in most VA hospitals. One is the chronic alcohol imbiber, and the second is the patient with major psychiatric problems. We know that the chronic alcoholic has abnormal zinc metabolism and I think Dr. Pfeiffer tomorrow is going to talk a little about some of the micronutrient abnormalities in some of the psychiatric states. Have you built this into your protocol allowing for this?

Dr. Hermann: No we have not. As I mentioned, zinc deficiency is a problem we find very difficult to define and therefore these are random variables that will be handled in this fashion. We will obviously look at this as time goes on. I am not too sure that many of these particular groups of patients that you mention will be a part of the study. At the moment it appears that the paraplegic patient will be the greatest number in the study and our other patients will be sort of distributed around chronic neurological disease, chronic brain syndromes, etc. So the psychiatric and the alcoholic patients will probably comprise a fairly small number although certainly some of them can be paraplegic or have chronic brain disease too. Are there any other questions?

Dr. Spencer: How will you standardize the ancillary therapy also given to your patients in five different hospitals?

Dr. Hermann: This is a hard nut to crack and it is very difficult to get any two doctors to agree on what the right method of treatment of any condition is, much less something as complex as this. We have attempted to provide certain guidelines which all of us have agreed to. We realize that the primary therapeutic effort for decubitus ulcers must be to prevent pressure and, therefore, this is the primary goal. We still see too many patients who are allowed to lie flat in bed for prolonged periods of time so that this is rigidly controlled. The other factor that we have attempted to control is to avoid the use of a wide variety of local treatments on the ulcer. We are sticking to saline dressings without the use of various ointments, or local antibiotics or things of this nature which would possibly confuse the picture. All the investigators have agreed to this, although obviously we are going to have to check to be sure that this is being followed.

Dr. Henkin: One of the problems that has disturbed me about the entire series of papers we have heard this afternoon on ulcers is that ancillary methods of treatment certainly are useful and, in fact, can be therapeutic. This statement was made by Dr. Haeger and was obviously shared by others. You mentioned that ancillary measures would be used in your study. I am concerned about the way in which you can handle these in five different hospitals—what you allow and what you do not allow, how vigorous the ancillary therapies are, and how you handle that problem in a double-blind study. It is a very diffuse base.

Chapter 17

PANEL DISCUSSION FOR SECTION C
ZINC AND HEALING

(Panel discussion was omitted because of lateness of the hour)

SECTION D

Chapter 18

SUPPLEMENTARY TREATMENT FOR ORAL TISSUE HEALING

JAMES F. SMITH

AND

JAMES BELL

THE INCIDENCE OF PROLONGED HEALING following oral surgery has been reduced by improved surgical methods and new knowledge of post-operative tissue response. However, some problems—such as localized osteitis or "dry socket"—persist regardless of the amount and quality of pre and postoperative care.

While much is still unknown about delayed healing, dietary supplements have proven to be of benefit in some instances. Vitamin C and the B Complex group have been used for years to improve healing, and recently interest has been revived in the possible healing value of zinc sulfate, particularly in difficult cases.

Some investigators feel that unless a vitamin deficiency is actually present, vitamin supplements are not needed and will not aid healing. This is erroneous; over a period of many years, a large number of well-documented cases have been reported in which supplementary vitamins and minerals have shortened healing periods and reduced various complications.[1]

Although little work has been done with the effects of zinc and healing in the oral cavity, much work has been done in regard to other pathological conditions. Abnormally low zinc levels, for example, have been linked to ectodermal and embryonic defects, Laennec's cirrhosis, poor skin graft acceptance, alcoholic cirrhosis, active tuberculosis, indolent ulcers, cystic fibrosis and myocardial infarct.[2]

The results of extensive research have led some scientists to conclude that a direct correlation exists between body zinc stores and the rate of wound healing, which would suggest that zinc may play a key role in the healing process. Studies have also indicated that a fall in plasma zinc levels occurs after acute tissue injury, regardless of origin,[3] and noticeable improvement in alveolar bone healing has been reported in zinc-supplemented hamsters which received experimental extraction wounds.[4]

Larson et al.[5], in discussing patients who had small chronic wounds with minimal epithelization and poor skin graft acceptance, stated there was an improvement after zinc therapy and the rate of epithelization was apparently faster and graft acceptance seemed better.

Halsted and Smith[6] found abnormally low zinc values in alcoholic cirrhosis, active tuberculosis, indolent ulcers, cystic fibrosis and myocardial infarct. Savlov et al.[4] showed by studies of radiozinc retention in experimental wound healing in rats with incised abdominal wounds, a preferential accumulation of radioactivity in the acute healing stage of incised wounds. Measurements made on the scar connective tissue of the excised wounds after one hundred days showed very low retention of radiozinc compared to the surrounding skin and hair.

Bottomley et al.[3] state that a direct correlation exists between body zinc stores and the rate of wound healing which suggests that zinc may play a key role in the healing process. They further state that their studies indicated that a fall in plasma zinc levels occurs after acute tissue injury, regardless of origin.[5] Prasad[6] presented an excellent history of the research on the metabolic role of zinc, which is worthy of careful reading by those interested in the role of zinc in healing.

Pories et al.[9] report that zinc is intimately involved in healing and that zinc deficient animals heal poorly. In their work, oral medication with 220 milligrams of zinc sulfate three times daily, resulted in the acceleration of healing by 43 percent in a well-controlled study of young men with granulating wounds.[5]

Sandstead et al.[10] in a study of zinc in wound healing found that histological examination of twelve-day postoperative incisions from zinc deficient controlled rats showed fewer fibroblasts in the region of the healing incision of the zinc-deprived animal and decreased density of the collagen. They concluded from their studies that tensile strength of healing incision is decreased by dietary deficiency of zinc.[11] Henzel et al.[12] in discussing zinc concentration in healing wounds, state that from the summated results of laboratory and clinical studies, it would appear that zinc participates in certain biochemical processes which precede or underlie histogenesis of wound repair and that the efficiency with which these processes are able to function during wound healing is probably dependent upon local sufficiency of zinc.

Because of these and other research efforts, we chose to treat a group of dental patients during pre- and post-operative stages with combined vitamin supplements and zinc sulfate. The compound selected contained, in each instance, 80 milligrams zinc sulfate, ascorbic acid, thiamine mononitrate calcium pantothenate, riboflavin, magnesium sulfate, and pyridoxine.* Patients were chosen who could be used as their own control by means of multiple surgical procedures.

*Kindly supplied by Meyer Laboratories as Vicon-C® capsules.

MATERIALS AND METHODS

We selected 25 patients, each of whom had had either a history of "dry socket" from extractions of teeth or who had presented some problem with delayed healing of oral mucous membranes. Each needed bilateral oral surgery.

In order to obtain comparisons, the corresponding teeth could be selected for removal on opposite sides of the mouth, or similar periodontal surgery could be performed.

One tooth was surgically removed or surgery performed on one side of the mouth, without pre or postoperative treatment, and healing time was observed, noted and recorded. Tissue from a site close to the healing area was biopsied at one-week intervals for 3 weeks.

On the opposite side, after a one month healing period, the patient was treated preoperatively with three zinc-vitamin capsules daily. This preparation was given morning, noon and night one month prior to surgery. The treatment was continued on the day of surgery and for two months postoperatively. Biopsies were performed by dentists who were not familiar with the patient nor his treatment and their evaluation and observations were recorded. The biopsy tissues were seen by an oral pathologist, who again was not familiar with the treated or untreated patients and he was asked to record his findings.

Three stains—hemotoxylin and eosin, Azan blue and elastin stain—were chosen in order to determine epithelization, connective tissue regeneration and inflammatory cell infiltrate.

All data were tested by Chi-square analysis.

RESULTS

The results of visual estimation of tissue healing evaluation (See Table 18-I) were as follows: Sixteen of twentyfive patients who had a previous history of poor tissue healing showed good tissue response when treated with Vicon-C.® Six showed fair tissue response in healing, which was an improvement over their previous healing history, while three showed no improvement in healing. The evaluations were made by three oral surgeons

TABLE 18-I

TISSUE HEALING EVALUATION

Healing	*Control*	*Treated*
Good	2	16
Fair	11	6
Poor	12	3

who did not know the history of the patient, and the visual evaluation was rated as good, fair or poor. We realize the limitations in this method of evaluation, but it was interesting to have the opinions of the observers in order to determine the comparison of these results with histopathological findings.

In the histological examination of these patients, the three who had shown clinically poor tissue healing were reported as having incomplete epithelization of the wound and a persistant inflammatory cell infiltrate. Of the sixteen who had been rated as good tissue healing, all sixteen were reported as having good epithelization, (See Tables 18-II and 18-III) evidence of good fibroblastic response and regeneration of supporting

TABLE 18-II

EPITHELIZATION EVALUATION

	Control	*Treated*
Good	2	16
Fair	13	6
Poor	10	3

TABLE 18-III

CONNECTIVE TISSUE EVALUATION

	Control	*Treated*
Good	2	16
Fair	16	9
Poor	7	0

subepithelial tissue with a limited number of inflammatory cells during the observation of the second biopsy, and few or no inflammatory cells at the third examination. Of those patients remaining, six were reported as having complete epithelization, but did not show fibroblastic response expected at this particular stage of their healing.

No dry sockets developed in the treated patients (See Table 18-IV). All of these patients had had previous experience with localized osteitis or "dry socket" after tooth extraction.

TABLE 18-IV

LOCALIZED OSTEITIS

Osteitis	*Control*	*Treated*
Extractions	17	17
Local osteitis	17	0

CONCLUSION

From the results we concluded that there was a definite improvement in the majority (64 percent) of the patients treated with the vitamin-zinc supplement. Another 24 percent demonstrated a fair degree of improved healing. From these initial findings we plan to work with the healing problems of the diabetic patient undergoing oral surgery procedures.

REFERENCES

1. Clark, J. W., Cheraskin, E., and Ringsdorf, W. M. Jr.: *Diet and the Periodontal Patient*. Springfield, Thomas, 1970, pp. 120-162.
2. Boyett, J. D., and Sullivan, J. F.: Zinc and collagen content of cirrhotic liver. *Am J Dig Dis, 15*(9):797, 1970.
3. Bottomley, R. G., Cornelisen, R. L., and Lindeman, R. D.: Zinc metabolism following acute tissue injury in man. *Clin Res, 17*:82, 1969.
4. Mesrobian, A. Z., and Sklar, G. T.: The effect of gingival healing of dietary supplements of zinc sulfate in the syrian hamster. *Periodontics, 6*:224, 1968.
5. Larson, D. L., Maxwell, R., Abston, S., and Debrkovsky, M.: Zinc deficiency in burned children. *Plast Reconstr Surg, 46*:13, 1970.
6. Halsted, J. A., and Smith, J. C., Jr.: Plasma zinc in health and disease. *Lancet i*:322, 1970.
7. Savlov, E. D., Strain, W. H., and Huegin, F.: Radiozinc studies in experimental wound healing. *J Surg Res, 2*:229, 1962.
8. Prasad, A. S.: A century of research on the metabolic role of zinc. *Am J Clin Nutr, 22*:1215, 1969.
9. Pories, W. J., Henzel, J. H., Rob, C. G., and Strain, W. H.: Acceleration of healing with zinc sulfate. *Ann Surg, 165*:432, 1967.
10. Sandstead, H. H., Lanier, V. C., Jr., Shepard, G. H., and Gillespie, D. D.: Zinc and wound healing: Effects of zinc deficiency and zinc supplementation. *Am J Clin Nutr, 23*:514, 1970.
11. Sandstead, H. H., and Shepard, G. H.: The effect of zinc deficiency on the tensile strength of healing surgical incisions in the integument of the rat. *Proc Soc Exp Biol Med, 128*:687, 1968.
12. Henzel, J. H., DeWeese, M. S., and Lichti, E. L.: Zinc concentrations within healing wounds. *Arch Surg, 100*:349, 1970.

DISCUSSION

Dr. Mesrobian: I would like to thank Dr. Woosley in the absence of Dr. Smith. I would like to know about the 17 extractions with 17 cases of localized osteitis or dry sockets, as otherwise known. I hope you don't mean that in each of these 17 extractions all had localized osteitis because the percentage is much lower than that.

Dr. Woosley: Yes, you are quite correct. These patients were selected for their history of poor healing and would be likely candidates for dry sockets.

Chapter 19

ZINC AND TASTE ACUITY: A CLINICAL STUDY INCLUDING A LASER MICROPROBE ANALYSIS OF THE GUSTATORY RECEPTOR AREA

Robert I. Henkin, Paul J. Schecter, Morton S. Raff, Diane A. Bronzert
AND William T. Friedewald

INTRODUCTION

Decreased taste acuity (hypogeusia) in man has been associated with several clinical disorders[1-6] and follows administration of some drugs (geusatoxicity), surgical procedures not necessarily involving the oral area, various malabsorptive states and acute illnesses of several types, usually including those influenza-like in origin. In general, patients with hypogeusia following surgery, various malabsorptive states or influenza-like illnesses exhibit significantly lower than normal concentrations of serum zinc and treatment with zinc ion has returned both their hypogeusia and serum zinc levels to normal.

This present paper will deal with a systematic study of 103 patients who developed hypogeusia and their treatment with either placebo or zinc ion in a single blind study. In addition a study of the localization of zinc in the tongue of rat and man will be discussed in an effort to demonstrate the role which zinc may play in the gustatory system.

CLINICAL HISTORY AND METHODS OF STUDY

Patients

The patients consisted of 48 males and 55 females with a mean age of 55 years (range, 25-81 yrs). The average duration of the illness at the time they were first seen at the N.I.H. Clinical Center was 3.5 years (range, 7 months-49 yrs).

The racial distribution of the patients was 102 Caucasians and one Negro. This distribution may not necessarily indicate an increased incidence of this syndrome in any one race but may reflect economic and social factors. During the evaluation and treatment periods each patient was required to travel to the N.I.H. on several occasions at his own expense and each had to be referred by his local physician who was willing to resume care of the patient when the diagnosis and/or treatment was established. Furthermore, since each patient commonly informed his own physician about the existence of this disease from his perusal of publications in the lay press, an awareness of this source of information was a common, unanticipated, requirement for evaluation and treatment. Since compiling these data, four additional Negro patients with this disease have been evaluated.

There is no apparent geographical localization of this syndrome as patients have come from all portions of the U.S.A. as well as from several European and one Asian country.

Onset Of Symptoms

The onset of this syndrome can be grouped into three patterns: 1) 57 percent (59 to 103) reported that their symptoms began during or shortly after an upper respiratory illness which was usually accompanied by a fever of at least 3 days duration (66 percent). Many patients experienced this febrile illness during the winter and spring of 1968 to 1969 and their disease was termed "Hong-Kong flu" by their local physicians. Thirty-one of these 59 had experienced decreased taste and smell acuity during previous upper respiratory illnesses with sensory acuity returning to normal within a few days after the illness had subsided. In the case of the last upper respiratory illness, however, normal acuity did not return, and the patients sought medical advice. 2) 33 percent (34 of 103) reported no illness or unusual event preceding their sensory loss. 3) The remaining patients (10 of 103) reported several events preceding the onset of symptoms. Three patients reported onset immediately following various uncomplicated surgical procedures unrelated to the head or neck. With the first oral intake post operation they noted alterations in taste. The operative procedures were a colectomy, a gastrectomy and a vagotomy and pyloroplasty. Seven patients reported loss of taste acuity after events which may be termed unusual in that they are not usually considered to affect taste acuity. One patient experienced loss of taste after a traumatic ear irrigation without puncture of the tympanic membrane. Two patients reported onset after excessive ethanolic intake, one reported onset after her local physician gave her a "cold shot", one after a disturbing event in her personal life, one after a local anesthetic was injected by his dentist for a routine tooth extraction with persistence of symptoms after analgesia had worn off, and one reported onset during the 7th month of an uncomplicated pregnancy with persistence of symptoms following delivery.

Eighty-four percent (86 of 103) reported a sudden onset of symptoms. With two exceptions, all patients with a preceding upper respiratory illness had a sudden onset of taste and smell loss. Thirteen of 15 patients with a gradual onset had no preceding illness or event prior to their taste or smell loss.

Thirty-six percent (37 of 103) reported some spontaneous variation in their level of taste acuity. At no time from the time of onset of symptoms until they were seen at the N.I.H. did these patients feel that their taste or smell acuity had returned to normal levels.

Associated Abnormalities

Sixty percent of the patients had no known allergies. Those patients who reported allergies were hypersensitive to a variety of substances and drugs but no consistent pattern could be established between allergic phenomena and onset or severity of symptoms.

Fourteen percent (14 of 103) had a history of hypertension which was discovered from 3 weeks to 20 years prior to their initial N.I.H. visit. In 11 cases the hypertension had preceded the onset of their hypogeusia from 6 months to 19 years. One patient developed hypertension many years after his loss of taste acuity and in two patients the onset of hypogeusia occurred apparently simultaneously with the hypertension. Three additional patients were found to have elevated blood pressures (i.e. diastolic B.P > 100 mm Hg) at their initial visit to our clinic.

Of 22 patients questioned, 6 (27 percent) noted a decrease in sexual libido which could be directly related in time to the onset of their symptoms of decreased taste and smell.

Description of Symptoms

TASTE: *Hypogeusia,* or a generalized decrease in taste acuity, was reported by 93 percent of the patients (96 of 103). Seven percent (7 of 103) did not complain of hypogeusia but complained either of dysgeusia, hyposmia or dysosmia.

Dysgeusia is a term used to describe any distortion of normal taste perception. This symptom was reported by 44 percent of the patients (45 of 103), three of whom were subjectively unaware of any decreased taste acuity. Forty-two of these patients noted subjective hypogeusia. Dysgeusia may be manifested in several different ways; three of these have been labeled by us *cacogeusia, phantogeusia,* and *heterogeusia.*

Cacogeusia is a term used to describe the abhorrent, obnoxious taste produced by the introduction and/or mastication of food in the oral cavity. This symptom was reported by 38 percent (39 of 103). Many foods were reported to produce this symptom although the subjective responses of the patients to specific foods were quite similar. Patients usually described the foods which elicited this symptom as tasting foul, rotten, rancid or spoiled. Foods which most commonly elicited this symptom were eggs, tomato products, meats, poultry, fish, onions, garlic, coffee, and most foods fried in oil or fat. Some patients reported that cold food was less offensive than the same foods when heated. Patients with this symptom usually limited their diets to bland cheeses and dairy products such as milk and ice cream, lettuce without dressing and a few other fresh vegetables and fruits.

Phantogeusia is a term used to describe the intermittent or persistent salty, sweet, sour, bitter or metallic taste perceived in the oral cavity independent of any external stimuli. This symptom of "phantom taste" was reported by 11 percent (11 of 103). Some patients reported that more than one taste sensation would occur either simultaneously or successively. Most commonly, however, this taste was described as being bitter-sour or metallic. This symptom was usually unrelieved by any measure and persisted throughout the day and night without significant fluctuation.

Heterogeusia is a term used to describe an inappropriate taste quality of consistent nature associated with the presence and/or mastication of specific items of food and drink. This taste quality was generally unusual and unexpected, but not foul or obnoxious. This symptom was reported by 4 percent (4 of 103). Two patients reported that all food tasted as if it were oversalted, one that all food had a medicinal or metallic taste and one that salt and sugar tasted bitter.

Six patients had symptoms of cacogeusia and phantogeusia while one had symptoms of cacogeusia and heterogeusia. No patient exhibited all three symptoms simultaneously.

Patients with hypogeusia but without dysgeusia reported that most foods tasted flat, similar to chewing sawdust, vasoline, or flour paste. When the taste loss first appeared the patients commonly ate many different and unusual foods in an effort to find a food which would produce any acceptable taste or in some cases, any taste at all. Four reported an increase in body weight (up to 15 lb) during the initial stages of this illness due to what they described as compulsive overeating. Patients reported that once they realized that most, if not all, food and drink were devoid of taste, or possessing an obnoxious taste quality, they subsequently limited their intake of food to those few in which either some slight amount of taste was present or to those foods which were least obnoxious or best tolerated. Subsequent weight loss was a common finding in patients with this disease. Twenty-six percent (27 of 103) reported significant decreases in body weight (5 to 40 lb) with 78 percent (21 of 27) reporting symptoms of dysgeusia.

Patients with hypogeusia reported that to obtain the salty or sweet taste preferred in their food they had to add an excessive amount of salt or sugar to their food. Forty-seven of 98 patients reported the occurrence of this phenomenon. Often they found it necessary to coat their food with a visible layer of salt or sugar to obtain the salt or sweet taste associated with the food prior to the onset of their illness.

Most patients with dysgeusia reported a sense of hunger at mealtime. The limitations of food intake was related mainly to the unpleasant or abhorrent quality of the food itself. When this symptom was not present they commonly stated that they ate without obtaining any flavor as if "from memory". Indeed, those patients without dysgeusia generally did not suffer from weight loss and ate regular, although limited, meals. A few patients with weight loss and hypogeusia without dysgeusia reported anorexia. They stated that the eating of tasteless material eventually became revolting to them and they ate only when forced to do so by their physician or family who were deeply concerned by their loss of weight.

SMELL: *Hyposmia*, or a generalized decrease in smell acuity, was subjectively reported by 85 percent of the patients (88 of 103). The onset of the smell loss was uniformly accompanied by hypogeusia.

Dysosmia is a term used to describe any distortion of normal olfactory perception. This symptom was reported by 47 percent of the patients (48 of 103). Of these 48, 3 had no subjective decrease in smell acuity. Dysosmia may be manifested in several different ways; three of these have been labeled by us *cacosmia, phantosmia,* and *heterosmia.*

Cacosmia is a term used to describe the abhorrent, obnoxious smell produced by the inhalation of odorants. This symptom was reported by 43 percent (44 of 103). The offensive odorants were similar for most patients. Perfumes, colognes, soaps, automobile exhaust, frying grease or fat, and the odors of most foods described as eliciting cacogeusia were described as rotten, tar-like, foul, or manure-like. Often these patients could not enter restaurants, food stores, drug stores, or their own kitchens when these odors were present. They avoided crowded places where they might come into close contact with individuals wearing perfumes. Some reported that these offensive odors lingered long after the source was removed.

Phantosmia is a term used to describe the intermittent or persistent odor, pleasant or unpleasant, perceived when no odorant was inhaled. This symptom was reported by seven percent (7 of 103).

Heterosmia is a term used to describe an inappropriate smell of consistent nature associated with specific odorants. This smell was generally unusual and unexpected, but not foul or obnoxious. This symptom was reported by one patient who stated that frying onions, lamb chops, bacon, perfumes, and colognes all smelled "metallic."

Two patients had symptoms of cacosmia and phentosmia simultaneously. No patient had all three symptoms simultaneously.

Objective Measurements of Taste

Taste acuity was measured in each patient by determining detection and recognition thresholds for representatives of the taste qualities of salt, sweet, sour and bitter. To do this, a forced choice three stimulus drop technique previously described[5] was employed. NaCl was used as representative of the salt taste quality; sucrose, of sweet; HCl, of sour; and urea, of bitter. The patient was required to detect which one of 3 drops placed consecutively on his tongue and tasted in the oral cavity was different from the other two. Two of the drops presented were distilled water, one of the drops was distilled water plus a given concentration of solute. In addition, the patient was required to describe the dissimilar drop as being either salty, sweet, sour or bitter. The lowest concentration of solute which the patient could consistently detect as different from water was called the *detection threshold;* the lowest concentration of solute consistently recognized correctly as salt, sweet, sour or bitter was called the *recognition threshold.*

In these tests NaCl and sucrose were presented at concentrations of 6, 12, 30, 60, 90, 150, 300, 500, 800, 1000, 3000 (NaCl only) mM and at saturation. HCl was presented at concentrations of 0.5, 0.8, 3, 6, 15, 30, 60, 150, 300, and 500 mm. Urea was presented at concentrations of 60, 90, 120, 150, 300, 500, 800, 1000, 2000, and 5000 mm. Taste thresholds were determined by 4 experimenters and, whenever possible, each patient was tested by more than one experimenter. Each patient was tested two to four times prior to any therapeutic measure and at least once during each treatment condition.

Results of the patients were compared with results from 150 control subjects to whom the same tests were administered. These subjects included normal volunteers and patients with various diseases but without any subjective abnormality of taste or known abnormality of metal metabolism. The subjects consisted of 62 Caucasian men and 88 Caucasian women aged 15 to 77 years (mean 33 years).

All patients included in the present study exhibited elevated detection and recognition thresholds for at least one taste quality.

Patient Evaluation

Each patient was evaluated clinically and by laboratory tests to establish whether or not any metabolic, neurological, or drug-induced abnormality might explain his loss of taste. Each patient underwent an extensive examination of the head and neck region with particular emphasis on the nasal, oral and pharyngeal areas. The following laboratory tests were included in this evaluation: a hematological examination including hemoglobin, hematocrit, RBC indices, WBC count with a differential count, reticulocyte and platelet counts and erythrocyte sedimentation rate; serum sodium, potassium, chloride, carbon dioxide, calcium, phosphorus, magnesium, blood sugar, urea nitrogen, creatinine, uric acid, alkaline phosphatase, liver enzymes, total protein, albumin, serum electrophoresis, and cholesterol; urine analysis with microscopic examination of the sediment; x-rays of the chest, skull including measurement of the volume of the sella turcica,[7] and sinuses; electrocardiogram; brain scan with technetium-99m; electroencephalogram; measurements of parotid salivary flow rates bilaterally. Results of these tests did not relate the hypogeusia to any underlying pathological state.

Serum concentrations of zinc and copper and 24 hour urinary excretion of these trace metals were determined in the patients with hypogeusia and in control subjects. These subjects included normal volunteers without disease and patients with various diseases, but without any subjective abnormality of taste or known abnormality of metal metabolism. The subjects consisted of 44 Caucasian men and 51 Caucasian women, aged 15 to 77 (mean, 39 years). Each subject took food and fluid *ad libitum.* The blood and urine samples were collected from patients and control subjects, in metal-free tubes and plastic containers, respectively, as described previously.[8] Measurements of zinc and copper were carried out by atomic absorption spectrophotometry on an IL Model 153 atomic absorption spectrophotometer by a method previously described.[8] Results from patients and control subjects who received estrogen or adrenocorticosteroid therapy were excluded from this analysis.

Treatment

After diagnosis patients were assigned to a single blind study. The design specified that without the patient's knowledge, but with the knowledge of the treating physician, he would be treated with placebo for periods of one week to 4 months, the patient being tested at least once during this period. Placebo was administered to 47 patients in clear gelatin capsules and given orally four times daily with food. This therapy was administered until one of the following criteria was met: 1) no significant change in taste thresholds had occurred; 2) no subjective change in taste acuity had occurred; or 3) subjective or objective changes which did occur remained the same for 2 successive measurement periods. Forty two of the 103 patients were then treated with zinc ion which was given in the form of zinc sulfate in clear gelatin capsules which were indistinguishable from the placebo capsules and were taken orally four times daily with food. This switch in therapy was accomplished by the treating physician without the knowledge of the patient. Zinc was initially given in two dosage schedules: 25 mg/day as Zn^{++} or 100 mg/day as elemental Zn^{++}. At 25 mg/day if no subjective change in taste or objective change in taste thresholds was evident after 2 to 4 months, the dosage was increased to 50 mg/day. If this dose failed to alter taste acuity subjectively or objectively in 2 to 4 months it was then increased to 100 mg/day. Following the entire treatment period with zinc each patient was placed, once again, on placebo without the knowledge of the patient for periods of two to four months and evaluated at the end of this period. Results of previous threshold data were available to two of the four experimenters.

Evaluation of the changes in the symptom of dysgeusia was made by subjective reports only. Eighteen subjects were questioned about this symptom at each visit to the clinic during treatment with zinc or placebo.

Data from only those patients treated with placebo or zinc for 2 to 4 months were included in the analysis of the effect of zinc administration on detection and recognition thresholds. Changes were calculated only from those thresholds which were above the normal range before treatment.

RESULTS

The median detection and recognition thresholds of 103 patients with idiopathic hypogeusia prior to any treatment are compared with similar thresholds of 150 control subjects in Table 19-I. Median detection and

TABLE 19-I

MEDIAN AND RANGE OF DETECTION AND RECOGNITION THRESHOLDS
FOR 4 TASTE QUALITIES IN 103 PATIENTS WITH IDIOPATHIC
HYPOGEUSIA AND 150 CONTROL SUBJECTS

Taste Quality	Patients		Controls	
	MDT/MRT	Range*	MDT/MRT	Range
	in mM/L		in mM/L	
NaCl	75/150	12-∞/30-∞	12/30	6-60/6-60
Sucrose	60/60	6-∞/12-∞	12/30	6-60/6-60
HCl	15/120	0.5->500/3->500	3/6	0.5-6/0.8-6
Urea	50/80	60->5000/90->5000	120/150	60-150/60-150

*-∞, inability to detect or recognize a saturated solution of solute.

recognition thresholds for salt, sweet, sour, and bitter in the patients were higher than in normals. Relative to the upper limits of normal recognition thresholds were elevated to a greater degree than detection thresholds.

By definition each patient had an elevation of detection and/or recognition threshold for at least one taste quality. Seventy-three percent of the patients (75 of 103) exhibited elevated detection and recognition thresholds for NaCl; 48 percent (49 of 103) exhibited elevated detection and recognition thresholds for sucrose. In spite of this, median detection and recognition thresholds for sucrose were the only ones in which these thresholds were within normal limits. Ninety-seven percent (100 of 103) of the patients exhibited elevated detection and recognition thresholds for urea and 98 percent (101 of 103) had elevated detection and recognition thresholds for HCl. Thirty-six percent of the patients (37 of 103) had elevated detection and recognition thresholds for all 4 taste qualities. One patient had ageusia; i.e. he was unable to detect or to recognize any concentration of solute presented.

Table 19-II illustrates the within patient variability of detection and recognition threshold measurements in 52 patients whose taste was tested

TABLE 19-II

VARIABILITY OF PRE-TREATMENT MEASUREMENTS ON
THE SAME INDIVIDUAL*

Taste Quality	Threshold	Estimated Std. Deviation
NaCl	Detection	1.0 bottles†
	Recognition	1.8 bottles
Sucrose	Detection	1.3 bottles
	Recognition	1.5 bottles
HCl	Detection	1.1 bottles
	Recognition	2.0 bottles
Urea	Detection	1.4 bottles
	Recognition	1.5 bottles

*For individuals measured more than once. There were 52 such individuals and 128 measurements of each threshold for these individuals.

†A "bottle" is the interval from one concentration of the tastant to the next stronger concentration used.

more than once prior to initiation of any treatment. For the purposes of this and subsequent statistical analysis, the term "bottle-unit" is used to indicate the interval from one concentration of tastant to the next stronger concentration presented. If the patient were ageusic for any tastant his detection and recognition thresholds were considered to be one "bottle-unit" beyond the highest concentration presented.

Analysis of variance for each of the 8 thresholds (detection and recognition threshold for 4 tastants) indicated that differences between patients were very much greater than differences among measurements in the same patient for each threshold ($p < 0.01$).

Total serum concentrations of zinc and copper and 24 hour urinary excretion of zinc and copper in patients with idiopathic hypogeusia prior to treatment are compared with similar values obtained in control subjects in Table 19-III. Mean total serum zinc concentration of the patients was significantly lower than control ($p < 0.001$) while urinary zinc excretion was slightly but not significantly higher. Mean total serum copper concentration was significantly elevated above normal ($p < 0.001$). No dif-

TABLE 19-III

SERUM CONCENTRATION OF AND URINARY EXCRETION OF ZINC AND
COPPER IN PATIENTS WITH IDIOPATHIC HYPOGEUSIA
AND IN CONTROL GROUPS

Metal	Idiopathic Hypogeusia mcg/100 ml	Control mcg/100 ml
Serum Zn	76 ± 1*† (N = 91)	99 ± 2 (N = 95)
Cu	114 ± 3†	100 ± 2
	mcg/24 h	mcg/24 h
Urinary Zn	460 ± 27 (N = 88)	419 ± 25 (N = 67)
Cu	34 ± 2	34 ± 3

*Mean ± 1 standard error of mean (SEM).
†$p < 0.001$ with respect to control.

ference was observed in the urinary excretion of copper between patients
and control subjects.

Figure 19-1 illustrates the differences between the distribution of total
serum concentration of zinc in 95 normal volunteers and in 91 patients
with idiopathic hypogeusia. It is clear that no patient with idiopathic
hypogeusia exhibited serum zinc concentrations above 110 mcg/100 ml while
10 control subjects had serum levels above that value. On the other hand,
total serum zinc concentration in the control subjects did not extend below
60 mcg/100 ml while values this low or lower were observed in 11 patients.

The effect of oral zinc administration on detection and recognition
thresholds of 4 tastants is given in Table 19-IV. Before and after placebo
administration differences in the 8 thresholds measured (4 detection, 4
recognition) were not statistically significant, i.e. placebo did not significantly lower any of the thresholds ($p > 0.15$, 1 sided t test). After the
smallest dose of zinc given (25 mg/day) 5 of 8 thresholds (salt recognition, sour and bitter detection and recognition) were significantly decreased

TABLE 19-IV

EFFICACY OF ZINC AT VARIOUS DOSES FROM SINGLE BLIND STUDY

Threshold*	Standardized Values of the Wilcoxon Rank-Sum Statistic	
	Zinc Dose	
	25	100
NaCl —Detection	1.38	3.77†
—Recognition	3.90†	4.15†
Sucrose—Detection	2.22	3.06†
—Recognition	2.35	2.52†
HCl —Detection	3.22†	2.83†
—Recognition	3.63†	3.65†
Urea —Detection	4.04†	4.85†
—Recognition	4.14†	4.46†

*Only patients with abnormal taste thresholds for the quality tested were included.
†$p < 0.05$, one-sided with due regard for the multiplicity of tests.

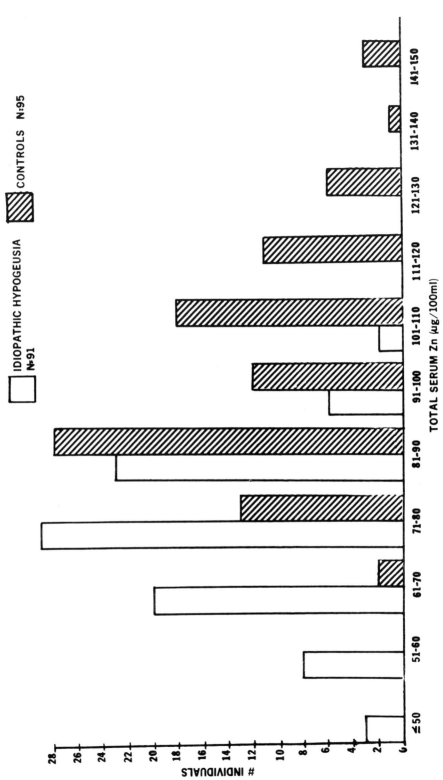

FIGURE 19-1. Total serum concentration of zinc in normal controls (hatched bars) and in patients with idiopathic hypogeusia (clear bars). Number of individuals within each bar is plotted on the ordinate, serum zinc concentration on the abscissa. Note the skewing of the distribution of the serum zinc concentrations of the patients to the left, in the direction of lower than normal concentrations of zinc.

(p < 0.05). After the largest zinc dose given (100 mg/day) significant decreases were noted in all thresholds (p < 0.05). The dose of 50 mg/day was given only to those patients who did not respond after 25 mg/day and it produced decreases in only two thresholds, recognition of salt and sour. Of the 47 patients treated with placebo, three exhibited a sustained return to normal detection and recognition thresholds for each taste quality without significant subjective improvement in their symptoms. One patient exhibited a spontaneous return to normal detection and recognition thresholds without any therapy.

Table 19-V describes further in detail the data from patients treated

TABLE 19-V

TASTE THRESHOLDS OF PATIENTS RECEIVING 100 MG ZINC ION
IN SINGLE BLIND EXPERIMENT

Threshold	Median Threshold Value			Fraction Who Are Normal After Treatment
	Before Treatment°	After Treatment°†	Change†	
NaCl —Detection	150	60	2	10/15‡
—Recognition	300	60	3	11/20
Sucrose—Detection	150	45	2½	6/10
—Recognition	300	60	3	6/10
HCl —Detection	30	15	1	8/17
—Recognition	150	22	3½	5/20
Urea —Detection	900	300	2½	8/18
—Recognition	1000	300	3	7/18

°Concentration in mM/L.
†In "bottle" steps. Changes of ½ bottle step were calculated as the midpoint between the upper and lower concentrations of the interval.
‡Each threshold was above normal prior to treatment.

with Zn^{++} 100 mg/day. Sixty percent of the patients had a restoration to normal (within normal median limits) of thresholds for sweet detection and recognition, 67 percent experienced a return to normal for salt detection, 40 to 50 percent for salt recognition, sour detection and bitter detection and recognition, and 25 percent for sour recognition.

Four of the 18 (22 percent) patients questioned reported a diminution of dysgeusia on placebo while 14 (78 percent) reported no change. On zinc therapy 12 (66 percent) patients reported a significant diminution in dysgeusia, one reported a slight worsening after zinc and 5 were unchanged.

Table 19-VI illustrates the changes in median detection and recognition thresholds of 21 patients with idiopathic hypogeusia before treatment with zinc ion, following treatment with zinc ion (100 mg daily) for two to four months and following administration of placebo for two to four months. These results indicate that median detection and recognition thresholds

TABLE 19-VI

MEDIAN DETECTION/RECOGNITION THRESHOLDS IN PATIENTS WITH
IDIOPATHIC HYPOGEUSIA AND IN CONTROL SUBJECTS

Taste Quality	Pre Zn mM	During Zn mM	Post Zn mM	Controls mM
NaCl	150/1K°	60/60	90/90	12/30†
Sucrose	150/150	30/60	60/60	12/30
HCl	30/150	6/6	15/30	3/6
Urea	1000/5000	150/150	500/800	120/150

°N = 21, †N = 150.

for each taste quality returned to normal during treatment with zinc ion and that following an equal time on placebo detection and recognition thresholds for NaCl, HCl and urea rose to levels above the upper limit of normal. However, the increase in thresholds for both detection and recognition was not to levels as abnormal as noted prior to therapy with zinc ion but rather to intermediate levels. Although the median detection threshold for sucrose increased neither median detection or recognition thresholds for this taste quality rose to levels above the normal range.

Table 19-VII illustrates the changes in serum and urinary zinc and copper in these same 21 patients measured at the same time that their threshold data were collected prior to treatment with zinc, during treatment with zinc and following treatment with zinc while taking placebo. Prior to treatment serum zinc concentrations were significantly below normal, as noted previously, while serum copper concentrations were significantly elevated above normal. At this time urinary zinc excretion was significantly elevated above normal. During treatment with zinc ion (100 mg daily) for two to four months serum zinc concentration increased significantly over pretreatment and control levels while serum copper levels decreased slightly over pretreatment levels. As expected, urinary zinc excretion increased significantly reflecting the changes in serum zinc concentration and the increased zinc administration. Withdrawal of zinc therapy and treatment with placebo resulted in a significant decrease of serum zinc concentrations in the patients toward their original, abnormally low levels and an increase in their serum copper levels. However, serum zinc concentrations did not fall to levels as low as noted prior to zinc therapy. Urinary zinc excretion, as expected, fell to levels significantly below those noted during zinc therapy.

Laser-Microprobe Studies

In an effort to localize the distribution of zinc in the oral cavity in an attempt to relate the results of administration of zinc ion with the taste

TABLE 19-VII

SERUM AND URINARY ZINC AND COPPER IN 21 PATIENTS WITH IDIOPATHIC HYPOGEUSIA AND IN CONTROL SUBJECTS

	Pre Zn μg/100ml	*During Zn* μg/100 ml	*Post Zn* μg/100 ml	*Controls* μg/100 ml
Serum Zn	68 ± 3* %	116 ± 6 Δ	79 ± 4%	99 ± 2 $
Cu	123 ± 7 %	116 ± 6 Δ	122 ± 6%	100 ± 2
	μg/24°	μg/24°	μg/24°	μg/24°
Urine Zn	580 ± 64 Δ	1661 ± 224%	486 ± 130	419 ± 25#
Cu	30 ± 3	33 ± 4	50 ± 7	34 ± 3

*Mean ± 1 SEM, $ N = 95, #N = 67

% (p<0.001 with respect to controls), Δ (p<0.05 with respect to controls)

receptor, laser microprobe analysis of the tongue and lingual papillae of a normal rat was carried out.[*]

By this technique a Q-spoiled Nd glass rod laser, which emits an intense beam of coherent light of 6944 Å, is passed through the objective of a conventional light microscope in reverse, by diverting laser radiation by a glass prism system in controlled pulses.[9,10] For these studies a laser beam was passed through a microscope objective focused on an area of approximately 25 μ of either an area of the surface of a normal rat tongue, a section of a vallate papilla from a normal rat, or a section of a circumvallate papilla from a patient with idiopathic hypogeusia before and after treatment with zinc ion, 100 mg daily for 3 months. The energy of the beam vaporizes any tissue placed on the microscope leaving a crater with a depth of approximately 12 μ. The luminous vapor, which is ionized by the laser beam rises from the crater in a plume and passes between two electrodes providing an electrical path from the charge stored on capacitors. The resulting spark discharge provides the excitation required for analyses by an emission spectrograph. The spectrum is recorded on film and read in a semi-quantitative fashion to evaluate the ions present. For this scale 0 was taken to represent the fact that an ion was not detected, 1^+, that an ion was detected as a trace constituent, 2^+, that an ion was detected as a minor constituent and 3^+, that an ion was detected as a major constituent.

Since the tissue studied can be viewed optically up to 400 X through the same light microscope used to transmit the laser beam it is possible to select the point of impact of the beam with reasonable accuracy and to observe the location of the crater.

A diagrammatic picture of the laser and the microscope is shown in Figure 19-2 while a photograph showing the entire experimental apparatus is shown in Figure 19-3. A typical plume of ionized vapor is shown in Figure 19-4 which leaves a crater in the tissue analyzed, as shown in Figure 19-5. A typical spectrographic pattern is shown in Figure 19-6.

For these studies two tissues served as the targets for the laser microprobe: the tongue of a normal Sprague-Dawley rat was excised, *in toto,* and placed immediately in dry ice; the vallate papilla from the tongue of a normal Sprague-Dawley rat was excised, embedded in glutaraldehyde, fixed in araldite, cut in 5 to 10 μ sections and fixed to a clear plastic slice. Taste buds could be clearly identified upon examination of the unstained sections of the rat vallate papilla through a light microscope.

[*]The authors wish to thank Mr. Frederick Brech, Director of Laboratories of Jarrell-Ash Division, Fisher Scientific Company, and his associates, for their assistance in the performance of these studies carried out at the Jarrell-Ash Laboratory, Waltham, Massachusetts. All results were obtained on a Mark I Laser Microprobe, Model 46-601, manufactured by the Jarrell-Ash Division, Fisher Scientific Company.

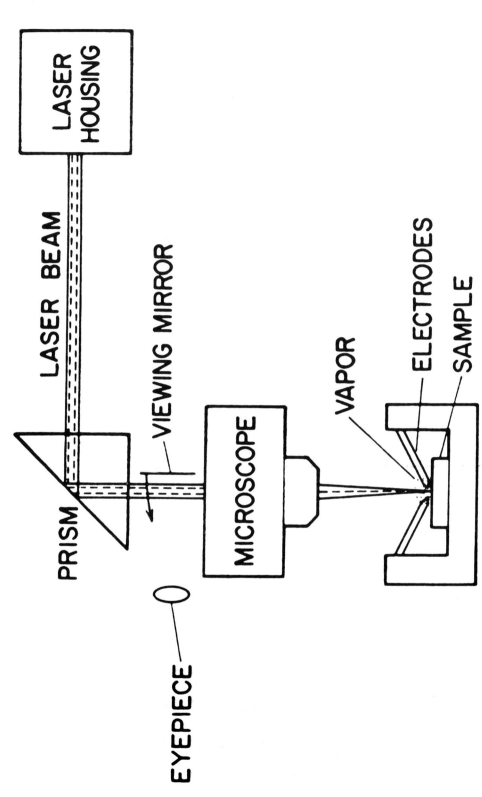

FIGURE 19-2. A diagram illustrating the equipment used to elicit ionized vapor from a tissue sample through the use of a focused laser beam.

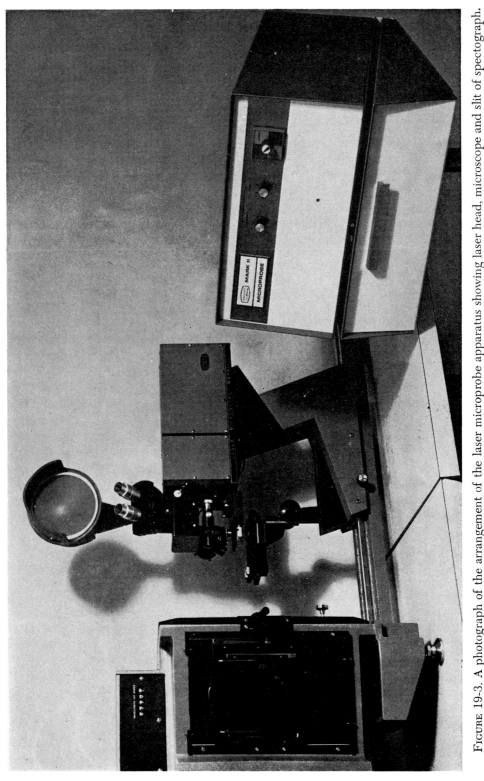

FIGURE 19-3. A photograph of the arrangement of the laser microprobe apparatus showing laser head, microscope and slit of spectograph.

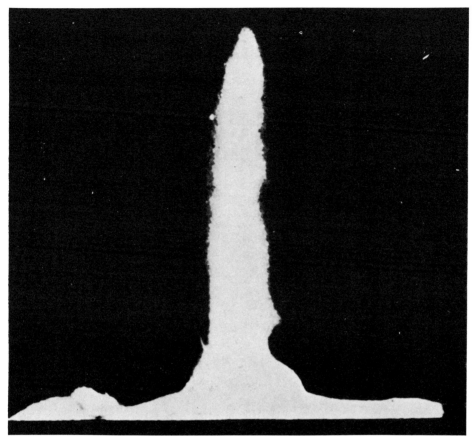

Figure 19-4. A photograph of the ionized vapor plume which is emitted from a sample following impact of a focused laser beam.

The results of the rat studies can be observed in Figure 19-7. Analyses of the spectrographic record indicates that zinc was found only in the area of the vallate papilla in association with strontium, barium and phosphorus. Upon sectioning of the tongue to expose a cross section of the vallate papilla zinc was again found, this time only in the epithelial area and in association with boron and aluminum. The amount of zinc identified was small in comparison with the amount of other ions noted. However, included in the vaporized area and subjected to analysis by spectroscopy was not only epithelial tissue of the vallate papilla but also taste buds.

DISCUSSION

Analysis of the taste bud from the patient with untreated idiopathic hypogeusia revealed no measurable zinc. However, analysis of the taste bud from the patient after treatment with zinc ion, 100 mg/day, when

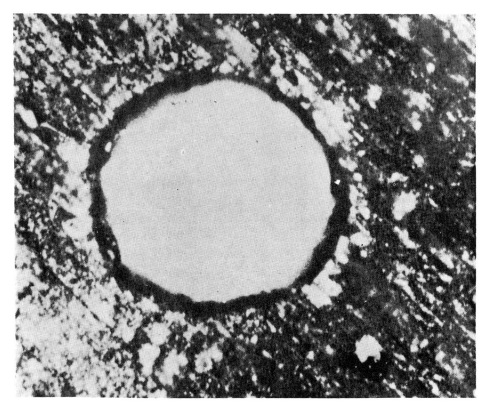

FIGURE 19-5. A typical crater left in the tissue following laser microprobe impact. This crater is approximately 25 μ in diameter and 10 to 15 μ in depth.

the patient's blood and urine reflected the administration of this ion, and the patient's taste acuity had returned to normal, revealed measurable zinc ion.

Idiopathic hypogeusia with dysgeusia, hyposmia and dysosmia appears to be a common disease. Over 4000 patients with these symptoms have written to the National Institutes of Health requesting evaluation and therapy and at the present time over 400 patients with this syndrome have been evaluated at the taste and smell clinic of the National Institutes of Health. The first 103 patients studied are reported in this work. At the National Institutes of Health, which has an employee population of approximately 10,000 people, 20 patients with idiopathic hypogeusia have been identified. On the basis of this sample the incidence of this disease in the population would be projected to be 1 in 500.

Although we have stressed the gustatory aspects of this syndrome the accompanying hyposmia is a constant and important symptom of this disease. The hyposmia is the primary factor contributing to the patients'

SPECTRA

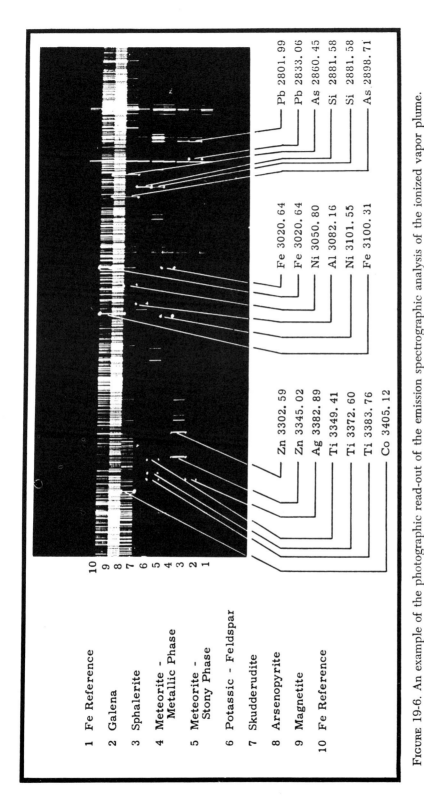

FIGURE 19-6. An example of the photographic read-out of the emission spectrographic analysis of the ionized vapor plume. 35 mm film strip showing spectra of several geological samples after laser microprobing. The excited vapor was focused on the slit of a Jarrell-Ash 1.5 Meter Wadsworth Spectrograph.

Slit Width: 35 microns
Slit Height: 2 mm

· Grating Dispersion: 11.4A mm in 1st order
Emulsion: 103-0, 35 mm film

1 Fe Reference

2 Galena

3 Sphalerite

4 Meteorite -
    Metallic Phase

5 Meteorite -
    Stony Phase

6 Potassic - Feldspar

7 Skudderudite

8 Arsenopyrite

9 Magnetite

10 Fe Reference

Zn 3302.59
Zn 3345.02
Ag 3382.89
Ti 3349.41
Ti 3372.60
Ti 3383.76
Co 3405.12

Fe 3020.64
Fe 3020.64
Ni 3050.80
Al 3082.16
Ni 3101.55
Fe 3100.31

Pb 2801.99
Pb 2833.06
As 2860.45
Si 2881.58
Si 2881.58
As 2898.71

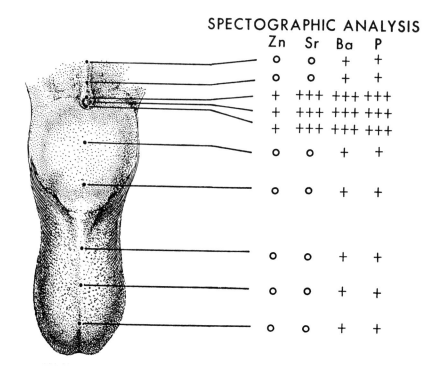

SPECTOGRAPHIC ANALYSIS

	Zn	Sr	Ba	P
	o	o	+	+
	o	o	+	+
	+	+++	+++	+++
	+	+++	+++	+++
	+	+++	+++	+++
	o	o	+	+
	o	o	+	+
	o	o	+	+
	o	o	+	+
	o	o	+	+

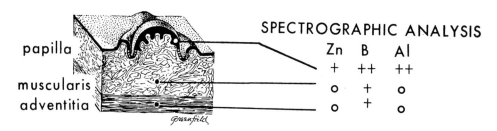

SPECTROGRAPHIC ANALYSIS

	Zn	B	Al
papilla	+	++	++
muscularis	o	+	o
adventitia	o	+	o

FIGURE 19-7. A drawing of the surface of a rat tongue (upper) and a cross section of this tongue through the vallate papilla (lower). A semiquantitative scale of the ions present following laser microprobe impact and emission spectrographic analysis is placed at the right. Each solid line extending to the left of the analysis indicates an area where a laser microprobe impact was made in the tissue. The scale was graded from 0 to +++; 0 indicates that ions were not detected, + indicates that a trace amount of that ion was detected. ++ indicates that these ions represent a minor constituent, +++ indicates that these ions represent a major constituent. Zinc, as a trace constituent, was identified only in the area of the vallate papilla and only in the epithelial layer, the area which contains taste buds. Zinc was always associated with other ions, as noted.

decreased appreciation of the flavor of foods. In addition, this symptom may leave the patients unable to differentiate between spoiled and fresh foods, to distinguish between cooked and uncooked foods and to detect escaping cooking or heating gas or the odor of burning food or fire. These problems are of special importance to women who experience this syndrome. Smell acuity in 35 of these patients has been reported elsewhere.[11]

Approximately half the patients with this syndrome have associated dysgeusia and dysosmia. These symptoms are particularly disturbing to the patients and usually caused them to alter their life styles and patterns of activity. In several patients these symptoms were so severe that they ceased gainful employment and suffered mental depression. Several expressed suicidal intent.

The role which abnormalities of zinc play in this disease is not at all clear. This is particularly apparent from knowledge of the complex nature of the equilibrium between body pools of zinc.[12-14] Thus, the decreases in serum zinc concentration must be evaluated within the context of a complex metabolic net whose major determinants are not yet known. Nevertheless, the interrelationships between trace metals and sensory processes is intriguing. Results from this laboratory have already shown that experimentally induced changes in trace metals or in thiol concentrations can alter taste acuity in humans and in animals[15] and a mechanism for this action has been proposed.[15,16] Further, it is of interest that a majority of patients studied with idiopathic hypogeusia reported some illness or event immediately preceding the onset of symptoms which has in the past been associated with changes in transition metal metabolism; i.e. infectious processes,[17,18] post-operatively,[19] and during pregnancy.[20] The relationships between these disease entities, zinc metabolism and taste acuity have not been securely established.

Although far from conclusive, the laser microprobe studies lend some credence to the concept that zinc may be a normal constituent of the taste bud. What role, if any, strontium, barium, aluminum or boron may play in this system is totally unknown. However, it is reasonable to assume that zinc, since it plays such an important role as a cofactor in DNA and protein synthesis,[21-23] should be involved in any cellular system that is undergoing rapid turnover. The epithelial cells of the gastrointestinal tract turn over rapidly as do the cells of the taste buds.[24] Thus, the requirement for zinc by cells of both of these tissues might be expected to be high. Any disease process which would interfere with the availability of zinc to this system may result in its malfunction. It is clear that the first sign of zinc depletion in rats is anorexia,[25] and it is also clear that administration of minute amounts of zinc to zinc-deficient rats results in the relief of their anorexia within a few hours of the administration of the zinc.[25] In children, zinc deficiency is manifested not only by growth retardation but also by hypogeusia and anorexia.[26] Administration of zinc to these children resulted initially in the disappearance of their anorexia and subsequent return of their hypogeusia to normal.[26] Thus, another role of zinc in the control of food intake appears to be through its relationship with anorexia, present in zinc deficiency and corrected following zinc administration. These observations lead to the hypothesis that the gustatory system may be considered to be an integral part of the gastrointestinal tract, acting as an important sensory system controlling intake.

These observations provide further evidence for the role of zinc as a factor in the control of gustatory acuity and food intake both in man and in other animals.

REFERENCES

1. Henkin, R. I.: Abnormalities of taste and olfaction in patients with chromatin negative gonadal dysgenesis. *J Clin Endocrinol Metab, 27*:1436, 1967.
2. Henkin, R. I.: Impairment of olfaction and of the tastes of sour and bitter in pseudohypoparathyroidism. *J Clin Endocrinol Metab, 28*:624, 1968.
3. Henkin, R. I.: Neuroendocrine control of sensation. In Bosma, J. F. (Ed.): *Oral Sensation and Perception II*, Springfield, Thomas, 1969, pp. 493-534.
4. Henkin, R. I. and Kopin, I. J.: Abnormalities of taste and smell in familial dysautonomia. *Life Sci, 3*:1319, 1964.
5. Henkin, R. I., Gill, J. R., Jr., and Bartter, F. C.: Studies on taste thresholds in normal man and patients with adrenal cortical insufficiency: The effect of adrenocorticosteroids. *J Clin Invest, 42*:727 1963.
6. Henkin, R. I., and Powell, G. F.: Increased taste and smell sensitivity in cystic fibrosis, *Science, 138*:1107, 1962.
7. DiChiro, G., and Nelson, K. B.: The volume of the sella turcica. *Am J Roentgenol, 87*:989, 1962.
8. Meret, S., and Henkin, R. I.: Simultaneous direct estimation by atomic absorption spectrophotometry of copper and zinc in serum, urine and cerebrospinal fluid. *Clin Chem, 17*:369, 1971.
9. Brech, F.: Current status and the potentials of laser excited spectrochemical analysis. Jarrell-Ash Company, Waltham, Massachusetts.
10. Snetsinger, K. G., and Keil, K.: Microspectrochemical analyser of minerals with the laser microprobe. *Am Miner, 52*:1842, 1967.
11. Henkin, R. I., Schechter, P. J., Hoye, R. C., and Mattern, C. F. T.: Idiopathic hypogeusia with dysgeusia, hyposmia and dysosmia: A new syndrome. *JAMA, 217*:434, 1971.
12. Cartwright, G. E., and Wintrobe, M. M.: Copper metabolism in normal subjects. *Am J Clin Nutr, 14*:224, 1964.
13. Vallee, B. L.: Biochemistry, physiology and pathology of zinc. *Physiol Rev, 39*:443, 1959.
14. Spencer, H., Rosoff, B., Feldstein, A., Cohn, S. U., and Gusmano, E.: Metabolism of zinc[65] in man. *Radiat Res, 24*:432, 1965.
15. Henkin, R. I., and Bradley, D. F.: Regulation of taste acuity by thiols and metal ions, *Proc Natl Acad Sci, 62*:30, 1969.

16. Henkin, R. I., and Bradley, D. F.: On the mechanism of action of carbohydrate-active steroids on tastant detection and recognition. In Sawyer, C., and Gorski, R. (Eds.): *Steroid Hormones and Brain Function*, Los Angeles, Calif Pr, 1971.

17. Wolff, H. P.: Untersuchungen zur pathophysiologie des zinkstoffwechsels. *Klin Wochenschr*, 34:409, 1956.

18. Pekarek, R. S., and Beisel, W. R.: Characterization of the injection-inducted endogenous mediator of serum zinc depression (Abstract). *Fed Proc*, 29:297, 1970.

19. Henzel, J. H., DeWeese, M. S., and Lichti, E. L.: Zinc concentrations within healing wounds. *Arch Surg*, 100:349, 1970.

20. Henkin, R. I., Marshall, J. R., and Meret, S.: Maternal-fetal metabolism of copper and zinc at term. *Am J Obstet Gynecol*, 110:131, 1971.

21. Williams, R. B., and Chesters, J. K.: The effects of early zinc deficiency on DNA and protein synthesis in the rat. *Br J Nutr*, 24:1053, 1970.

22. Lieberman, I., and Ove, P.: Deoxyribonucleic acid synthesis and its inhibition in mammalian cells cultured from the animal. *J Biol Chem*, 237:1634, 1962.

23. Rubin, H.: Inhibition of DNA synthesis in animal cells by ethylene diamine tetracetate and its reversal by zinc. *Proc Natl Acad Sci*, 69:712, 1972.

24. Beidler, L. M., and Smallman, R. L.: Renewal of cells within taste buds. *J Cell Biol*, 27:263, 1965.

25. Chesters, J. K., and Quarterman, J.: Effects of zinc deficiency on food intake and feeding patterns of rats. *Br J Nutr*, 24:1061, 1970.

26. Hambridge, K. M., Hambidge, C., and Jacobs, Baum, S. D.: Low levels of zinc in hair, anorexia, poor growth, and hypogeusia in children. *Pediat Res*, 6:868, 1972

DISCUSSION

Dr. Spencer: I would like to ask you whether these patients have any other basic disease because if they have zinc deficiency they wouldn't just have hypogeusia; maybe they have some other symptoms. The second question is, inasmuch as this is a problem of the oral cavity, do these patients have any periodontal disease?

Since zinc is secreted in saliva, do these patients have less or more zinc in saliva than other patients? And are some of your patients alcoholics, because Dr. Sullivan has shown for many years now that these patients excrete a great deal of zinc in the urine and also have low plasma levels of zinc.

Dr. Henkin: We measure salivary flow rate and some electrolyte concentrations in most of our patients. Salivary flow rates and electrolyte concentrations (e.g., sodium, potassium or magnesium) appear to be normal. However, the techniques we are now using are not entirely adequate to measure salivary zinc concentrations and we are in the process of setting up a more elaborate way of looking at this. Although we cannot measure salivary zinc levels in all patients with untreated idiopathic hypogeusia, we can easily measure zinc in their saliva after these patients are successfully treated with zinc ion (i.e., in those whom taste acuity returned to normal subjectively and by objective measurement of taste thresholds). The problem is that the levels of zinc in saliva are so low in normal individuals that it is difficult at present to evaluate the meaning of these changes.

As in other diseases, idiopathic hypogeusia is called idiopathic because there are no other diseases that go along with it. In other words, any patient who has any other clinical abnormality that could be related to zinc metabolism has been excluded from the study. There was no periodontal disease associated with any of the patients in the present study.

Dr. Sullivan pointed out many years ago, as you mentioned, that alterations in zinc metabolism occur in patients with liver disease. We have reported that patients with hepatitis have decreased smell acuity (hyposmia) and have dysgeusia, dysosmia and hypogeusia, as well. In addition, we described the specific changes in zinc metabolism which occur in these patients with hepatitis over the course of their disease. There is no question that there is a relationship between zinc and taste in several clinical situations.

Chapter 20

ORAL ZINC SULFATE IN THE MANAGEMENT OF SEVERELY BURNED PATIENTS

Duane L. Larson

O PTIMAL WOUND HEALING is extremely important to the burned patient. If the burn is extensive, donor sites are few in number; therefore, graft take should be excellent. Furthermore, donor sites must heal rapidly so that additional grafts can be removed in ten to fourteen day intervals. Poor wound healing often leads to chronic unhealed wounds which develop increased collagen deposition and, ultimately, in scar contracture and unstable scars. It is imperative that wound healing be optimal at all times in the burned patient for it may be a deciding factor as to whether that patient lives or dies.

METHODS

Analysis of zinc concentrations were made on a Perkin-Elmer atomic absorption spectrophotometer (Model #303) with a standard burner atomizer and a varicord recorder (Model #43). Zinc levels were determined at a wave length of 213.9 Å with a special slit width of 5, using a zinc hollow cathode lamp and a lamp current of 15 ma. Contamination was avoided by the use of disposable needles, plastic syringes and plastic tubes. Sodium-heparin was used as an anticoagulant. The plasma was diluted 1:6 with triple distilled water for analysis. Zinc standards of 0.5, 0.1, 1.5, and 2.0 ppm were prepared and a new calibration curve was run with each determination. The equipment used to determine tissue levels of zinc was the same as that utilized for determining plasma levels. Wet ashing with 1:1 mixture of nitric and perchloric acid for digestion was preferred over dry ashing. Dry ashing should be used only if it is carefully established that no losses occur. Losses can occur especially in samples rich in chloride.

RESULTS

Correlation of plasma and tissue levels of zinc were analyzed in 73 acutely burned patients with 62 patients having good correlation. There was fair correlation in 8 patients who had moderately high tissue levels with slightly lower plasma levels. There was very poor correlation in one determination in 3 patients; 2 had high tissue levels and low plasma levels, whereas, the third patient had the reverse. Although there was good correlation between plasma and tissue levels of zinc, red blood cell and plasma zinc levels correlated very poorly. The plasma zinc levels were often low with a corresponding normal level of zinc in the red blood cells.[1]

Zinc Levels in Unburned Children

To determine the normal zinc levels of plasma, 100 children returning for reconstructive surgery were examined. The average zinc level in plasma was between 90 and 120 mcg percent. Tissue levels in 70 children admitted for reconstructive surgery varied from 11 to 20 ppm with the majority falling between 14 to 19 ppm.

Zinc Levels in Burned Children

Plasma zinc levels determined in 200 burned children revealed levels between 20 and 80 mcg percent with the majority being 50 to 70 ug percent. Normal plasma zinc levels greater than 90 mcg percent were found in 28 patients; all of these patients were burned less than 20 percent of their body surface or were primarily partial thickness injuries.

A number of children with extensive partial thickness burns revealed normal plasma zinc levels, whereas those children with full thickness injuries had low plasma zinc levels.

Tissue zinc levels were determined in 73 burned children by analyzing skin removed for autografting. Therefore, the earliest tissue levels were obtained approximately four weeks after the accident. Fifty children, or 68 percent, had tissue levels greater than 11 ppm, (i.e. 12 to 20 ppm with the majority falling between 14 and 19 ppm.) Twenty-three children, or 32 percent, had tissue levels below 11 ppm. The low tissue levels in 9 of these children gradually rose to normal levels without showing any significant gross changes in wound healing. Fourteen of the children had persistent low tissue levels associated with poor wound healing. In other words, in analyzing 73 burned children for tissue zinc levels, 19 percent had persistent low tissue levels associated with poor wound healing.

Prophylactic ZnSO₄ Therapy in 14 Acutely Burned Children

Plasma zinc levels were determined in 228 patients with only 28 having normal levels of about 90 mcg percent. Those that were normal during the first three weeks following the accident were minor or partial thickness injuries. Because the majority of burn patients were found to have low plasma zinc levels, a protocol was set up to study 14 acutely burned children receiving prophylactic $ZnSO_4$ orally. ZnSO was given in liquid or capsular form with milk as soon after the accident as possible; 220 mg t.i.d. to those children weighing over 30 kg; 110 mg t.i.d. to those between 10 and 30 kg.

Thirteen of the fourteen acutely burned children receiving prophylactic supplemental zinc sulfate orally responded with an increase in plasma zinc levels.[2] The one child which did not respond received 110 mg t.i.d by mistake rather than 220 mg t.i.d. which she should have had due to her weighing over 30 kg. Unfortunately, the rate of wound healing was extremely difficult to measure in the burned patient because there are so many factors that influence this, (i.e. depth of the burn, circulation, nutrition, infection, and local wound care to name a few.) The fourteen patients were observed to have no gross changes in their clinical course or rate of wound healing compared to those patients receiving no supplemental zinc therapy.

Wound Healing with ZnSO₄ Therapy

During the past four years, 39 children were observed to have decreased rate of wound healing. This diagnosis was usually made between 2 and 7 months following the injury. Zinc sulfate therapy was given as described except that some of the older children required an increase from 220 mg t.i.d. to 220 mg q.i.d. before evidence of increased plasma and tissue zinc levels as well as rate of wound healing was observed. Therapy was usually continued from two to four months, although normal zinc levels were usually reached between two and four weeks after starting zinc sulfate therapy. Of these thirty-nine burned children, fourteen or ⅓, had an obvious increase in wound healing following oral supplementation of zinc sulfate. Twenty-five, or ⅔, of the children so treated revealed no gross increase in the rate of wound healing. The latter group had zinc plasma levels greater than 90 mcg percent and tissue levels greater than 13 ppm; whereas, the former group had very low plasma and tissue levels prior to supplemental zinc sulfate therapy.

DISCUSSION

The burned patient is a most difficult one to study because of the many internal and external variables that are present and constantly changing. An example of one of these variables is the different types of local treatment. Epidermal regeneration in the rabbit's ear can be retarded from 15.5 days to 39.5 days by the local application of Sulfamylon®. This can be corrected by the administration of zinc sulfate orally.[3] Six of the children exhibiting an increase in wound healing following zinc sulfate therapy were receiving Sulfamylon®. However, eight of the others exhibiting an increase in wound healing were receiving silver sulfadiazine, locally. Silver sulfadiazine prolongs wound healing in the rabbit's ear by only 2.5 days, (i.e. from the control of 15.5 days to the treated 18 days.)[3] Dr. Edward Kentish, in his book "Essay on Burns" written in 1797, stated this problem very well: "It falls to the lot of few men to appreciate properly the effects of various modes of treatment in a particular disease, for if the patient recovers whatever was the treatment whether good or bad, we flatter ourselves it was the effect of our superior merit in conducting the disease; but future experience may convince us that the recovery of which we so vainly boasted was a victory of nature over the malpractice of art."

The severely burned patients are deficient in zinc for a number of reasons. There is a considerable loss of zinc in the wound exudate; our measurements in 10 patients revealed the zinc concentration in wound exudate to be 2 to 4 times that of the plasma. An increase in urinary excretion of zinc is also present.[4] The diet is often insufficient in zinc because of the poor oral intake and the administration of zinc-poor intravenous fluids. A relative preponderance of total biological zinc is concentrated within the skin (20 percent) and this is lost with the eschar. These facts plus our initial studies revealing the plasma and tissue levels of zinc in burned patients to be low, prompted this gross clinical study. It was readily apparent that the zinc levels in plasma in the burned patients were always low during the first month following the burn, except in those patients burned over less than 20 percent of their body surface, or those with partial thickness injury. The zinc levels in the red cell and plasma are correlated very poorly for the red cell zinc levels continue to be high even in the face of very low plasma zinc levels. Tissue and plasma zinc levels, however, correlated quite well. The tissue levels were determined from the skin removed at the time of autografting; consequently, the first values obtained were approximately four weeks after the accident.

At the time of the first grafting, 58 (or 68 percent) of the 73 children had normal tissue levels of zinc; 23 (or 32 percent) of the patients had low tissue levels. However, only 14 of these, or 19 percent of the total number of children studied, had persistent low tissue levels associated with poor wound healing. The other nine showed no discernible decrease in wound healing and their low levels rose to normal range without therapy. These 14 children who revealed a persistent low tissue zinc level showed an improvement in rate of wound healing following supplemental zinc sulfate therapy. The 14 acutely burned patients who received prophylactic zinc sulfate therapy and the 39 patients who were treated because of poor wound healing revealed no discernible toxic symptoms from the orally administered zinc sulfate therapy in the doses as described. From these initial studies, it appears that approximately 1/5 of the severely burned children have persistent low tissue levels of zinc which are associated with a decrease in the rate of wound healing. This data would indicate that a burned patient exhibiting a decrease rate in wound healing may benefit from the oral administration of zinc sulfate; consequently, these patients should have a two week trial of therapy. Whether or not the acutely burned patient should receive prophylactic zinc sulfate therapy during his initial stage remains to be determined.

SUMMARY

Zinc concentrations were determined in plasma, red blood cells, wound exudate and the skin of burned children. Those children with extensive thermal injuries revealed prolonged low plasma zinc levels and initial low tissue zinc levels. About one fifth of these children studied revealed persistent low plasma and tissue levels associated with minimal epithelization and/or poor skin graft acceptance which improved after oral zinc supplementation. Those patients with normal zinc levels and decreased wound healing did not improve with zinc supplemental therapy. However, there are so many variable factors involved in wound healing in burn patients that no definite conclusions can be established from these studies, except to recommend oral zinc sulfate supplementation in those patients exhibiting decrease wound healing associated with low zinc, plasma and tissue levels.

REFERENCES

1. Larson, D. L., Dobrkovsky, M., Abston, S., and Lewis, S.: Zinc concentrations in plasma, red blood cells, wound exudate and tissue of burned children. In Matter, P., Barclay, T., and Knoickova, Z. (Eds.): *Research in Burns.* Bern, Stuttgart, Vienna, Hans-Huber, 1971.
2. Larson, D. L., Maxwell, R., Abston, S., and Dobrkovsky, M.: Zinc deficiency in burned children. *Plast Reconstr Surg, 46*:13, 1970.
3. Wisner, H. K., Lynch, J. B., Larson, D. L., and Lewis, S. R.: Correction of retarded epidermal regeneration due to Sulfamylon by administration of oral zinc. In Matter, P., Barclay, T., and Knoickova, Z. (Eds.): *Research in Burns.* Bern, Stuttgart, Vienna, Hans-Huber, 1971.
4. Henzel, J. H., DeWeese, M. D., and Lichti, E. L.: Zinc concentrations within healing wounds. *Arch Surg, 100*:349, 1970.

DISCUSSION

Dr. Flynn: Yesterday, Dr. Pories introduced some of our preliminary work on adrenocortical hormones and zinc metabolism, as studied in hemodynamically stressed rats (*Science 173*:1035, 1971). To compliment this study and the report given by Larson on zinc metabolism in major burns, we have recently completed the monitoring of several major burn patients who have been treated with pharmacological doses of glucosteroids. As has been reported here and in many other burn studies, body zinc levels gradually deteriorate over the first month after a major burn to markedly deficient values. Yet, in patients receiving massive doses of glucosteroids as vasodilators, according to the procedure described by Dietzman *et al.* (*Chest* 57:440, 1970), rapid large declines were measured in blood serum zinc.

Two patients are of particular interest for discussion here: One, a 65 year-old male with 65% third-degree burns, received vasoactive cortico-steroid therapy (equivalent to 800 mg cortisone, I.V., q.i.d.). A rapid drop of 42 mcg per 100 ml serum zinc was determined after the initial administration of steroids, the fall in serum zinc occurring within two hours of the beginning of drug treatment. As shown in Figure 20-1, during the first three days post-burn, substantial subnormal zinc levels were measured with the continuation of the corticosteroid therapy. Only after discontinuing the course of glucosteroids, and administering corticotrophin did blood serum zinc levels rise to approximately normal values. A second case, which is also indicative of the involvement of a proper pituitary-adrenal relationship in zinc metabolism, was a vascular surgery patient who presented with low cardiac output syndrome after massive hemorrhage. This 52 year-old male had undergone surgery for a femoralpopliteal bypass the day prior to the first serum zinc sample. Serum zinc before corticosteroid therapy was elevated, 160 mcg per 100 ml, in this hemodynamically stressed patient. A single massive I.V. dose of dexamethasone phosphate, 200 mg (equivalent to 8 gm cortisone), was given the patient as supplemental vasoactive therapy. Forty-five minutes after the administration of the potent synthetic glucosteroid, serum zinc levels fell 85 mcg per 100 ml, as illustrated in Figure 20-1. The effects of this single steroid treatment on serum zinc values was short-lived, however, for within 24 hours the serum zinc levels had again returned to abnormally high values.

These brief clinical findings, as well as much additional animal and patient data, have indicated to us an important role for the secretion of the adrenal cortex in the maintenance of blood serum zinc. The accumulated results tend to implicate adrenocortical steroids in the overall balance of body zinc stores. Two implications are to be noted: First, the rapid changes in serum zinc levels in the two patients discussed illustrate a lack of reliability of serum zinc to accurately indicate the body zinc stores. Second, the delaying effect of steroids on wound healing that has been known for twenty years may be related in part to the effects of glucosteroids on zinc metabolism. Of course, to prove this relationship of steroid delayed healing to impaired zinc metabolism will require much further work. We feel, however, that the steroid: zinc relationship is of considerable import in considering the clinical courses of major trauma patients.

Dr. Henzel: A comment with respect to the ACTH levels is that again, looking at skin, the lowest levels that you find in skin, particularly in dermatology patients, are patients who receive steroid therapy for skin con-

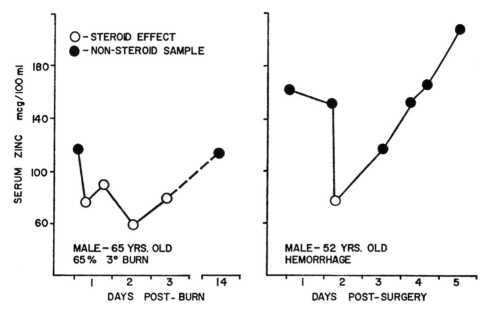

FIGURE 20-1. Serum zinc changes in patients receiving pharmacological doses of glucosteroids.

ditions over a long period of time. I can't give you the exact reference, but one of our residents prior to going into the service at Fitzsimmons about three years ago, looked at a large number of these patients.

Dr. Petering: It is well known that when one gives contraceptive drugs, estrogens, you get a diminished zinc plasma level as well as an elevated copper level and I wonder whether anyone has looked at the copper levels in the patients getting these amounts of zinc for a long period of time. And the other point is that it is also known that zinc given to animals will diminish or reduce the amount of hematopoiesis or at least reduce red cells. And I wonder whether or not you have any information on the actual situation with respect to the amount of hematopoiesis in these patients because these things might all be involved in some of the failures as well as some of the good results.

Dr. Larson: Burned patients all require blood about once a week. These patients are losing blood continuously and so it would be very difficult to determine. There would be no way for us to really determine this. It would have to be done in another type of patient. But I can say, that with those who were receiving zinc required no more blood than those who did not. But the burned patient is a very poor patient to study because there are so many variables going on constantly that you can't run a good study.

Dr. Woosley: One quick comment that interested me about the report on ACTH and steroids and that is the problem you see when you give steroids to asthmatic children. For years you see a syndrome of dwarfism almost identical to the findings in Iran with delayed growth and maturation, and it would be of interest to see if you could prevent this with the administration of zinc.

Dr. Larson: May I close and just say when I made the comment that I felt it was malpractice not to use zinc, I was just trying to jar the audience a little bit. I do feel that one thing we have learned in taking care of these burned children is that if you do have one that is difficult in wound healing, go ahead and try zinc sulfate. You will be surprised how often this will get you out of trouble. I don't know what the answer is, but there is a block, at least in burn patients and it is a very common block in their late burn period. Epithelization just doesn't seem to occur and they will sit there for months and months before finally you get tired of looking at him and you send him home and then over a period of many months he will finally heal. But the zinc does make a difference, a very great difference in that particular area.

Chapter 21

ORAL ZINC AND VITAMIN THERAPY FOR LARYNGOTRACHEAL TRAUMA AND SURGICAL AFTERCARE

Fredric W. Pullen, II

INTRODUCTION

ALTHOUGH THE EFFICACY OF ORAL ZINC SULFATE in wound healing has been well documented in many fields of medicine,[1,2,3,4,5] it has only recently been explored in the field of Otolaryngology.[6]

In a preliminary communication,[6] the use of zinc in laryngotracheal trauma and laryngeal contact granulomas was reported. This paved the way for further exploration in Otolaryngologic patients with delayed healing.[7] The following case reports illustrate the effectiveness of zinc therapy in laryngeal trauma.

CASE REPORTS

Case 1

Thirty-three year old white female who was first admitted to JMH in March, 1968 with a history of ingestion of a large quantity of barbiturates. An endotracheal tube and respirator was maintained for five days. Approximately two weeks later she noted slight dyspnea and a physical examination at that time revealed a small granuloma subglottically on the left. The vocal cords were otherwise normal.

The granulomas enlarged and the patient was admitted to the hospital with severe dyspnea. She was placed on steroids, voice rest and antibiotics. However, two weeks later a tracheostomy was performed because of marked edema in the subglottic area as well as granuloma formation.

The disease continued with increasing tenderness as well as pain around the area of the cricoid cartilage. Tomograms revealed complete occlusion of the airway due to subglottic edema and granulation tissue. Culture was taken showing *pseudomonas aeruginosa* as the offending organism and the diagnosis of chrondritis of the cricoid cartilage was made. Treatment consisted of several courses of ampicillin, colymycin and steroids.

The tracheostomy was continued and on November 8, 1968 the patient had had no subglottic airway for approximately two months. At that time she was receiving ascorbic acid, 250 mgs daily, colymycin, 75 mgs b.i.d., and ampicillin, 500 mgs q.i.d. She was begun on zinc sulfate (U.S.P.) on November 8, 220 mg t.i.d. On the next day she was able to speak with a fairly normal voice. Within one week she was able to breath with the tracheostomy tube plugged, and the tube was permanently removed three weeks after the institution of zinc therapy.

The tracheostomy tube has been out since that time and the patient has done well; the granulation tissue in the trachea has disappeared and she has been able to lead a relatively normal life.

Case 2

Sixty-six year old white female who was hospitalized in October, 1968 with metabolic encephalopathy, with endotracheal intubation for 48 hours. The endotracheal tube was removed, and three days later dyspnea was noted and examination showed acute laryngeal edema.

One month later she was found to have large posterior vocal cord granulomas and marked hoarseness. In December, one month later, the granulomas were still present and remained unchanged until January 15, 1969 when the patient was started on zinc sulfate (U.S.P.), 220 mg three times daily by mouth (Fig. 21-1).

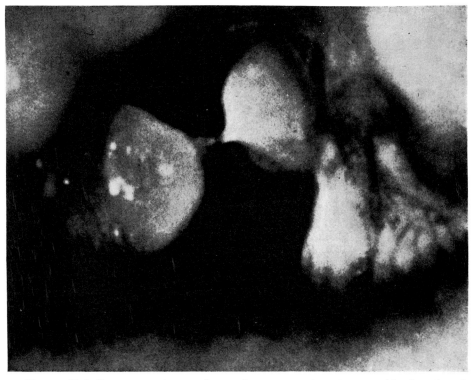

FIGURE 21-1. Large posterior vocal granulomas in a sixty-six year old white female prior to treatment with oral zinc sulfate, 200 mg., t.i.d.

Two weeks later the patient's voice was improved and the granulomas were smaller. On the 24th of February a small subglottic granuloma was noted only on the left vocal cord. The zinc was continued for a total of two months until there was no further evidence of any laryngeal pathology (Fig. 21-2).

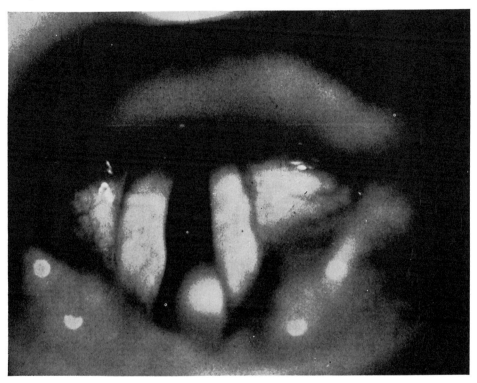

FIGURE 21-2. Essentially normal posterior vocal cord in the same sixty-six year old white female with no evidence of larygeal pathology after two months treatment with oral zinc sulfate, 220 mg., t.i.d.

DISCUSSION

Since the original cases were reported, 10 cases of laryngotracheal granulation secondary to traumatic endotracheal intubation have been treated with the use of zinc sulfate (U.S.P.), 220 mg t.i.d. Eight of these 10 cases have needed no further therapy and have healed without sequelae.

Contact ulcers and granulations occurring spontaneously are a serious problem in Otolaryngology that heretofore have been resistant to medical treatment. The typical history of contact granuloma is fraught with repeated surgical excisions as well as many months of unsuccessful treatment. Steroids as well as antibiotics have proven useless in this disease.

At the present time eight cases of contact ulcers and granulomas have been treated with oral zinc sulfate and several in combination with ascorbic acid, 250 to 500 mg daily. Five of the 8 cases healed with no further recurrence of the lesions after varying periods of treatment up to five months. Two healed cases were patients of other physicians, Dr. J. Ryan Chandler[8] of Miami and Dr. Paul Holinger[9] of Chicago. Previously all of these patients had had multiple excisions of the contact granulomas which recurred even after these excisions.[7]

In a recent investigation an attempt was made to discern the effectiveness of zinc in postoperative Otolaryngologic patients who had undergone tonsillectomies. A double blind controlled study was performed comparing a placebo to a combination of multiple vitamins and zinc (Vicon-C®) to the immediate postoperative period. Comparisons were made between the healing rate, which was measured by eschar formation and retention; the presence or absence of pain; and the return to a normal diet. Daily logs were kept by each of the patients over a period of 3 to 4 weeks and these were compared. Clinical evaluations were performed at weekly intervals to note the presence of eschars, edema, bleeding, pain and dietary intake. Each patient was given two capsules three times daily or a daily total of 477 mg of zinc. Table 21-I summarizes the findings.

TABLE 21-I

HEALING RATE AND PAIN IN POST-TONSILLECTOMY PATIENTS

Postop Week	Healing Rate (Eschar Disappearance)		Pain	
	Vitamin-Zinc Group	Placebo Group	Vitamin-Zinc Group	Placebo Group
I	11	5	12	10
II	10	8	10	8
III	3	9	2	4

Healing rates were determined by the presence of eschar formation in the tonsillar fossa. Postoperatively the presence or absence of an eschar was noted at weekly examinations. In the vitamin-zinc group 21 of 24 patients or 88 percent had healed completely at the end of two weeks. Whereas, in the placebo group only 13 of 22 patients or 59 percent exhibited this healing rate. Nine patients of 22 receiving the placebo, or 41 percent still had eschars present at the end of the third week. These are highly significant figures and equate with a $p < 0.01$.

Each patient was asked to keep a daily log of pain on swallowing and the date the pain disappeared was the end point for pain. In 22 of 24 patients in the vitamin-zinc group the pain disappeared within three weeks, as opposed to 18 of 22 patients in the placebo group. Essentially no difference was found between these groups, nor was there any difference noted with respect to dietary intake.

The use of a vitamin mineral preparation including zinc sulfate in the postoperative tonsillectomy patient showed a significant increase in the healing rate. The average otolaryngologic patient in the postoperative period has minimal oral intake and the vitamin-zinc therapy restored these essential elements. The results are even more striking when one realizes that these tonsillectomies were performed in otherwise healthy individuals and not those with cirrhosis, or other debilitating diseases. One interesting note—8 patients in the placebo group were dropped from the study because of "reactions" to the medication, while only 3 of the drug group stopped the medication.

It should be evident that postoperative patients have certain needs for various vitamins and minerals and that those needs must be met if the body stores become depleted. Further study is of course necessary in ascertaining the mode of action of zinc in healing, however it is very apparent that zinc is a necessary ingredient within the healing mechanism.

SUMMARY

Otolaryngologic patients in the postoperative period usually have poor oral intake and vitamin mineral supplementation of their diet is recommended therapy.

Laryngotracheal trauma has successfully been treated with oral zinc sulfate and has been reported previously. A recent double-blind controlled study showed a significant increase in the rate of healing of tonsillectomy patients when they were given a vitamin-mineral zinc capsule as compared to those given a placebo. Further studies must be initiated to elucidate the mechanism of action of zinc and it is hoped that these clinical studies will give impetus to this research.

REFERENCES

1. Savlov, E. D., Strain, W. H., and Huegin, F.: Radiozinc studies in experimental wound healing. *J Surg Res*, 2:209, 1962.
2. Sandstead, H. H., Lanier, V. C., Jr., Shepard, G. H., et al: Zinc and wound healing: Effects of zinc deficiency and zinc supplementation. *Am J Clin Nutr*, 23:514, 1970.
3. Halsted, J. A., and Smith, J. C., Jr.: Plasma zinc in health and disease. *Lancet*, i:322, 1970.
4. Husain, S. L.: Oral zinc sulphate in leg ulcers. *Lancet*, i:1069, 1969.
5. Pories, W. J., Strain, W. H., Peer, R. M., and Landew, M. H.: Zinc deficiency as a cause for delayed wound healing. In Zuidema, G. D., and Skinner, D. B. (Eds.): *Current Topics in Surgical Research*. Vol. I, New York, Acad Pr, 1970, vol. I.
6. Pullen, F. W.: Postintubation tracheal granuloma. *Arch Otolaryngol*, 92:340, 1970.
7. Pullen, F. W., Pories, W. J., and Strain, W. H.: Delayed healing: the rationale for zinc therapy. *Laryngoscope 81*:1638, 1971.

8. Chandler, J. R.: Personal communication. 1971.
9. Holinger, P. H.: Personal communication. 1971.

DISCUSSION

Dr. Duane Larson: Why did the granuloma disappear? Is it due to the epithelial growing over the granuloma and grafting down, or what is the reason?

Dr. Pullen: No. Basically these people report that the granuloma—that they start spitting out chunks of it. It just falls apart. Granulomas in the past, just don't disappear in general, the majority of them stay and are just real problems and after repeated months and months of therapy they are still there.

Dr. Pfeiffer: Have you ever looked at prepubertal laryngeal polyps?

Dr. Pullen: Yes. It has no effect whatsoever on laryngeal polyps. Laryngeal polyps is an entirely different disease. A polyp itself is not an inflammatory disease. Polyps that cause hoarseness and huskiness especially in children are usually due to vocal abuse and are nothing more than a callous that has formed on the vocal cords.

Chapter 22

LONG-TERM ORAL ZINC SULFATE IN THE TREATMENT OF ATHEROSCLEROTIC PERIPHERAL VASCULAR DISEASE: EFFICACY OF POSSIBLE MECHANISM OF ACTION

John H. Henzel, Edgar L. Lichti, William Shepard and Joseph Paone

Some four years ago, in a presentation at the Second Annual Conference on Trace Substances in Environmental Health,[1] we expressed a conviction that with respect to the trace substances-environmental health interrelationship fruitful investigation, as well as interpretation and application of study results, would require a uniquely-cooperative interdisciplinary approach, based on an awareness of and respect for what each of us has to contribute. This statement remains as true today as it was four years go. Those of you in this audience represent many disciplines; your training, capability, experience and varied interests constitute phenomenal potential for unraveling the mystery to preventing atherosclerosis and other major ecologic-health care problems. A clinician's potential is relatively limited; the majority of our efforts are directed towards treating disease which is already present. The potential of your combined abilities is unlimited; your efforts are oriented toward prevention.

Many of the topics which have been amalgamated for this symposium take their origin from an observation which Dr. Strain made nearly 20 years ago. In no small measure, he and our Program Chairman have been key figures in igniting and enkindling the comprehensive, unified interdisciplinary approach to micronutrient research. Albeit the time was ripe, with terms like biosphere, ecology and pollution saturating the news media. Nonetheless, productive fruition of a concept requires involvement, interaction and leadership. These two individuals have provided these in the past; this conference is mute evidence of their continuing involvement.

In providing us with a specific title for this presentation, I'm certain that Dr. Pories expected us to summarize for you the current status of our ongoing investigation of the role of zinc sulfate in atherosclerosis. Approximately five years ago we initiated a Clinical Research Unit Study which was specifically designed to answer whether oral zinc sulfate constitutes effective therapy for certain patients with severely symptomatic atherosclerosis. It does, and in attempting to answer how, we've focused in on small vessel perfusion and zinc enzyme activity within skin and muscle of the severely ischemic limb. Our findings are presented in the hope that they will serve as a stimulus for additional and more sophisticated efforts at the cellular and sub-cellular level.

STUDY POPULATION AND METHODOLOGY

Results of long-term $ZnSO_4$ administration to patients with severely-symptomatic inoperable atherosclerosis have been reported previously.[2] About three-and-a-half years ago, as soon as preliminary observations supported the efficacy of oral zinc in certain treated patients, effort and methodology were specifically reoriented to acquire definitive objective evidence to support the subjective improvement which we were witnessing. Toward this end, techniques were implemented for monitoring low-level perfusion and for measuring activity of zinc and specific zinc-enzymes, within ischemic limbs of patients who responded, or failed to respond, when medicated with $ZnSO_4$. Prior to describing our methodology and results, it is pertinent to look at those criteria which we accepted as evidence of zinc-associated improvement, and to understand that from the outset we ignored all subjective impressions which could not be substantiated by patient-performance, measured improvement of perfusion, or expert observation. In other words, subjective impression of improved hair growth or increased warmth in an atherosclerotic extremity constituted acceptable evidence of improvement only when study project physicians documented the former, and ultrasonic flow probe confirmed the latter. Table 22-I outlines the criteria which were considered as supportive evi-

TABLE 22-I

OBJECTIVE EVIDENCE OF IMPROVED BLOOD SUPPLY TO ISCHEMIC LIMBS

1. Doubling of treadmill-exercise performance.
2. Complete healing of previously-refractive (before $ZnSO_4$) ischemic ulcers.
3. Increased resting ankle pressure in association with unchanged (or lower) arm pressure.
4. Appearance of previously-undetectable digital flow.
5. Early post-exercise appearance of previously delayed (or absent) reactive hyperemia.
6. Improved distal limb flow following doubled exercise tolerance.
   A. Shortened rebound of exercise-precipitated drop in ankle pressure, frequently with overshoot.
   B. Increased flow velocity, in some cases during and following worsened ankle pressures.
   C. Accelerated recovery of exercise-precipitated drop in ankle pressure, associated with a doubling of original exercise tolerance.

dence of enhanced limb perfusion. The parameter which we assess most critically is the last one listed in this table. Thorough and accurate evaluation of *distal extremity perfusion* may be accomplished by means of innovated and standardized use of the transcutaneous ultrasonic flowmeter, an instrument which has proven of immense value in evaluating these study patients.

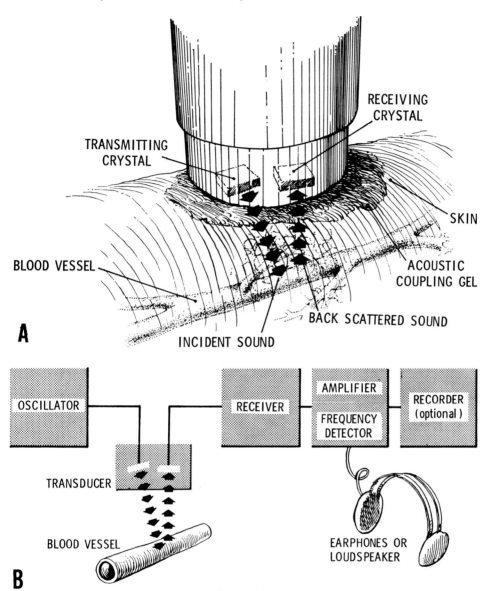

FIGURE 22-1
DOPPLER PRINCIPLE AND CIRCUITRY

A—Principle of Flow Detection by Ultrasound: One of 2 piezoelectric crystals within the tip of the flow probe transmits ultrasound, while the second detects and receives the ultrasonic waves which are reflected back from the particulate cellular components of flowing blood. The resulting frequency shift in sound is transmitted through appropriate circuitry (below) such that pulsatile flow is transformed into audible sound.

B—Doppler Flowmeter Circuitry: Backscattered sound is filtered and amplified such that changes in flow-velocity are perceived as audible sound.

A brief description of flow-pathology and instrumentation is essential at this point, since an understanding of and appreciation for the flow-improvement which we documented in subjectively improved zinc-treated patients requires a base-line knowledge of vascular hemodynamics, relative to the manner in which the ultrasound flowmeter permits dynamic evaluation of pressure and flow in vascular channels. In patients with moderately-severe occlusive arterial disease, exercise precipitates a reduction in blood flow to working muscle, and prolongation of the hyperemia which follows the muscular effort. The overall response depends upon numerous variably-present and variably-active factors, two of the most critical of which are extent and severity of occlusive involvement, and the presence of patent collateral secondary channels. When extensive disease is present, as was the case with 90 percent of the patients in the zinc-treated population, exercise produces a painful, cadaveric limb in which little evidence of flow can be detected for some minutes following the muscular work. In these patients, hyperemic activity may be negligible and limb recovery, evidenced by return of color and resolution of pain, may be markedly prolonged. In order to assess and sequentially monitor blood flow in the severely atherosclerotic limb, one needs sensitive instrumentation which is atraumatic, economical, accurate and sufficiently portable that pressure and perfusion can be measured within seconds after exercise. Figure 22-1 schematically illustrates the principal behind the Doppler ultrasonic flowmeter. In essence, flow-velocity is detected by sensing and amplifying the frequency-shift which occurs when ultrasound is transmitted through moving blood by one piezo-electric crystal and received back by a matching crystal. This instrument has wide applicability, as evidenced by a recent comprehensive review of our own clinical experience with this modality.[3]

Doppler Principle

Summarized in somewhat oversimplified fashion, the ultrasound reflected back from streaming elements within a specific vessel is directed through appropriate circuitry, such that changes in flow-velocity are filtered, amplified and perceived as audible sound. Although the ultrasound signals may be graphically displayed via an audiospectrum analyzer, the human ear is equally discriminating in its ability to differentiate frequency (pitch) and intensity (amplitude) relative to time. Any sudden change in the amplitude or frequency of the velocity-shift signal, indicates a change in either the velocity pattern or the direction of flow relative to the incident beam of ultrasound. Collateral vessels arising from an artery proximal to an occlusion change the direction of flow relative to the flow probe, which of course changes the frequency of the velocity signal. Figure 22-2 graphically illustrates why sound interpretation alone, particularly when the

FIGURE 22-2
SCHEMATIC ILLUSTRATION OF DOPPLER SOUND ENCOUNTERED AS
AN ULTRASONIC FLOWPROBE PASSES ALONG (SUPERIOR TO INFERIOR)
NORMAL, STENOTIC AND TOTALLY OCCLUDED ARTERIAL SEGMENTS.

When the flowprobe passes a patent collateral takeoff; or as it approaches, passes directly over and arrives beyond a stenotic or occluded area, characteristic changes occur in sound frequency (perceived as pitch) and intensity (perceived as amplitude). In addition, diminution in or disappearance of the second pulse sound, discontinuity (separation) of pulse waves and water-hammer thumping become audible. Pulsatile flow-velocity sounds are sufficiently distinctive that normal and abnormal can be recognized and differentiated.

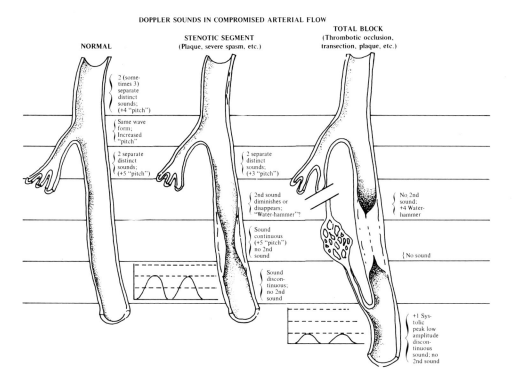

listener is adept with a stethoscope, is entirely adequate for acoustically detecting and evaluating normal and pathologic flow. In trying to describe the Doppler principle and applicability in a few sentences, we recognize that the significance of being able to detect and qualify normal and abnormal flow may remain totally perplexing. Figure 22-3 may not clarify

FIGURE 22-3. Doppler sound-frequency profiles of digital flow before and immediately after smoking an early a.m. cigarette. Before smoking (left) pulsatile flow resulting from each cardiac stroke is audible as 2 separate distinct sounds characterized by continuous wave-form, +4 pitch and booming amplitude. After smoking (right), the second sound diminishes or may disappear (becoming continuous with the first), while pitch increases and amplitude is blunted.

matters, but it will at least stimulate the smokers in this audience to do a little outside homework. The two audiospectrums illustrate what your ear would hear and what the audiospectral analyzer would record when the flow probe was positioned over the tip of the index finger before, and immediately following, a medium-sized panatela cigar. The outstanding value of the Doppler flow probe, excluding our own data acquisition, has been its effectiveness in providing previously-refractive patients with the motivation necessary to stop smoking. When a patient listens to his digital flow just before his night-time soporific, and notes the difference before his first A.M. cigarette 8 hours later, he has gained a conceptual grasp of what the cigarettes are doing to his already-marginal flow.

Oral Zinc Medication

As will be seen below, by sequentially evaluating patients before and immediately following standardized treadmill exercise, we documented increased flow in the ischemic extremities of nearly all those who experienced subjective improvement during medication with oral zinc. Evidence suggests that perfusion-improvement occurs via collateral channels. However, the magnitude and flow-velocity characteristics of improvement associated with oral zinc differs from and exceeds the optimal "flow-takeover" which occurs through "adequate" collateral channels in untreated symptomatic patients, and in treated but unimproved patients, who have extensive major vessel occlusive disease.

Throughout this study, it has been evident that positive responders among zinc-treated patients, exhibit direct and indirect evidence of improved tissue metabolism (Table 22-II) within the ischemic extremity.

TABLE 22-II

OBJECTIVE EVIDENCE OF ENHANCED TISSUE METABOLISM IN ZINC-TREATED, IMPROVED PATIENTS

1. Healing of previously-refractive ischemic ulcers (skin and granulation tissue of which usually characterized by increased zinc concentration).
2. Increased hair growth on and "pinkness" of ischemic extremities (documented by pre- and post-treatment photographs).
3. Increased warmth.
4. Increased pO_2 of femoral vein blood (2 patients) following exercise.

One's initial reaction is that all of these observations may be secondary to and directly associated with the improved perfusion documented by Doppler. However, there are three reasons which fail to support this possibility. First, a few zinc-treated patients have improved subjectively and exhibited evidence of enhanced tissue nutrition, *but still experience claudication and/or exhibit unchanged or worsened perfusion.* Second, a few patients demonstrated enhanced tissue nutrition and experienced resolution of claudication, *but perfusion remains the same or decreases.* Third, the pathophysiology underlying claudication is thought to be related to metabolic toxic-product buildup, rather than impaired oxygenation. A major focus of recent research endeavor has been evaluation of aerobic and anaerobic metabolism in working ischemic cardiac and skeletal muscle, and it is at this level that we have concentrated an important phase of our investigation. Early results support our early thesis that zinc medication may indirectly enhance metabolism in ischemic tissue,[2] and lower or eliminate a lactate-pyruvate dependent claudication threshold. Postulating that activity of the zinc enzyme, which regulates lactate-pyruvate interchange (lactic dehydrogenase), may directly or indirectly affect claudication-threshold, we have implemented spectrophotometric and histochemical methodology to quantify the presence and activity of zinc and zinc enzymes within skin and gastrocnemius muscle of improved and nonimproved patients who are medicated with $ZnSO_4$.

Zinc content of skin and muscle obtained by biopsy (or following amputation) is determined by the methods previously reported.[4] LDH activity is quantitatively determined by spectrophotometry of homogenized tissue,[5] and qualitatively assessed by histochemical staining.[6]

RESULTS

Table 22-III summarizes the flow-augmentation data for objectively-confirmed, subjectively-improved patients who were medicated with zinc sulfate. Figure 22-4 graphically compares pressure-flow phenomena observed in normal patients, untreated severely-symptomatic patients, and treated improved patients. All patients designated "improved" were either

TABLE 22-III

SUMMARIZED OBJECTIVE EVIDENCE (DOPPLER) OF INCREASED
PERFUSION WITHIN ISCHEMIC LIMBS FOLLOWING
MEDICATIONS WITH $ZnSO_4$

1. Increased resting ankle pressure (with unchanged or lower arm pressure).
2. Appearance of audible digital flow which wasn't present prior to $ZnSO_4$.
3. Shortened rebound* from exercise-precipitated drop in ankle pressure.
4. Accelerated recovery† of exercise-precipitated drop in ankle pressure.
5. Increased flow velocity, in some cases with worsened ankle pressures.

Rebound* and recovery† are shown schematically below:

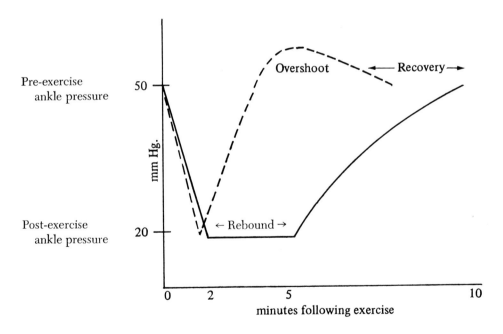

FIGURE 22-4. Comparison pressure-flow phenomena before and after exercise to illustrate rebound, overshoot and recovery phases as elaborated in the text.

totally free of claudication or else had persisting but less symptomatic claudication immediately after doubling their pre-zinc treadmill exercise performance. In only 2 of 15 subjectively-improved patients were we unable to document increased perfusion. However, 5 of the 13 improved patients who exhibited increased perfusion had residual claudication. Table 22-IV outlines the preliminary findings for zinc and lactic dehydrogenase activity in muscle from study patients, the significance and implications of which will be discussed below.

TABLE 22-IV

LDH AND ZINC ACTIVITY IN GASTROCNEMIUS MUSCLE OF MEDICATED
AND NON-MEDICATED SYMPTOMATIC PATIENTS

Patient Group	Muscle Zn (ppm)	LDH (quant.)	LDH (histo-stain)
Untreated	<2	462	+1
Treated	29	684	+3

DISCUSSION

Administration of $ZnSO_4$ to over 100 patients with symptomatic atherosclerosis, including nearly 60 who have been definitively studied for periods exceeding 24 months, has been associated with objectively-confirmed subjective improvement in about one third of the patients. In a previous review,[2] which outlined the parameters that are used to sequentially evaluate patient progress, we also expressed cautious optimism about the value of monitoring limb perfusion with the ultrasonic Doppler. We postulated that the diminution in claudication experienced by improved patients might be related to zinc-enzyme "control" of those metabolic by-products which physiologists feel underlie the characteristic pain that exercise precipitates within ischemic muscle.

The Doppler has provided us with a sensitive instrument, with which we are able to sequentially assess subnormal (indeed near-absent) flow rapidly, atraumatically and accurately. Although early models of this ultrasonic device, limited by their inability to reflect retrograde flow (which constitutes a significant fraction of total flow in certain areas of the body) were not able to quantitate flow, the new models (the prototype of which we've had for nearly 3 years) have separate outputs for antegrade and retrograde flow. The qualitative-quantitative flow assessment provided by this instrument is limited only by the auditory accuity, experience and vested interest of the listener. In order to obtain maximum yield of dynamic flow data, more often than not from extremities in which flow was barely detectable, a standardized evaluation protocol was designed in which exercise-induced pressure changes were quantified (at four levels), pressure-drop end points were timed, and return-rates were determined. With the Doppler, it is possible to monitor digital flow, auscultate arterial pressure as low as 20 mm Hg, and to detect disappearance (and/or appearance) of digital flow at even lower levels of arterial pressure. Although it is possible to record flow velocity (cps), combined use of the ear's ability to differentiate continuous and discontinuous sound and to discriminate pitch and intensity—together with a stopwatch and an arterial pressure cuff—allow the type of perfusion assessment which is summarized in Table 22-III.

Tissue Nutrition

Most of those treated patients whose subjective improvement was confirmed by documentation of objectively increased perfusion, also demonstrated evidence of enhanced tissue nutrition, but this was not universally the case. We indicated above that in a few subjectively-improved patients (claudication diminished significantly or completely), distal extremity perfusion either worsened or remained unchanged. All of these patients exhibited pink, warm skin with increased hair-growth and, in two patients, the pO_2 of femoral vein blood, following enhanced treadmill performance, was significantly greater than post-exercise values which were documented before $ZnSO_4$ was initiated. At present, certain observations suggest that perfusion *and* tissue metabolism are effected by $ZnSO_4$, (but whether in an inter-dependent or variably-independent fashion is anyone's guess at this point). First, diminution or resolution of claudication (a symptom of toxic-byproduct buildup within working ischemic muscle) was observed when perfusion remained unchanged or worsened. Second, in some patients previously-refractive ischemic ulcers healed despite decreased perfusion. Third, improved color, warmth and hair growth was observed in all subjectively-improved patients, irrespective of whether perfusion improved or worsened. Finally, two subjectively-improved patients whose perfusion decreased, exhibited increased venous oxygen concentration within an ischemic limb; an observation which supports a zinc-related "tissue effect."

If improvement in tissue nutrition were related solely to enhanced perfusion, one would not expect to observe the latter unless perfusion had increased. The fact that improved tissue nutrition and diminished claudication occurred in the face of progressively decreased pressure and perfusion supports the thesis of zinc-related enhancement or optimization of energy processes within ischemic skin and muscle. How might this occur, and how would one go about investigating this thesis? Since two of the most important "tissue-respiration" enzymes are zinc-dependent, and since catalytic activity of these two enzymes is dependent upon availability and sufficiency of their specific metallo-component, a logical starting point would be to sequentially monitor zinc LDH and carbonic anhydrase activity in skin and muscle of ischemic extremities. Since we have just finished standardizing methodology for the second enzyme, our discussion today will be limited to zinc and lactic dehydrogenase. First, however, it is pertinent to realize how the pathophysiology of claudication also fits into the "tissue-nutrition" picture. This symptom, which is characterized by sequentially occurring fatigue, pain, numbness and paresis, is felt to be related to buildup of metabolic by-product(s) within ischemic muscle. The "by-products" which remain under prime consideration are pyruvate and lactic acid, and most investigators feel that claudication is directly related to accumulation of one or both of these two metabolic intermediates whose interconversion is catalyzed by LDH. A brief review of the physiology of working muscle will elucidate the rationale for investigating the zinc-LDH related formation (and accumulation) of these two metabolic by-products.

Muscle contraction requires energy which is supplied by ATP via either aerobic or anaerobic pathways. Depending upon the magnitude of muscle work, and O_2 availability-sufficiency during this work, ATP energy production occurs via either aerobic glycogen breakdown (Krebs cycle) or anaerobic glycolysis (Cori pathway). The aerobic pathway generates pyruvate which is cycled through the Krebs route to CO_2 and water as long as sufficient O_2 continues to be available. When muscular activity outruns available O_2, two pertinent events transpire. First, existing pyruvate (which can no longer traverse the "stalled" Krebs cycle) either accumulates, or is enzymatically converted to lactic acid *by LDH* at the expense of NAD reduction. Second, ATP energy production continues, but in anaerobic fashion via a much less-efficient glycolytic pathway which generates lactic acid in the process. In the absence of O_2, the only "escape route" for this product (irrespective of whether it has been generated indirectly from Krebs cycle pyruvate, or directly from Cori pathway glycolysis), is mechanical diffusion through the cell wall, following which it can be transported to the liver for conversion into glycogen. As long as the muscle is ischemic, pyruvate-to-lactate interconversion is weighted to the right until reoxidized NAD permits resumption of the lactate-to-pyruvate interchange. When O_2 is again available, the reduced NAD co-enzyme can be oxidized and LDH (with oxidized NAD) can convert lactic acid to pyruvate, thereby providing the muscle cell with a second mechanism for "eliminating" this undesirable by-product; viz. Krebs cycle breakdown into CO_2 and water.

Lactate Dehydrogenase Activity

Awareness that the zinc enzyme LDH is one of two principal factors controlling the pyruvate-lactate ratio in ischemic muscle—the other being NAD—and that claudication resolved in certain zinc-medicated patients who failed to exhibit enhanced perfusion, was not our only reason for looking at zinc and LDH activity in ischemic tissue. Not only does LDH simultaneously catalyze the interconversion of pyruvate and lactate, and of reduced and oxidized NAD, it is the *only* enzyme in mammals capable of catalyzing the formation and degradation of lactate when O_2 shortage prevents Krebs cycle conversion of pyruvate to CO_2 and H_2O. In addition, by catalyzing the reversible reaction between NAD and NADH, LDH primes glycolysis. The fact that there are five isoenzymes of LDT complicates monitoring tissue activity of this enzyme; however, there are certain reasons why it is essential to do so. Not only do specific isoenzymes of LDH predominate in certain tissue (LDH-5 in skeletal muscle), there is also evidence that specific catalytic activity of the different isoenzymes varies. Although space doesn't permit comprehensive review of the important discoveries which have been made in this area during the past three years,[7] it is pertinent to point out that recently acquired information lends support to the thesis that biologic adequacy and local sufficiency of the LDH metallo-component (viz. zinc) may in some fashion gear pyruvate-lactate interchange away from that threshold ratio at which claudication occurs. First, under the anaerobic conditions in which lactate accumulates in skeletal muscle, pH's in the 6.4 to 6.8 range occur, and may be considered physiologic. Second, while it appears that physiologic concentrations of pyruvate and lactate do not inhibit *substrate* activity of the important skeletal muscle isoenzymes LDH-1, and LDH-5, investigators have demonstrated a difference in the degree of inhibition between these two isoenzymes by the *end-product* lactate. Third, it appears that the concentration of reduced NAD is rate-limiting for the LDH reaction. LDH-1 and LDH-5 function have been studied and confirmed for those combinations of pyruvate-lactate-pH and NAD-NADH values which occur within ischemic muscle. Summated current thinking suggests that if tissue-specific LDH isoenzymes are present, they should be able to perform their function.

Since 1969, investigations have focused on the dynamics of synthesis, degradation and stability of the LDH isoenzymes within working ischemic cardiac and skeletal muscle, reasoning that availability and reaction-capacity of this critical enzyme may be an important factor underlying functional reserve of these muscles. To us, this approach suggests the possibility that a process which we've termed "demand-adaptation" may come into play with respect to synthesis, degradation and stability of the LDH isoenzymes. In other words, the LDH-5—LDH-1 ratio needed for optimal function of chronically ischemic muscle may be different from the specific isoenzyme ratio which functions in the usually-aerobic environment of normally-perfused muscle. If chronic ischemia does evoke a change in the proportion of LDH isoenzymes, a concomitant change in metallo-component requirement probably also occurs. Such a sequence could well explain observed improvement in or resolution of pyruvate-lactate dependent claudication, particularly since clinical improvement was invariably time-dependent. If activity of existing isoenzymes had been effectively enhanced by supplementation of metallo-component, one would expect to observe improvement in hours or days. Instead, definite diminution of claudication required weeks or months, a duration of time suggestive of major change in homeostatic metabolism. The implications of zinc availability come into sharper focus when one considers that a specific characteristic of the relationship which exists between an enzyme and its metallo-activator is the variable nature of metal binding at the active site. The qualitative physical characteristics of this binding variably affects synthesis of new enzyme, as well as activity and degradation of existing enzyme.

Recent studies have shown that during zinc deficiency, certain zinc enzymes become susceptible to structural changes which increase their vulnerability to degradation.[7] Therefore, a number of factors (decreased synthesis, structural instability, accelerated breakdown, increased turnover) which may underlie decreased or suboptimal enzyme activity, may have the same etiologic denominator, viz. subnormal or suboptimal amounts of specific metallo-ion. Recognizing all of the above factors, that LDH isoenzymes exhibit tissue specificity, that working ischemic muscle places greater demands on anaerobic energy production, and that claudication diminished or resolved in improved treated patients, it becomes essential to ascertain whether a change occurs in the proportion of individual LDH isoenzymes, in response to a chronically-present anaerobic pyruvate-lactate environment. If such a change does occur, biologic zinc levels which were sufficient for LDH isoenzyme synthesis, stability and activity under predominantly aerobic conditions, may not be sufficient for generating or supporting the anaerobic LDH isoenzyme pattern, or for meeting the demands of "handling" the increased pyruvate-lactate levels associated with anaerobic muscle contraction.

Subsequent to overcoming numerous stumbling blocks, we are currently able to quantitate and histologically examine LDH activity in muscle and skin. Observations in a still small group of patients reveals enhanced LDH activity within the gastrocnemius muscle of patients with symptomatic atherosclerosis who are medicated with $ZnSO_4$. Thus far we have observed noticeably greater enzyme activity in muscle from those patients whose claudication diminished or resolved during medication with $ZnSO_4$. Concentration of zinc within the muscle increases in most treated patients, but thus far the positive correlation seems to be between patient-improvement and enhanced enzyme activity, rather than between patient-improvement and increased tissue zinc concentration. Table 22-V outlines

TABLE 22-V

EVIDENCE SUPPORTING ALTERATION OF LDH ISOENZYME PATTERN
WITHIN CHRONICALLY ISCHEMIC MUSCLE

1. Observed enhancement of gastrocnemius-muscle LDH activity during $ZnSO_4$ medication.
2. Fact that this significantly-enhanced LDH activity becomes definite only after a prolonged interval of time.
3. Enhanced LDH activity appears to occur in muscle and/or skin of most atherosclerotic patients medicated with $ZnSO_4$, but the highest levels of enhancement were evident in the gastrocnemius muscle of those patients whose claudication resolved in association with $ZnSO_4$.
4. Objective improvement in claudication can rarely be documented before 6 to 12 weeks of $ZnSO_4$, a time interval prior to which distinct enhancement of gastrocnemius LDH activity is not usually evident.
5. Awareness that synthesis-stability-degradation-activity relationship exists between isoenzymes and their activator ion, relative to observation that LDH enhancement was not evident in non-treated patients, was slow to develop in medicated patients, and was most intense in improved patients.

those observations which support the thesis that adaptive change in LDH isoenzyme "population" and activity (toward a population "better suited" for function within the predominantly anaerobic environment of chronically ischemic muscle), may account for part if not all of the resolution of claudication which occurred in $ZnSO_4$-treated *and improved* patients. This thesis would explain all of our observations to date, particularly the time-delay which is universally observed before improvement occurs. Does medication with $ZnSO_4$ stimulate change in LDH isoenzyme pattern? Probably not - - -. Recognizing that syntheses, structural degradation and turnover are adversely affected when activator-ion sufficiency is "less-than-optimal", medication with $ZnSO_4$ probably facilitate "demand-adaptation" by assuring that adequate metallo-ion is available for increased and optimal syntheses, structure and activity of a different isoenzyme pattern.

Confirmation that the resolution of claudication which occurs in certain zinc-medicated atherosclerotic patients is related to alteration of LDH isoenzyme pattern and function (toward a pattern and activity-level which is better suited for minimizing lactate-pyruvate accumulation in an anaerobic environment) demands further investigation. Toward this end, our own ongoing efforts are monitoring LDH isoenzyme patterns, zinc concentration and pyruvate-lactate concentrations within calf muscle of improved and unimproved, medicated and nonmedicated patients who have severely symptomatic atherosclerosis.

SUMMARY

More than three years ago, shortly after initial results of a long-term study confirmed the efficacy of oral $ZnSO_4$ in patients with severely symptomatic atherosclerosis, investigational effort and methodology was re-oriented to acquire answers which would reveal how, as well as why, objective improvement was related to this particular micronutrient. Toward this goal, instrumentation and techniques were implemented for monitoring flow dynamics associated with standardized exercise, and for measuring activity of zinc and specific zinc-enzymes within calf muscle of patients who responded, or failed to respond, during $ZnSO_4$ medication.

Sequential evaluation of pressure-perfusion characteristics with the Doppler ultrasonic flowmeter, before and immediately after standardized treadmill exercise, disclosed increased *perfusion* in the ischemic extremities of nearly all patients who experienced subjective improvement during medication with oral zinc. The magnitude and flow-velocity characteristics of perfusion improvement associated with $ZnSO_4$ differs from and exceeds the optimal "flow-takeover" which was observed through "adequate" collateral channels in untreated symptomatic patients, and in treated but unimproved patients who have extensive occlusive vascular disease. Most treated patients whose subjective improvement was confirmed by documentation of objectively increased perfusion, also demonstrated evidence of *enhanced tissue nutrition*, as did certain subjectively improved patients in whom perfusion either decreased or remained unchanged. Additional presented evidence for a zinc-related "tissue effect", separate from the observed "perfusion effect", supports a thesis of zinc-related enhancement or optimization of energy processes within ischemic muscle. Recognizing that two of the most important "tissue respiration" enzymes (LDH and carbonic anhydrase) are zinc-dependent, and that function of these two enzymes is dependent upon availability and sufficiency of their specific metallo-component, methodology was implemented to sequentially monitor zinc LDH and carbonic anhydrase within skin and muscle of ischemic extremities. The pathophysiology underlying claudication, and energy-metabolism of ischemic muscle constitute additional reasons for focusing on this area. Review of the physiology of working muscle elucidates that accumulation, ratio and interchange of the two metabolic by-products which are felt to underlie claudication (viz. pyruvate and lactic acid) are zinc-LDH regulated. Moreover, zinc-activated LDH is the only enzyme in mammals capable of catalyzing the formation and degradation of lactate in the predominantly anaerobic environment which characterizes ischemic muscle.

Our own observations in this investigation, evaluated in light of recently-discovered knowledge about the LDH isoenzymes, lends support to a thesis that biologic adequacy and local sufficiency of LDH metallo-component (viz. zinc) may in some fashion gear pyruvate-lactate interchange away from the threshold ratio (or level) at which claudication occurs. During the past two years investigators have been interested in LDH isoenzyme patterns and functions within working ischemic cardiac and skeletal muscle. Preliminary results suggest that availability and reaction-capacity of the isoenzymes of this critical enzyme may be an important factor underlying functional reserve of these muscles. Awareness of this observation, and assessment of our own early muscle zinc and LDH data, suggests the possibility that a metallo-component related process which we've termed "demand-adaptation" may come into play with respect to synthesis, degradation and stability of LDH isoenzymes, when chronic ischemia necessitates anaerobic metabolism in a previously aerobic environment. If LDH isoenzyme pattern does change in response to predominantly anaerobic conditions, "enriched" activator ion availability may be needed, as evidenced by known relationship between these ions and synthesis, structural stability and degradation of their specific enzyme. Certain observations made in recently studied patients support the possibility that provided with a suitable activator-ion millean, and a chronically-present anaerobic lactate-pyruvate environment, adaptive change in isoenzyme pattern may ensue. Ongoing investigation should confirm (or refute) whether the resolution of claudication which occurs in certain zinc-medicated atherosclerotic patients, is related to alteration of LDH isoenzyme pattern and function (toward more optimal control of lactate-pyruvate accumulation) which can occur when sufficient activator-ion is present.

REFERENCES

1. Henzel, J. H., Holtmann, B., Keitzer, W. F., DeWeese, M. S., and Lichti, E.: Trace Elements in Atherosclerosis, Efficacy of Zinc Medication as a Therapeutic Modality. *Trace Substances in Environmental Health II.* Columbia, University of Missouri Press, 1969, pp. 83-99.
2. Henzel, J. H., Lichti, E. L., Keitzer, W. F., and DeWeese, M. S.: Efficacy of Zinc Medication as a Therapeutic Modality in Atherosclerosis: Followup Observations in Patients Medicated Over Prolonged Periods. *Trace Substances in Environmental Health IV.* Columbia, University of Missouri Press, 1970, pp. 336-341.
3. Henzel, J. H., Lichti, E. L., and DeWeese, M. S.: Diagnosis and localization of acute vascular injury by ultrasonic Doppler. *South Med J, 64*:882, 1971.
4. Henzel, J. H., DeWeese, M. S., and Lichti, E. L.: Zinc concentrations within healing

wounds: significance of postoperative zincuria on availability and requirements during tissue repair. *Arch Surg, 100*:349, 1970.

5. Wuntch, T., Chen, R. F., and Vessell, E. S.: Lactate dehydrogenase isozymes: kinetic properties at high enzyme concentrations. *Science, 167*:63, 1970.

6. Fritz, P. J., Morrison, W. J., White, E. L., and Vessell, E. S.: Comparative study of methods for quantitative measurement of lactic dehydrogenase isoenzymes. *Anal Biochem 36*:443, 1970.

7. Vessell, E. S., and Fritz, P. J.: Factors affecting the activity tissue distribution, synthesis and degradation of isoenzymes. In Recheigl, M. Jr., (Ed.). *Enzymes, Synthesis and Degradation in Mammalian Systems.* Baltimore, Univ. Park Pr., 1971, pp. 339-374.

Chapter 23

A STUDY OF ZINC & MANGANESE DIETARY SUPPLEMENTS IN THE COPPER LOADED SCHIZOPHRENIC

CARL C. PFEIFFER

AND

ALLAN COTT

❧❧❧

INTRODUCTION

I N 1967 WHEN WE FOUND that some schizophrenics were low, while others were high, in their blood histamine levels, we turned to trace metal studies to see if abnormalities might be present and account for these differences. This possibility was encouraged by the reports that histamine occurs in the mast cells with zinc and that the highest brain level of zinc (other than the pineal gland) occurs in the hippocampus, possibly in connection with terminal vesicles of the mossy fibers where again histamine may be stored. Also diaminoxidase (histaminase) is one of the well known copper containing enzymes of the body. Zinc and copper are well known biological antagonists since in animal studies any dietary excess of one will lead to a depletion of the other. A few reports indicate that zinc and manganese are biological synergists, and manganese poisoning results in Parkinson's Disease—the symptoms of which may be mimicked as a side effect of any of the presently used antischizophrenic drugs. Manganese has many functions in the body, but it is specifically needed for the action of choline acetylase and also for normal thyroid function.

Excess copper blood levels have been recorded frequently in groups of schizophrenics, and these reports would be easier to catagorize if the worker had studied the biochemical types of schizophrenics rather than schizophrenia as a homogeneous entity. Good precedence for this concept exists since seven clinical and biochemical syndromes have been separated from "schizophrenia" since 1900.[3] The concept that metals, now called trace elements, may be deficient in some types of schizophrenia is not entirely new.

HISTORY

The trace elements known to be essential to animal life are copper, iron, manganese, zinc, chromium, molybdenum, cobalt, tin, vanadium, iodine and selenium. Others, such as sodium, potassium, magnesium and calcium are needed in large daily amounts, so they are not usually included as trace elements.

The elements which may be low in the schizophrenic are zinc, manganese, chromium and molybdenum. Those that may be high are copper, iron, cadmium, mercury and lead. The last three are of course poisons, but the poisoning may produce symptoms which mimic those of schizophrenia. This has been documented for mercury and lead. For the porphyric schizophrenic, the suggestion of a need for extra dietary zinc goes back to 1929 when Derrien and Benoit[4] found a high level of zinc in the urine of a porphyric patient. They suggested that zinc deficiency might be the cause of the abnormal psychiatric symptoms. The excess loss of zinc via the chelating action of uroporphyrin has been confirmed by Watson and Schwartz,[5] Nesbitt[6] and Peters.[7]

In 1965 Kimura and Kumura[8] found that brain autopsy specimens from schizophrenics contained approximately half the zinc of that of brains of patients dying of other causes. Henkin and co-workers[9] find zinc deficiency to be one of the etiological factors in loss of normal taste. This sometimes occurs after a severe virus infection such as "Hong Kong Flu." The taste disperception (dysgeusia) is relieved by therapy which includes extra zinc each day. Pecarek and Beisler[10] find that endotoxins will produce a quantitative reduction in the serum zinc levels of the rat. Pories[11] and Henzel[12] plus others find that zinc is necessary for maximal healing of wounds and the stress of an operation frequently depletes the bodies' stores of zinc. Caldwell and co-workers[13] find that offspring born of zinc deficient rats and mice have learning deficits. Hurley[14] finds birth anomalies in zinc deficient rats. She reports that the use of a zinc-free diet will cause a 38 percent drop in serum zinc levels of the rat within 24 hours. This indicates a lack of easily mobilized zinc reserves in body tissues so the daily intake of some zinc may be of great importance.

Plasma or serum zinc levels do not, in our experience, provide a valid index to the tissue zinc levels or the degree of deficiency which may exist. However, plasma zinc levels are significantly reduced in serious liver disease, active tuberculosis, indolent ulcers, myocardial infarction, Down's syndrome, cystic fibrosis, growth retardation, pregnancy and in women with oral contraceptive therapy.[15]

A possible relationship between serum polyamines and trace metals may exist and be reflected in changes in RNA synthesis. Dawson and co-workers,[16] and Swenerton et al.[17] ascribe congenital malformations after zinc deficiency to impaired DNA synthesis, and Weser and co-workers[18] find that zinc increases thymidine incorporation into DNA in zinc deficient rats. Cox[19] finds zinc necessary for RNA synthesis and also need for adrenal corticoid action involving protein synthesis. Gregoriadio and Sourkes[20] find copper accumulation in the liver of adrenalectomized rats. Thus severe adrenal insufficiency may be accompanied by increased tissue copper which would antagonize zinc.

Since hypoglycemias occur frequently in psychic disorders and are misdiagnosed as schizophrenias, one should always consider the possibility that the patients may be zinc deficient since insulin and pancreatic action requires zinc.

Other than indirect copper studies, very few studies of trace metals appear in the literature on schizophrenia. In fact, the use of trace metals as a possible treatment method in schizophrenia started in 1929. At that time W. M. English[21] of Brockville, Ontario, used manganese chloride intravenously in 181 schizophrenic patients and found that half of them improved. As with chlorpromazine and reserpine therapy, English reported a gain in weight in those patients who responded to manganese therapy. (Intravenous manganese produced a cutaneous flush like that of niacin!) This study was in part repeated by R. G. Hoskins[22] of the Worchester Foundation who published in 1934, but instead of using manganese chloride intravenously he used, for the most part, suspended manganese dioxide given intramuscularly. In the first instance the intravenous route was unnecessary with water soluble and easily absorbed manganese chloride. In the second instance manganese dioxide is a nonabsorbable form which was deposited intramuscularly where it probably stayed for a very long time. Hoskins found no improvement in the few schizophrenics injected with manganese dioxide.

Of the trace metals which theoretically should produce some benefit in the schizophrenic, manganese is a likely prospect since it increases the activity of acetylcholine acetylase. We know that drugs that increase the acetylcholine effect in the brain will benefit schizophrenia. For example, reserpine (which produced symptoms of acetylcholine overdosage, i.e. drooling and tremor) might be called the prototype of antischizophrenic drugs.

In many instances other elements may substitute for a given trace element. The function of the enzyme is then either enhanced or depressed. We suggest that in the schizophrenic copper or iron may be present in excess rather than the normal zinc and manganese.

METHODS

In general the methods used in this study have all been detailed in previous publications. A Perkin-Elmer 305 Atomic Absorption Spectrophotometer was used to determine serum and urinary iron, zinc and copper. Serum manganese was determined by the same method of using 4 ml of concentrated serum. Hair analyses for trace metals were done by a commercial laboratory.*

Urinary excretion of trace metals was determined for a six hour period which ran from 9:00 A.M. to 3:00 P.M. In this way accurate collections could be obtained in a 7.5 hour work day. These patients and normal subjects usually had a quantitative electroencephalogram taken every 10 minutes out of each hour for a six hour period after the control run.

Normal subjects were laboratory personnel, reformatory inmates and others who passed a psychiatric interview and who also had a normal score on the Experiential World Inventory (EWI).[23] Outpatients with schizophrenia were referred by physicians mainly to determine their type in regard to high or low blood histamine level. Most patients had been hospitalized one or more times for their schizophrenia. Patients who had not been hospitalized were given the EWI and Minnesota Multiphasic Personality Inventory to ascertain their degree of psychopathology.

Various treatments were used to improve the psychiatric status of the patients. These were the conventional antischizophrenic drugs, vitamin supplements, lithium therapy to the level of 1.0 meq/l and a trace element dietary supplement consisting of 10 percent zinc sulfate and 0.5 manganous chloride in distilled water. When used at the level of 5 drops A.M. and P.M., this solution provides half of the zinc and manganese which should be present in an ideal normal diet.

Patients were studied at 5 week intervals over a period of 1 to 3 years. A 30 ml blood sample was taken at each visit. Two ml of whole blood was taken for histamine and polyamine determinations. The remaining serum was used for lithium, creatine phosphokinase, trace metal and other determinations. In most instances a sample was frozen for future reference.

RESULTS

The results are tabulated in the form of tables and figures wherein an attempt has been made to have completely explanatory legends. Some tables represent several years of study on 300 schizophrenic out-patients with a trace metal report on a longitudinal study of 240 patients. The results are collected in Tables 23-I to 23-XIV.

Trace metal urinary excretion and plasma levels have been done on six hospitalized patients and six to 30 schizophrenic out-patients. In most instances the trials have been repeated to determine the variability of a given patient and to increase the actual number of trials. Urinary excretion of the trace metals studied varies widely. Thus a series of 25 trials is sometimes necessary to produce a reasonably low standard deviation.

*Albion Laboratory, Clearfield, Utah 84015.

TABLE 23-I

URINARY EXCRETION OF COPPER, ZINC, AND IRON[a]
(Total mcg/6 hr)

Medication and oral dose	Patients				Normals			
	No Trials	Cu	Zn	Fe	No Trials	Cu	Zn	Fe
Placebo	18	1.7	152	16	26	4.6	148	20
Ca lactate, 2.0 gm	9	1.5	163	33	—	—	—	—
Cr acetate, 5 mg	8	1.4	155	14	—	—	—	—
NH_4 molybdate, 5 mg	12	1.2	146	10	—	—	—	—
$ZnSO_4$, 50 mg	11	2.3	204	20	16	2.1	115	13
ZnAc, 35 mg	13	3.7	108	22	10	3.6	138	15
$MnCl_2$, 3 mg	11	5.5	137	47	10	1.2	325	12
ZnMg[*], 70 mg	18	6.6	140	10	10	15.7	133	20
ZnMgMn[†], 70 mg	21	7.8	108	13	—	—	—	—
B-6, 50 mg	21	3.9	89	15	14	7.4	105	10
ZnMn, 50/3 mg	12	11.0	147	15	12	9.1	154	15
ZnMn B-6, 50/3/50 mg	14	20.0	224	16	13	3.0	186	6
$CuSO_4$, 5 mg	16	2.5	126	36	15	1.4	151	42
$MgCl_2$, 200 mg	10	2.3	141	28	10	3.1	116	34
$FeSO_4$, 900 mg	9	0.4	262	116	13	6.5	123	21
Na_2SO_4, 200 mg	18	7.3	118	19	12	6.7	116	8
CPZ[‡], 150 mg	27	9.3	122	19	—	—	—	—

[a]Urinary excretion over a 6 hour period of copper, zinc and iron after the oral administration of small amounts of various trace elements. Schizophrenics compared with normal male subjects. Schizophrenics excrete less copper and iron. Zinc increases copper excretion but zinc-manganese with B-6, 50 mg results in the greatest increase in copper excretion. The sulfate ion and chlorpromazine also increase copper excretion. In both schizophrenics and normals pyridoxine (B-6) tends to conserve zinc insofar as urinary excretion is concerned. Both calcium and magnesium increase iron excretion as does also copper. Added iron causes increased iron excretion in schizophrenics but not in normals.

[*]1 Vicon-C

[†]1 Vicon-C plus $MnCl_2$ 3 mg

[‡]Chlorpromazine

TABLE 23-II

EFFECT OF A STARCH PLACEBO ON 13 NORMAL SUBJECTS

Element	0 Hr.	6 Hr.
Zinc	1.05 ± 0.05	0.83 ± 0.11 (—21%)[*]
Copper	0.93 ± 0.09	0.93 ± 0.14 (0%)
Iron	1.40 ± 0.4	1.33 (—5%)

Changes in serum, zinc, copper and iron after a starch placebo tablet. The zinc levels decrease significantly in the six hour test period while copper and iron remain much more constant. This may indicate the need for regular zinc intake with each meal. Henkin[36] has found similar changes in a balanced dietary intake and refers to the daytime drop in zinc as a circadian rhythm.

[*]Change significant at the 1 in 20 level of confidence.

TABLE 23-III

HUMAN QUANTITATIVE EEG AFTER ZINC SULFATE 50 MG ORALLY

	Trials		Control	Hours after dietary supplement					
				1	2	3	4	5	6
Patients	(11)	MIA	100	92	83°	90	93	85	85
		CV	9.0	12.6	16.9°	14.1	12.4	17.0	11.7
Normals	(10)	MIA	100	102	100	102	96	95	96
		CV	20.8	18.7	21.9	16.1	22.8	26.4	21.0
50 mg + B6 50 mgm									
Patients	(15)	MIA	100	97	87°	85°	94	95	96
		CV	12.0	14.1	19.1°	18.9°	13.1	14.7	14.0

MIA = Mean Integrated Amplitude.   CV = Coefficient of Variation.

In patients Zn decreases MIA and increases CV which changes occur with antianxiety drugs. In the normals where the CV is higher no significant change occurs. This may indicate that zinc is needed in the schizophrenic because of deficiency. The addition of pyridoxine (B-6) accentuates the response of the patients to zinc sulfate. Zinc is needed for the normal action of B-6.

°Significant change from control level $P<0.05$.

TABLE 23-IV

EFFECT OF ZINC + B-6 ON HISTAMINE, SPERMIDINE, AND SPERMINE LEVELS OF BLOOD°

Date		Serum			Whole Blood		
		Cu	Fe	Zn	H	Spd	Sp
7/14	0 hr	.92	1.38	.82	21.7	.62	1.08
7/14	6 hr	.94	1.04	.64			
7/15	6 hr	.94	1.04	.64			
7/16	6 hr	.80	1.04	.78			
7/17	6 hr	1.02	0.88	1.04			
7/18	6 hr	.96	1.64	1.00			
7/20	6 hr	1.06	.96	.92	30.8	1.09	1.63

°E.E., (Normal ? Male, age 27, ZnSO₄ + B-6, 50 mg of each/day. The zinc dietary supplement raises serum zinc level. The rise in histamine and polyamine levels is also of interest, in that this (normal ?) subject had abnormally low levels.

TABLE 23-V

ZINC DIETARY SUPPLEMENT—24 MALES AND FEMALES WITH LOW ZINC.

	Control	1	Visit				
			2	3	4	5	6
EWI	52	52	43	29°	34	47	36
Cu	1.22	1.29	1.37	1.31	1.43	1.44	1.53
Zn	0.73	1.10°	0.97°	0.99°	1.09°	0.92°	0.88°
Fe	1.05	1.23°	1.16	1.18	1.45°	1.20	1.28°

°Significant change from control level $P<0.05$.

Note that the serum zinc level rises and stays up for the 6 month period covered by the six visits. Serum copper and iron also rise. The EWI decreases.

TABLE 23-VI

ZINC DIETARY SUPPLEMENT IN HIGH-COPPER MALE PATIENTS

			Visit			
	Control	1	2	3	4	5
EWI	60	66	56	58	35	47
Copper	1.44°	1.25	1.19	1.26	1.30	1.32
Zinc	1.23	1.31	1.06	1.08	.96	1.05
Iron	1.18	1.22	1.26	1.21	1.25	1.11

°The high serum copper level (normal 1.0 mcg/ml) may decrease promptly in high-copper patients (14 in sample). This is accompanied by improvement in psychiatric symptoms (EWI).

Source: Hurley, *J Clin Nutr*, 22:1332, 1969.

TABLE 23-VII

ZINC DIETARY SUPPLEMENT WITH RISING COPPER RESPONSE°

			Visit		
	Control	1	2	3	4
EWI	43	45	46	43	34
Copper	1.10	1.34	1.38	1.35	1.28
Zinc	1.06	1.10	0.96	0.98	1.01
Iron	1.31	1.24	1.15	1.26	1.35

°Data drawn from 28 male and female subjects. While no significant changes from the control occur, the copper rises for 3 months and then falls. This is accompanied by a decrease in the EWI. The normal zinc level does not increase.

Source: Lee, Jr., and Matrone, *Proc Soc Exp Biol Med*, 130:1190, 1969.

TABLE 23-VIII

RISING COPPER AND IRON AFTER ZINC DIETARY SUPPLEMENT IN OUTPATIENT SCHIZOPHRENICS°

			Visit (monthly)				
	Control	1	2	3	4	5	6
EWI	49	46	42	42	42	36	40
Copper	1.13	1.21	1.24†	1.27†	1.27†	1.31†	1.32†
Zinc	1.05	1.15†	1.01	1.00	0.98	1.03	1.04
Iron	1.18	1.42†	1.42†	1.40†	1.29	1.28	1.38†

°Data drawn from 72 subjects, male and female. With this type of serum trace-metal change the individual patient may get worse mentally before getting better. This may account for the slow decrease in the EWI.

†Significant change from control level ($p<0.05$).

TABLE 23-IX

ZINC DIETARY SUPPLEMENT IN SUBJECTS WITH LOW IRON°

			Visit				
	Control	1	2	3	4	5	6
EWI	51	65	62	65	60	59	29
Copper	1.25	1.39	1.23	1.22	1.45	1.61†	1.43
Zinc	0.90	1.13†	0.87	1.04	1.01	0.89	0.90
Iron	0.55	0.78†	0.97†	1.06†	1.00†	1.04†	0.84†

°Data drawn from 16 male and female subjects with low iron. Note that Zn supplement increased iron level of the serum. Over a longer period (5 months) the copper reached a peak. Zinc levels did not change.

†Significant change from control level $p<0.05$.

TABLE 23-X

SUMMARY BLOOD SERUM TRACE METAL STUDIES
240 SCHIZOPHRENIC OUTPATIENTS

	No. Subjects	*Percentage*
Low zinc° (>0.80 mcg/ml)	27	11
High copper (<1.20 mcg/ml)	47	20
Low iron (>0.60 mcg/ml)	18	8
High iron (<1.50 mcg/ml)	29	12
Changes After Zinc Dietary Supplement		
Increased copper and iron	76	32
Increased copper	43	18
No change	48	20

°Only 11% + 20% = 31% of the patients could be classified as low in zinc or high in copper, but with zinc supplementation the rise in copper (or both copper and iron) indicates many more may have excess copper and iron in their tissues.

TABLE 23-XI

EFFECT OF PLACEBO OR D-PENICILLAMINE ON SIX-HOUR URINARY
EXCRETION OF COPPER, ZINC AND IRON°

	Normals (8)	*Schizophrenics (11)*
	After Placebo (mcg ± S.E.)	
Copper	4.46 ± 1.69	0.2
Zinc	128.00 ± 24.78	143.90 ± 27.28
Iron	31.12 ± 7.03	16.18 ± 2.39°
	After 500 mg. D-Penicillamine (mcg ± S.E.)	
Copper	178.00 ± 37.96	174.00 ± 37.37
Zinc	299.71 ± 41.27	525.87 ± 132.66
Iron	9.28 ± 3.86	11.62 ± 3.08

°The normal excretes more copper and less zinc. Penicillamine greatly increases copper excretion, but zinc excretion is also more than doubled. Iron excretion is decreased.

TABLE 23-XII

SIX HOUR URINARY EXCRETION OF COPPER, ZINC AND IRON AFTER
VARIOUS INACTIVE TRACE METALS

Metal	*Trials*	*Dose (grams)*	*Urinary Excretion (mg)*		
			Cu	*Zn*	*Fe*
Placebo	18	—	1.7	152	16
Ca Lactage	9	2.0	1.5	163	33
Cr Acetate	8	0.005	1.4	155	14
NH₄ Molybdate	12	0.005	1.2	146	10
		Normals			
Placebo	26	—	4.6	148	20

Calcium acts like magnesium to increase the urinary excretion of iron. Note that copper excretion in the schizophrenic is consistently below that of the normal.

TABLE 23-XIII

ZINC AND COPPER CONTENT OF THE HAIR

	Females (ppm—means)			
	Zinc		*Copper*	
Age (years)	*Normals°*	*Schizophrenic†Outpatients*	*Normals*	*Schizophrenic Outpatients*
15	190	240	20	105
30	160	220	28	64
40	160	109	22	54
50	160	143	45	31
70	140	257	26	21

	Males (ppm—means)			
	Zinc		*Copper*	
Age (years)	*Normals*	*Schizophrenic Outpatients*	*Normals*	*Schizophrenic Outpatients*
12	147	44	34	25
15	180	161	33	77
30	150	150	18	44
39	150	132	18	31

°Data on normals from Petering, Yeager, and Witherup, *Arch Environ Health*, 23:202, 1971.

†Data on schizophrenics from Allan Cott, personal communication.

This preliminary comparison of 2 groups numbering 100-150 individuals shows copper to be high in the hair of schizophrenics aged 15 to 30 years. For females zinc is also high, but in males zinc is low in the adolescent years.

TABLE 23-XIV

CORRELATION COEFFICIENTS—r and *p* VALUES

		N	*Slope*	*Intercept*	*r*	*p*
Females	Ca/Age	44	5.5	13.2	+0.71	<0.001
"	Mn/Age	44	−0.68	18.3	0.02	N.S.
"	Zn/Age	44	0.00	18.1	0.001	N.S.
"	Mg/Age	44	0.79	6.8	+0.66	<0.001
Males	Mn/Age	50	−2.2	−25.4	−0.54	<0.001
"	Mg/Age	50	−0.09	22.6	0.02	N.S.

During the menarche ages 10 to 50 the hair calcium increases in females. This is highly significant and could only occur by chance, 1 in 1,000 times. The same is true for magnesium in the hair of females.

For males, but not for females, the manganese content decreases significantly with age. This could occur by chance only 1 in a 1,000 times.

TABLE 23-XIV

IMPORTANT TRACE ELEMENT LOSSES IN BREAD-MAKING°

Wheat Product	Manganese	Copper	Zinc	Magnesium
Wheat, common hard	38	5	24	1800
Wheat, common soft	35	4.5	22	1590
Wheat, durum	32	4.8	30	1860
Processed wheat foods				
Flour, cake	1.7	0.8	2.3	220
White bread	5.5	2.1	8.9	420
Whole wheat bread	41	5.1	27	1950
Doughnuts	3.5	1.7	6.5	320

°Note that each of these trace metals, expressed here as p.p.m., may be decreased in the milling process. Since doughnuts are made from cake flour, which is lowest in important trace elements, anyone who tries to get by on a "coffee and doughnut diet" is headed for nutritional deficiencies and mental health problems. These are selected data from Zook, Greene, and Morris, *Cereal Chem*, 47:720, 1970.

TABLE 23-XV

BIOCHEMICAL DIFFERENTIATION TO PROVIDE MORE EFFECTIVE
TREATMENT OF THE SCHIZOPHRENIAS

A) Thought disorder	B) Overstimulation
Histapenia (50%)	*Histadelia (20%)*
1) Grandiosity	1) Blank mind
2) Paranoia	2) Suicidal depression
3) Hallucinations	3) Compulsions
4) Mania	

Effective Treatments

Folic Acid—B12	Methionine (methylates?)
Niacin (Increases tissue histidine)	Calcium (releases)
Vitamin C	Dilantin (antifolate)
Zinc-Manganese	Methadone (releases)
	Zinc-Manganese

The mean excretion of zinc, copper and iron as given in Tables 23-I, 23-XI and 23-XII does provide trends on which to base working hypotheses on the interactions of trace metals in man. In the 4 year period covered by this study, many normal subjects have been run to provide comparative data.

Most of the trace metals have been cautiously tried for the effect on zinc, copper and iron excretion and quantitative EEG stimulation or sedation. In addition, the amino acids which may chelate trace metals have been explored for their effect on the excretion of zinc, copper and iron. In general copper, chromium and cobalt are stimulant to the brain while

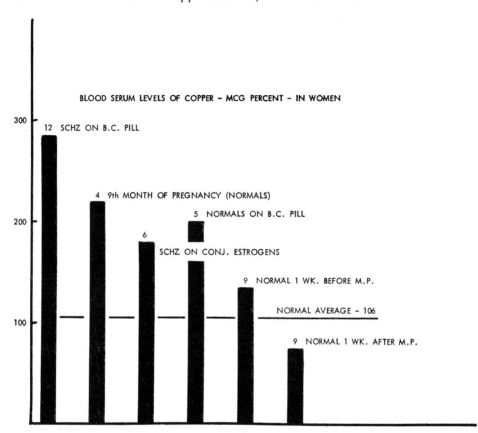

FIGURE 23-1. Serum copper levels of various categories of schizophrenic patients and normal females. The numbers at top of bar graphs indicate number of patients or normals. The schizophrenic on the contraceptive pill (B. C. Pill) has a great increase in serum copper which is greater than the 9th month of pregnancy in normals. Both rises are ascribed to estrogens which indicates the great estrogenic potency of the contraceptive pill. Premenstruation is also different from postmenstruation because of the normal variation in estrogen level. The high copper level coincides with the time of greatest emotional depression.

zinc, manganese, vanadium and molybdenum are sedative. Fluorine and selenium are without effect on the quantitative EEG at the low doses tested. The amino acids of present interest are ornithine, methionine, lysine, histidine and tryptophane.

DISCUSSION

It has been said that zinc deficiency in animals was not evident until the galvanized animal cages were replaced by stainless steel cages. One can now suggest that zinc deficiency in man was not evident until galvanized water pipes were replaced by modern copper plumbing! The rats obtained their needed zinc by gnawing the cages, and we can obtain zinc by drinking water which has coursed through zinc lined iron (galvanized) pipes. With copper plumbing and acid water we may get an excess of copper which antagonizes any zinc which may be in our food.

Some trace metals are known to compete with each other in biological systems so an excess of copper could block other more effective trace metals from an active enzyme site.[25,26] Cox and Harris[27] summarize previous studies on the displacement of copper from tissue by excess dietary zinc. In addition they studied rats given a diet containing 0.6 percent zinc which produced copper deficiency anemia in 3 weeks. This was corrected by the addition of 0.01 percent Cu to the diet. The addition of 0.08 percent Fe was less effective than copper. Liver and kidney copper levels were not reduced by this large zinc intake, but iron levels were significantly reduced.

Trace Element Correlates

Lee and Matrone[28] find in rats that high zinc diets produce a precipitous drop in ceruloplasmin levels within one week. This is restored towards normal by copper or copper/iron injections. The diet contained 1.4 percent zinc carbonate which is an enormous dose. Studies by Rimai and Heyde[29] show that adenosine triphosphate combines with Ca^{++} and Mg^{++} at the phosphate ionic bond while Zn^{++} and Mn^{++} complex both with the phosphate bond and the adenine base. McCormick and co-workers[29] report the stability constants of Fe^{++}, and especially Cu^{++}, with tridentate amino acids to be much higher than that of Zn^{++} or Mn^{++}. If these amino acids are involved in trace metal enzyme action, one could predict that excess copper would dominate zinc and manganese in tissue enzyme action.

The research use of the copper chelating agent penicillamine in schizophrenia is an attempt to decrease the copper level in the treatment resistant schizophrenic patient. Careful checks on serum levels and urinary excretion of copper are made on the patient with Wilson's disease, whereas penicillamine has been used in schizophrenics without the benefit of any objective trace metal tests. Fister and co-workers[30] suggested that the patient on this therapy be given extra trace metals (except copper) once each week. This regime was also followed by Nicolson and co-workers.[31] Others have ignored the finding that penicillamine chelates and may deplete zinc as well as copper.[32] One of the side effects of penicillamine is the loss of the sensation of taste which is a sign of zinc deficiency.[33] We can confirm the fact that penicillamine chelates zinc out of the body as well as copper. Urinary iron excretion is decreased, however (Table 23-XI). This confirms Walshe and Patston[34] who found no effect on serum iron. Penicillamine also complexes with pyridoxine (B-6) so that many workers have recommended 50 mg of B-6 per day as a supplement. If the penicillamine is given after meals to prevent nausea, then the B-6 (25 mg) should be given before breakfast and 25 mg before supper to minimize interaction with the penicillamine.

As cited previously, Henkin et al.[9] finds zinc deficiency to be one of the etiological factors in loss of normal taste. This sometimes occurs after a severe virus infection such as "Hong Kong Flu." The taste disperception is relieved by therapy which includes 100 mg of zinc sulfate per day. Pecarek and Beisel[10] find that endotoxins will produce a quantitative reduction in the serum zinc levels of the rat. Pories[11] and Henzel[12] plus others find that zinc is necessary for maximal healing of wounds, and the stress of an operation frequently depletes the bodies' stores of zinc. Caldwell and co-workers[13] find that offspring born of zinc deficient rats and mice have learning deficits. Hurley[14] finds birth anomalies in zinc deficient rats. She reports that the use of a zinc-free diet will cause a 38 percent drop in serum zinc levels of the rat within 24 hours. We find a 21 percent drop in serum zinc in a 6 hour period (Table 23-II). This indicates a lack of easily mobilized zinc reserves in body tissues so the daily intake of some zinc is of great importance.

Plasma or serum zinc levels do not, in our experience, provide a valid index to the tissue levels or the degree of deficiency which may exist. Plasma zinc levels are significantly reduced however in serious liver disease, active tuberculosis, indolent ulcers, myocardial infarction, Down's syndrome, cystic fibrosis, growth retardation, pregnancy and with oral contraceptive therapy.[15]

As mentioned previously, if one considers porphyric schizophrenia as one of the schizophrenias (frequently overlooked) zinc deficiency in schizophrenia can be traced back to 1929 when Derrien and Benoit[4] working at Montpelier in France discovered that uroporphyrin chelated zinc and thus depleted *zinc.* They postulated that some of the psychic and neurological symptoms could be precipitated by the zinc deficiency. The excess loss of zinc via uroporphyrin was confirmed by Watson and Schwartz.[5] Nesbitt[6] again suggested that the mental symptoms of porphyria might be caused by a zinc deficit. Peters[7] found an increase in zinc and also copper in patients with acute attacks of porphyric schizophrenia. Perhaps the main cause is added copper ingestion or absorption which then displaces zinc and both are excreted excessively. Peters also suggests another trace metal deficiency (which might be that of manganese). Pyridoxine deficiency as suggested by Metzler[35] could also be a precipitating factor. In any event, the mauve factor is now known to be a pyrrole derivative[36] which may come from the breakdown of myoglobin or hemoglobin. Thus mauve positive patients may be mild porphyrics.

Dietary and Environmental Factors

For copper and iron one can find many environmental factors which may overload the human system. These may have a varied degree of significance with each individual patient. Owing to vitamin publicity many patients unwittingly take vitamins with iron and copper. Frequently the only clue to the presence of iron and copper is the letter *M* after the brand name. When vitamin C is present, iron is better absorbed. This may also be true for copper. Many American families pump their own household water from the soil. In shale soils the water may be high in sulfur dioxide (sulfurous acid), and in marshy soils excess carbonic acid may be present. Either or both of these acids will remove copper from the pipes to produce water as high as 2 ppm of copper. By contrast New York City water has 0.02 ppm. Estrogenic action raises serum copper, and the schizophrenic is more susceptible to this effect. Birth control pills may thus raise copper levels to extremes greater than those found in the ninth month of pregnancy (Figure 23-1). Finally, zinc and/or manganese deficiency may allow copper and iron to accumulate in the tissues, so any depletion of zinc or manganese from our diet may allow copper and iron excess to occur. The treatment of green vegetables with the chelating agent EDTA prior to the freezing process reduces zinc and manganese to 20 percent of the expected normal range. The processing of flour decreases zinc, manganese and magnesium (Table 23-XIV).

With some impoverished or deficient soils the level of trace element may be definitely less in the food plants. Finally, a high grain diet with its high content of phytate may sequester trace metals so that they are not available to the body economy. Conversely, high doses of vitamin C keeps many trace metals in the reduced state so that excess absorption (as of iron) may occur.

The usual method for study of a metabolic need in man of a vitamin, essential amino acid, or a trace metal involves the establishment of a metabolic ward or dormitory wherein patients or stalwart young males are imprisoned to determine their intake tissue level, and output of the essential nutrient in question. This, in balance, gives answers which apply specifically to the accuracy of the biochemical diagnosis of the patient or to the need of stalwart young males for a nutrient which their bodies obviously conserve or they wouldn't be stalwart, healthy young volunteers. The action of stress, growth or pregnancy is seldom studied in the metabolic ward. The metabolic ward is limited by funds and nursing care to 8 to 16 beds, so the accumulation of statistically reliable data is frustratingly slow and expensive. However, if one considers each patient as a biochemical unknown and uses the available tests (at each visit) to see what changes may occur, then the possibility evolves that meaningful and prognostic changes may occur in the biochemical measurements if they have been carefully chosen to test a pertinent hypothesis. This method does not have the painstaking accuracy of a metabolic ward, but it does provide some challenging data relating to the subdivision of the schizophrenias on the basis of blood histamine levels and the serum levels of copper, zinc and iron.

Schizophrenia Studies

One may ask why a double-blind study has not been planned and executed before this report. Double-blind studies are only valid to compare homogeneous populations. The schizophrenias are biochemically very heterogeneous as shown by these exploratory biochemical studies. Trace metal serum levels show low zinc patients, high copper patients and patients who get a rise in copper and iron when zinc and manganese is given. In addition, some patients are high or low in blood histamine while others may be low in spermine and very high in spermidine. The agitated patient is high in blood serum creatine phosphokinase, a muscle enzyme which leaks out with muscle exertion or excess stimulation. Faced with these biochemical abnormalities, some of which may be very psychiatrically signfiicant, one can only study the individual schizophrenic and put the similar biochemical categories together. The search for biochemically similar schizophrenic patients is exactly what we have attempted in this exploratory study and report.

For example, *if* we had no knowledge of the anemias, vitamin B-12 would have scored poorly when used in a double-blind experiment to determine its effectiveness in the relief of lassitude in pale people even if the best of our presently available mood questionnaires or interviewers were employed. However, when the simple objective criterion of erythrocyte counts is added as a yardstick, then only a few anemia patients would respond to vitamin B-12 while most would not. Finally, when the anemia is hypochromic macrocytic, a distinct category, then vitamin B-12—folate is highly specific for this small percentage of anemias. A double-blind study has yet to be done on pernicious anemia since with objective diagnostic criteria such studies are less pertinent. At present everybody understands the double-blind study but few are interested in longitudinal biochemical changes by which one can select biochemically similar mental patients for future double-blind studies on homogeneous populations.

SUMMARY OF EXPLORATORY STUDIES ON TRACE METAL BALANCE IN SCHIZOPHRENICS

1) Serum zinc levels of normal subjects decrease significantly in a six hour period while copper and iron do not.

2) Zinc, with or without pyridoxine, produces an EEG "anti-anxiety effect" in schizophrenics but not in normals.

3) Urinary copper excretion is consistently less for schizophrenics than for normals.

4) Zinc increases urinary copper excretion as also does manganese, but Zn/Mn in dietary doses is most effective in increasing copper elimination.

5) D-Penicillamine increases urinary excretion of zinc as well as that of copper. Therefore, dietary supplement of zinc should be provided during P therapy.

6) Approximately 11 percent of 240 schizophrenic outpatients had a low serum zinc level (less than 80 mcg %), 20 percent had elevated copper levels (greater than 120 mcg %), 8 percent had low iron (less than 60 mcg %), and 12 percent had high serum iron (greater than 150 mcg %).

7) The serum level may not reflect the tissue level since with Zn/Mn dietary supplement 50 percent of the patients had a rise in serum copper and iron over a period of 4 to 5 months.

8) Of the dietary supplements used in the schizophrenic out-patients, the best results were obtained with zinc sulfate 10 percent plus manganous chloride 0.5 percent.

9) The lowest serum copper level occurs one week after the menstrual period while the highest level occurs the week before the period. Estrogens raise copper levels and the schizophrenic appears to be more susceptible to this hypercupremia since copper levels may exceed those of the ninth month of pregnancy. Hypercupremia can aggravate depression and other symptoms in the schizophrenic.

10) Trace metals which have not been explored adequately in the schizophrenias are chromium, manganese, molybdenum and selenium.

11) Because of zinc metal contamination (or addition in tableting), megavitamin therapy may in part be zinc dietary supplement.

12) Patients who have high serum copper levels, tremor of the hands, ataxia and intermittent symptoms of schizophrenia should be studied as potential victims of mercury poisoning.

13) Analyses of hair shows male schizophrenics to be low in manganese and high in copper. Females are high in copper. A probable factor in some of the schizophrenias is a combined deficiency of zinc and manganese with a relative increase in iron or copper or both.

REFERENCES

1. Pfeiffer, C. C., Iliev, V., Goldstein, L., and Jenney, E. H.: Serum polyamine levels in schizophrenia and other objective criteria of clinical status. In Sivankar, D. V.

(Ed.): *Schizophrenia Current Concepts and Research.* Hicksville, PJD Publications, 1969.

2. Pfeiffer, C. C., Iliev, V., Goldstein, L., Jenney, E. H., and Schultz, R.: Blood histamin polyamines and schizophrenias: Computer correlations of the low and high blood histamine types. *Res Commun Chem Pathol Pharmacol, 1*:247, 1970.

3. Pfeiffer, C. C., Ward, J., El-Meligi, M., and Cott, A.: *The Schizophrenias: Yours and Mine.* Moonachie, Pyramid Books, 1970.

4. Derrien, E., and Benoit, C.: Notes et observations des les urines et des quelques organs d'une femme morte en crise de porphyrie acuité. *Arch Soc Sc Med Biol Montpelier, 8*:456, 1929.

5. Watson, C. J., and Schwartz, S. J.: The excretion of zinc uroporphyrin in idiopathic porphyria. *J Clin Invest, 20*:440, 1941.

6. Nesbitt, S.: Acute porphyria. *JAMA, 124*:286, 1944.

7. Peters, H. A.: Trace minerals, chelating agents, and the porphyrias. *Fed Proc, 20(3)*:227, 1961.

8. Kimura, K., and Kumura, J.: Preliminary reports on the metabolism of trace elements in neuropsychiatric disease. I. Zinc in schizophrenia. *Proc Japan Acad, 41*:943, 1965.

9. Henkin, R. I., Graziadei, P. P. G., and Bradley, D. F.: Preliminary reports on the metabolism of trace elements in neuropsychiatric diseases. I. Zinc in schizophrenia. *Ann Intern Med, 71*:791, 1969.

10. Pecarek, R. C., and Beisel, W. R.: Effect of endotoxin on serum zinc concentrations in the rat. *Appl Microbiol, 18*:482, 1969.

11. Pories, W. J., Henzel, J. H., Rob, C. G., and Strain, W. H.: Acceleration of healing with zinc sulfate. *Ann Surg, 165*:432, 1967.

12. Henzel, J. H., DeWeese, M. S., and Lichti, E. L.: Zinc concentrations within healing wounds. Significance of postoperative zincuria on availability and requirements during tissue repair. *Arch Surg, 100*:349, 1970.

13. Caldwell, D. F., Oberleas, D., Clancy, J. J., and Prasad, A. S.: Behavioral impairment in adult rats following acute zinc deficiency. *Proc Soc Exp Biol Med, 133*:1417, 1970.

14. Hurley, L. S.: Zinc deficiency in the developing rat. *Am J Clin Nutr, 22*:1332, 1969.

15. Halsted, J. A., and Smith, J. C., Jr.: Plasma-zinc in health and disease. *Lancet i*:322, 1970.

16. Dawson, E. B., Cravy, W. D., Clark, R. R., and McGarrity, W. J.: Effect of trace metals on placental metabolism. *Am J Obstet Gynecol, 104*:953, 1969.

17. Swenerton, H., Shrader, R., and Hurley, L. S.: Zinc-deficient embryos: Reduced thymidine incorporation. *Science, 166*:1014, 1969.

18. Weser, U., Seeber, S., and Warnecke, P.: Reactivity of Zn^{2+} on nuclear DNA and RNA biosynthesis of regenerating rat liver. *Biochim Biophys Acta, 179*:422, 1969.

19. Cox, R. P.: Hormonal induction of increased zinc uptake in mammalian cell cultures: Requirement for RNA and protein synthesis. *Science, 165*:196, 1969.

20. Gregoriadis, G., and Sourkes, T. L.: Regulation of hepatic copper in the rat by the adrenal gland. *Canad J Biochem, 48*:160, 1970.

21. English, W. M.: Report of treatment with manganese chloride of 181 cases of schizophrenia, 33 of manic depression, and 16 of other defects of psychoses at Ontario Hospital, Brockville, Ontario. *Am J Psychiatry, 9*:569, 1929.

22. Hoskins, R. G.: Manganese treatment of "schizophrenic disorders." *J Nerv Ment Dis, 79*:59, 1934.
23. Osmond, H., and El-Meligi, A. M.: *The Experiential World Inventory.* New York, Mens Sana, 1971.
24. Lifschitz, M. D., and Henkin, R. I.: Circadian variation in copper and zinc in man. *J Appl Physiol, 31*:88, 1971.
25. Habermann, H. M.: Reversal of copper inhibition in chloroplast reactions by manganese. *Plant Physiol, 44*:331, 1969.
26. Nicholson, G. A., Greiner, A. C., McFarlane, W. J. G., and Baker, R. A.: Effect of penicillamine on schizophrenic patients. *Lancet, i*:344, 1966.
27. Cox, D. H., and Harris, D. L.: Effect of excess dietary zinc on iron and copper in the rat. *J Nutr, 70*:514, 1959.
28. Lee, D., Jr., and Matrone, G.: Iron and copper effects on serum ceruloplasmin activity of rats with zinc-induced copper deficiency. *Proc Soc Exp Biol Med, 130*:1190, 1969.
29. Rimai, L., and Heyde, M. E.: An investigation by Raman spectroscopy of the base-proton dissociation of ATP in aqueous solution and the interaction of ATP with Zn^{++} and Mn^{++}. *Biochem Biophys Res Commun, 41*:313, 1970.
30. McCormick, D. B., Sigel, H., and Wright, L. P.: Structure of Mn^{2+} and Cu^{2+} complexes with L-methionine, S-methyl, L-cysteine, L-threonine, and L-serine. *Biochim Biophys Acta, 184*:318, 1969.
31. Fister, W. P., Boulding, J. E., and Baker, R. A.: The treatment of hepatolenticular degeneration with penicillamine; with report of two cases. *Can Med Assoc J, 78*:99, 1958.
32. McCall, J. T., Goldstein, N. P., and Randall, R. V.: Comparative metabolism of copper and zinc in patients with Wilson's Disease (Hepato-lenticular degeneration). *Am J Med Sci, 254*:35, 1967.
33. Henkin, R. I., Schecter, P. J., Hoye, R., and Mattern, C. F. T.: Idiopathic hypogeusia with dysgeusia, hyposmia, and dysosmia. A new syndrome. *JAMA, 217*:434, 1971.
34. Walshe, J. M., and Patston, V.: Effect of penicillamine on serum iron. *Arch Dis Child, 40*:651, 1965.
35. Metzler, D. E.: Metal binding by pyridoxal derivatives and possible relationships to tryptophan metabolism. *Fed Proc, 20(3)Pt 2*:234, 1961.
36. Irvine, D. G., Bayne, W., Miyashita, H., and Majer, J. R.: Identification of kryptopyrrole in human urine and its relation to psychosis. *Nature, 224*:811, 1969.

DISCUSSION

Dr. Flynn: I would like to know, in the patients who are deficient, does their therapy include other tranquilizer-type drugs? The reason I bring this up is that we did some studies on animals with chlorpromazine which is a phenothiazine type tranquilizer that suppresses the zinc level. I was wondering if you had seen anything like this in your patients. Have you studied any of the effects of this in normal vs your treated patients?

Dr. Pfeiffer: Well, we have now treated twenty-seven patients with chlorpromazine to determine the effect on Cu, Zn and Fe excretion, and the excretion of Cu is increased by chlorpromazine. The excretion of zinc is less. We did twenty-seven with 150 mg orally in order to get a statistically reliable answer. The excretion is so variable that one needs an "n" of somewhere between 25 and 30 in order to be sure. To answer the first part of your question, most of these patients were on an antipsychotic therapy because we see in an outpatient setting, patients referred from all over the state of New Jersey and other places so that they are difficult patients usually to treat and they haven't responded to the usual antipsychotic therapy.

Dr. Flynn: Have you ever done any serum zincs with chlorpromazine?

Dr. Pfeiffer: Yes we have, and the Cu in the serum usually goes down. One interesting thing about chlorpromazine is that it tends to bring the histamine that is low up to a normal level and brings a high histamine down to a normal level. So that everything will fit in with the theory that they should have a fairly normal histamine level in order to be brought home.

Chapter 24

PANEL DISCUSSION FOR SECTION D
ZINC AND HEALING II

Moderator: Walter J. Pories
Panelists: Henkin, Henzel, Larson and Pfeiffer
Discussants: Hurley, Spencer, and Woosley

~~~~~~

Dr. Pories: Are there comments from any members of the Panel about any parts of the discussion?

Dr. Spencer: I have one question for Dr. Pfeiffer. You mentioned that when you gave estrogen that the serum Cu increased very much. I would like to ask you what happened to the serum zinc.

Dr. Pfeiffer: We don't have a reliable decrease in the zinc, but this is reported in the literature and there are several such reports on so-called normal women. But insofar as our schizophrenic females are concerned, the zinc does not go contrary to the Cu.

Dr. Spencer: I have another question to the Panel whoever would like to answer. This is general. When you give zinc for a prolonged period of time did you notice any change in the serum alkaline phosphatase and in LDH?

Dr. Henkin: We have given varying doses of zinc, 25, 50 and 100 mg of elemental zinc, for as long as one and one-half years, to patients with idiopathic hypoguesia without any significant alteration, and this is now a number of patients who would be looked at, would be about 50 without any significant alteration in serum alkaline phosphatase or LDH.

Dr. Hurley: May I ask one more question, you mentioned in your presentation that you gave 100 mg elemental zinc q.i.d., four times a day?

Dr. Henkin: No. 100 mg elemental zinc daily, that is 25 mg of elemental zinc q.i.d. Do you have any other questions?

Dr. Woosley: I have a question for Dr. Henkin.

There is an antihistamine now approved by the FDA for the stimulation of appetite, cyproheptidine. I wonder if this antihistamine, especially in the light of associations between histamine and zinc, should now be looked at to see if they have an effect on taste and if this could be responsible for their effect on appetite?

Dr. Henkin: I am afraid I don't know that drug. I have not had any experience with it. However, in the literature you will see rather frequent references to drugs which are affecting taste and we have not sincerely been able to document any changes in metals. For example, griesofulvin produces dysgusia, hyposmia and dysosmia to a severe degree as do a number of other drugs that people are using and this is not necessarily in relationship to any alteration in metal metabolism.

Dr. Woosley: One other question also for Dr. Henkin. Many people feel that the secretions of Brunner's glands are related to taste and since there is possibly a pH gradient there, I wonder if anyone has looked at the concentration of carbonic anhydrase in this gland.

Dr. Henkin: To the best of my knowledge no systematic studies have been done. However, the pH relationships in terms of metals are very important factors.

SUBJECT INDEX

A

Ageusia, 212

Alcoholism, chronic, zinc deficiency and, 113-118

zinc metabolism, 193

see also Zinc deficiency and chronic alcoholism

Alcoholism, trace metals in, 113-114

Amino acids, enhancement of catabolism of, 88

skin collagens in zinc-deficient rats, incorporation into, 47-48

skin proteins in zinc-deficient rats, incorporation into, 43, 45-46, 54

amino acid-^{14} C, 45-46

amino acid reutilization, 46

cystine-^{35} S, 43

decrease in, 43, 45, 46, 54

L-arginine-^{14} C, 46

tissue proteins in zinc-deficient rats, incorporation into, 43-45

cystine-^{35} S, 43-45

methionine-^{14} C, 45

Amino acid catabolism, in zinc-deficient rats, 48

protein synthesis, alteration in rate of, 48-49

Amino acid oxidation, 48-49

Anemia, due to magnesium deficiency, 89

Anencephalus, 61

Anorexia, 208, 225, 226

Appetite, enhancement of, 124

Atherosclerosis, symptomatic, zinc therapy for, 243-260

see also Zinc sulfate therapy, long-term

Atomic absorption spectrophotometry, 20, 22, 101, 153, 170, 210, 229, 262

Atrophy of the testes, in zinc-deficient rats, 59

see also Zinc deficiency, in non-pregnant rats

B

Biomembranes, damage of, 79

stabilization by zinc, 75-84

see also Zinc, biomembranes

Bone, resorption of, 68

Brain, malformation of, 61

Burned patients, blood loss in, 235

donor sites, 229

glucosteroid treatment of, 233-234

blood serum zinc, 234

body zinc levels, 233

graft take, 229

local treatment, types of, 231

optimal wound healing for, importance of, 229

vasoactive corticosteroid therapy for, 234

zinc deficiency in, reasons for, 232

see also Zinc sulfate therapy, in burned patients

Burns, zinc deficiency in, 144

C

Cacogeusia, symptoms of, 206-207

Cacosmia, symptoms of, 208

Cadmium, and healing, 149-150

antagonism to zinc and iron, 149-150

chemical castration, 149

tissue damage, 150

Cadmium toxicity, 149, 150

Calcium deficiency, bone resorption, 68

see also Zinc deficiency, and calcium deficiency

Central nervous system, asynchronous development of, 63

pathology of brain, chord, eye and olfactory tract, 63-64

malformations of, 61

Cirrhosis of the liver, 170

plasma zinc values, 170

Cobalt, and healing, 150

tissue damage, 150

Collagen, and healing, 156-157

Collagen deposit, increase in, 229

Collagen synthesis, 47-48

insulin treatment in zinc-deficient rats, 48

zinc involvement in, 47

Controlled clinical trial, concept of, 181

features for the formulation of, 181

of oral zinc therapy, 181-194

AUTHOR INDEX

297